Praise for *Dream Yoga*

"Andrew Holecek's book is a real treat. It covers all of the necessary information—which is still quite new to most people, often even to Buddhists. But it also contains numerous experiential exercises and practices—which are quite effective—so that you can directly experience these profound states for yourself. When you do so, you will literally never be the same again, I can assure you! Don't miss your opportunity to realize some of the very deepest and highest of all human potentials, from a real master of these realms!"

KEN WILBER, author of *The Fourth Turning*

"As Andrew Holecek writes, dream and sleep yoga are 'about bringing light into the darkness of any aspect of life.' His valuable book presents a wide variety of Eastern and Western practice techniques, drawing from many authentic sources. Between his words one can sense a deep enthusiasm that comes from personal experience with the practice. This informative book will be very beneficial for dedicated dream yoga practitioners."

TENZIN WANGYAL RINPOCHE,
author of *The Tibetan Yogas of Dream and Sleep*

"In *Dream Yoga,* Andrew Holecek has skillfully integrated the deeply philosophical and spiritual tradition of Tibetan dream yoga with the psychological methods and insights of the modern discipline of lucid dreaming. At once profound and pragmatic, traditional and contemporary, this is a fine contribution to the growing literature on ways of exploring the nature of the mind and its role in nature by way of awakening to our dreams."

B. ALAN WALLACE, author of *Dreaming Yourself Awake*

Andrew Holecek has written a comprehensive and much-needed book on the interface between lucid dreaming and dream yoga. His own long-term dharma practice and rigorous training in the Western scientific tradition helps us to clearly understand the remarkable opportunities that await us each night. Dream yoga practices have been used for centuries in Tibet, leading many beings to awakening. This book will help secure this important practice in the West and will introduce many to the wonders of our nocturnal meditations.

TSOKNYI RINPOCHE, author of *Open Heart, Open Mind*

"In *Dream Yoga*, Andrew Holecek invites us to relate to our experience while sleeping with the same intention we bring to our spiritual path work while awake. How can we use our dreaming, in practical and effective ways, to see through appearance and consciously participate in our most fundamental nature of awareness? How can we become aware of awareness? Andrew seamlessly moves from theories to practices to possible benefits and back again, all arising from his decades of personal work and study. His writing has a wonderful transparency, an offering that's at once profound while not taking itself too seriously. My experience of dreaming has already changed, just reading this book."

BRUCE TIFT, psychologist and author of *Already Free*

2/19

Dream Yoga

Dream Yoga

*Illuminating Your Life Through Lucid Dreaming
and the Tibetan Yogas of Sleep*

ANDREW HOLECEK

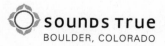

SOUNDS TRUE
BOULDER, COLORADO

Sounds True
Boulder, CO 80306

Published 2016

Cover design by Rachael Murray
Book design by Beth Skelley
Illustrations © 2016 Charlie Tomich

The poem "Out Beyond Ideas" by Jalal al-Din Rumi, translated by Coleman
Barks and published in *The Essential Rumi: New Expanded Edition* (New York:
HarperSanFrancisco, 2004), is reprinted by permission of the translator.

Printed in the United States of America

Library of Congress Cataloging-in-Publication Data
Names: Holecek, Andrew, 1955- author.
Title: Dream yoga : illuminating your life through lucid dreaming and the
    Tibetan yogas of sleep / Andrew Holecek.
Description: Boulder, CO : Sounds True, Inc., 2016. |
    Includes bibliographical references and index.
Identifiers: LCCN 2015044686 (print) | LCCN 2016006373 (ebook) |
    ISBN 9781622034598 | ISBN 9781622035519
Subjects: LCSH: Lucid dreams. | Yoga. | Sleep.
Classification: LCC BF1099.L82 H65 2016 (print) | LCC BF1099.L82 (ebook)
    DDC 154.6/3—dc23
LC record available at http://lccn.loc.gov/2015044686

Ebook ISBN 978-1-62203-551-9

10 9 8 7 6 5 4 3 2 1

To Cindy Wilson, for sharing the dream.

Contents

Foreword by Stephen LaBerge, PhD

FORWARD! To the lucid exploration of the dreamworlds and beyond within! But which way is forward? Consider that when you are walking upright in your dreamworld you are typically lying down in the physical world. So what is straight ahead in your dream is at right angles in physical reality. And consider this: suppose you find yourself explicitly conscious that you are dreaming (that is, "lucid"). Suppose that you decide you want to visit your physical body. You might remember perfectly well that your physical body is asleep in a bed somewhere in Silicon Valley, but in the dream you don't know the way to San Jose! That's because it isn't in any direction you can point to from your dreamworld; there's no direction you can walk to get there, however "far." You can't get there from here except one way—and that is to Wake Up!

But the "oneirony" of it is that you can't take that way when you don't know you're dreaming. Our dream experiences seem so real to our sleeping minds that it is usually only after we awaken that we recognize our dreams as the mental experiences they are. However, as mentioned above, there is a significant and felicitous exception: "lucid dreaming," in which we take explicit note, or *cognizance,* of the fact that we *are* dreaming while remaining asleep to the external world. This means that we know we are dreaming, and we also *know* that we know it. That allows us to direct our dreams in the direction of our goals and—importantly—our ideals, which cannot be sought except consciously.

I have devoted my scientific career to the exploration of this extraordinary state of consciousness. Research done by my colleagues and me at Stanford University has proven the objective reality of lucid dreams, delineated their basic types and psychophysiological characteristics, and led to the development of new techniques and technology for more effectively inducing them. I have also learned how to voluntarily access lucid dreams and have found them wonderfully educational in the deepest sense. That is, as a means of bringing forth what is within.

Of course, as Walt Disney said, "It's kind of fun to do the impossible," and this is one obvious answer to why people find lucid dreaming rewarding. There also seems to be something intrinsically rewarding about the enhanced mindfulness and presence associated with *remembering*. But more deeply meaningful for me have been the experiences of integration of shadow figures, which result in increased compassion, understanding, and wholeness. This process of integration is a form of dream yoga, and its practice leads to experiences of transcendence, which might be recognized as having similarities with the Tibetan dream yoga that is the subject of this book. That is no accident. I have had significant contacts with the Tibetan Buddhist tradition, starting with a workshop with Tibetan lama Tarthang Tulku at Esalen in 1972. In *Exploring the World of Lucid Dreaming* (coauthored with Howard Rheingold), I described this encounter as marking the inception of my venture of awakening to "this dream." Although I never became a Tibetan Buddhist, I have always respected the tradition and been grateful for what I have learned from it. Twenty-five years after that, I began teaching programs on lucid dream yoga in partnership with Western followers of the Tibetan tradition, starting with B. Alan Wallace and, most recently, Andrew Holecek.

I met Andrew at our annual "Dreaming and Awakening" retreat in Hawaii in 2012. (You can learn more about this at my website, lucidity.com.) I found Andrew to be a delightful person—warm and witty with a wonderfully developed sense of humor. By that I mean he laughed at all my jokes. (He will laugh at this one too.) I liked him immediately and asked him back as a guest teacher, mainly because I wanted to get to know him better. I am very glad that I did. Six months ago, we co-taught a program at Shambhala Mountain Center in Colorado, and Andrew and his wife, Cindy, generously hosted me in their home for several days before the program began. I felt blessed to share their dwelling, which embodied so clearly the luminous love of the dwellers. Over the course of our week together, I experienced numerous instances of those little acts of kindness and love that Wordsworth declared "the best portion of a good man's life." One of note: Andrew performed an impromptu piano recital for us, beautifully playing a selection of classical works from memory. I experienced music in a new way. I was touched. Andrew has hidden depths.

Implicit in lucid dreaming is the knowledge that you are dreaming, which is to say that you are not awake. Yet this is the paradox: as the beginning of wisdom is "to know that you know nothing," so too the beginning of awakening is to know that you are not awake. If we suppose we already are awake—as we do implicitly in most dreams, explicitly in those dreams called "false awakenings," and in those we do not call dreams at all but presumptively term "waking life"—how can we even frame the possibility of waking up? We already are awake. Or so we believe. This is a special case of the general problem of how thinking you already know blocks learning of what you only think you know. A part of learning how to learn is starting with the only thing you know—which is that you know nothing. But at least you know that you know. This truth is one level up from just knowing nothing. It's still nothing, but you can see it better.

So it may be better to think of yourself as asleep rather than awake, and instead of enlightened, endarkened. By accepting your original state, rather than dazzling yourself with imagined illumination, you can get to know the darkness and perhaps find the hidden treasure. Remember the story in which the character Nasrudin is under a streetlight outside his house searching for his lost key? A neighbor helps him look for a while—fruitlessly—then asks, "Where, exactly, did you lose your key?" Nasrudin answers, "In my house." The neighbor exclaims, "Then why in the world are we looking out *here!*" Coolly logical, Nasrudin replies, "Because there's more light here."

The outside world may have more light, but it isn't where the Key was lost and hence might be found: that is, inside, in the darkness within, our innermost home, beyond the self, in the beginning of all. And so Andrew Holecek has chosen to search where the Key was lost, following the path of dark wisdom. His book's prologue begins and ends with a quote from Rilke: "I believe in the night." In the context of the poem, which ends with this credo, Rilke says that he prefers the darkness from which he was born to the candle's circle of light that divides the world. But the darkness is the undivided whole, accepting all, allowing all potential being.

You will perhaps have noticed in the foregoing the frequent images of remembering, finding what has been lost, hidden treasure, and so on. I ended my most recent book, *Lucid Dreaming: A Concise Guide to Awakening in Your Dreams and in Your Life,* with a story called "The Precious Jewel." In a remote realm of perfection, the son and daughter of a king undertake a mission to descend into another world and seek, and bring back, a precious Jewel. They journeyed in disguise to a strange land whose inhabitants almost all lived a dark existence. Such was the effect of that place that they soon lost touch with each other and with all memory of their origins and mission. Wandering in an increasingly deep sleep, they soon took their reveries to be the only reality. When the king heard of his children's plight, he sent this reminder: "Remember your mission, awaken from your dream, and remain together." With this message they roused themselves and braved the perils surrounding the Jewel, and with its magical aid they returned to their realm of light, where they remain in increased happiness evermore.

If it weren't likely to be considered precious by some, and blasphemous by others, I'd call Andrew *Rinpoche,* the Tibetan honorific meaning "Precious Jewel." But I can use an American honorific metaphor and say that *Andrew is a jewel.* And that, in a *tigle,* is why I wrote this foreword. May this book help you to know him—and to find the Jewel within yourself.

I believe in the night.

RAINER MARIA RILKE, *Rilke's Book of Hours: Love Poems from God,* translated by Anita Barrows and Joanna Macy

Prologue

EVERY HUMAN BEING on this planet sleeps and dreams. It's a silent unifying feature of all humanity. Everybody knows what it feels like to fall into tranquil sleep, and everybody knows what it's like to be jolted awake. We've all had nightmares, blissful dreams, or difficulty with sleep. Right now, as you read this, about half of the people on Earth are sleeping and dreaming, snuggled into a mysterious state of consciousness. If you could stand on a stationary point in space and look at our planet for twenty-four hours, you would see the blanket of darkness drape across the globe. The front end of this comforter would be tucked around billions of people (and countless trillions of animals) as they fell into sleep, while the back end would be pulled off to arouse billions of others to the rays of the morning sun. And so we spend our lives, day after day and night after night, succumbing to the power of the cosmos as the spin of our planet forces us into its circadian rhythm—and into states of consciousness we know very little about.

Have you ever wondered what's going on when you sleep and dream? What are these shadowy states of consciousness we all share? Is there a way to use the night and bring sleeping and dreaming onto the path of psychological and spiritual growth? Can we use the process of sleep to "wake us up"? This book will show you that *yes,* you can. In the following pages you will discover an amazing world waiting for you in the stillness of the night. This world is full of wonder, mystery, and infinite profundity. It's the world of the inner space of your own mind, a dimension of reality that's as deep and vast as the outer space of the cosmos.

We spend more time in bed than any other single place, dead to the outer world, but potentially alive to an exciting inner world. About a third of our lives is lost in this inner space, and up to six years is spent in the dream world. From the cozy cradle to the nestled grave, some of the most momentous events of life occur on the mattress: we have ecstatic sex, give joyful birth, get miserably sick, and often die in bed. But the opportunities for psychological and spiritual evolution that are available in bed are even more momentous. Given the proper tools, turning off outer experiences allows us to turn on breathtaking inner ones.

I stumbled into this inner world nearly forty years ago and have been exploring it ever since. Like you, I've been dreaming my entire life, and some of the most remarkable experiences I've ever had occurred in my dreams. In my early twenties, one such experience changed my life.

I had just completed an exhausting five-year double-degree undergraduate program in music and biology, and I took a year off before going to graduate school. I spent the first half of this year working in a maximum-security federal prison. My job was to supervise inmate construction crews: motley gangs of killers, rapists, extortionists, and thieves. It was a gritty introduction to the shadow side of life. As I befriended these tough guys, I saw that their crimes for the most part were just surface expressions; I came to see these men as people who were just like me but who had lost their way.

For the second half of that year I worked as a surgical orderly. My job was to prep patients for surgery, deliver them to the operating room, and later take them into the recovery room. It involved intimate care and led to stark discoveries about the harsh realities of illness and death. Because I was thinking about going to medical school, I became the teacher's pet to a number of surgeons. They allowed me to watch countless operations and ask endless questions.

It was a marvelous opportunity to learn about life and death. As a young man, I experienced these two jobs as a sobering introduction to the human condition.

During that year I was also becoming interested in the ideas associated with the burgeoning New Age movement. I had started a practice of Transcendental Meditation (TM) two years earlier and was getting involved with other spiritual practices. TM showed me that there were dimensions of reality deeper than my external world, a surface world that was slapping me in the face with these two job experiences. I was also reading a great deal, things like *The Seth Material,* Edgar Cayce, pop psychology, and quirky books about dreams. The juxtaposition of heavenly spiritual experiences and hellish introductions into psychological, social, and physical disease shook me to the core. How could I reconcile my blissful spiritual states with the harsh realities of the prison and the hospital?

About six months into the year, I started having dreams that seemed to foreshadow something. These recurrent dreams, which increased in frequency, generated an ineffable sense of anticipation. I knew something was about to happen. One day, while deeply contemplating one of my New Age books, my mind suddenly broke open. In an instant I was flooded with insights and visions of an entirely new world. It was as if a huge spiritual hammer slammed down on top of my skull and split me apart. Words defy me even decades later. This new world was a kaleidoscope of electrifying perceptions, like having eyelids peeled back on eyes I never knew I had. I felt awake for the very first time, jolted from the slumber that had been my life.

I remained in this ecstatic state for two weeks, convinced that this is what it meant to be spiritually reborn, or mystically awakened. Two aspects of the experience stood out, one related to the night and the other to the day, both of which were connected to dreams. The first was that my dream life exploded. I had dozens of powerful dreams, many of which were lucid (which means I realized I was dreaming while still remaining in the dream), while others were prophetic. Many of these dreams were hyper-real, more intense and real than waking experience. I started a dream diary and within those two weeks had filled several notebooks. It was as if my deepest unconscious mind erupted and a volcano of dreams burst forth. Some of those dreams still guide my life today.

The second aspect was that my daytime experience became very dreamlike. My world had become fluid, illusory, and groundless. I saw everything as a transparent symbol. When I walked along the shore of Lake Michigan near my house, the waves were teaching me about the rising and falling of thoughts in my mind. When the sun broke through the clouds, it was a teaching about the awakened mind shining through the gaps between my thoughts. A rainbow was showing me the transient and ephemeral nature of things. Everywhere I looked, it was as if the world was sending me a message. I was treading a fine line between metanoia and paranoia (that is, deriving spiritual meaning from my world versus imputing excessive meaning to it). In addition to my burgeoning dream diary, I also filled several notebooks with insights delivered during the day. I was thrust into a dazzling and highly surreal experience. It's impossible to convey the impact of these miraculous weeks, which remain the most transformative of my life.

Because my daytime experience was becoming more dreamlike and my nighttime dreams were becoming more real (clear and stable), I had a hard time determining if I was awake or asleep. There were times when my dreams felt super-real and waking experience became the dream. These previously separate worlds were mixing together.

This was entertaining at first but became progressively disconcerting. An experience that started out so fresh became frightening. Where was my solid and secure world? I was losing my grip on reality. Instead of asking myself, "Is this enlightenment?" I began to panic and ask, "Is this madness?" My thrill in being spiritually awake was replaced with my fear of being insane.

I felt that if I went to a therapist, I would probably be medicated, or even institutionalized. The contemplative psychiatrist R. D. Laing said, "Attempts to wake before our time are often punished, especially by those who love us most. Because they, bless them, are asleep. They think anyone who wakes up, or who, still asleep, realizes that what is taken to be real is a 'dream' is going crazy."[1] In a desperate attempt to reestablish some sense of ground, and therefore sanity, I shut the experience down. I jumped into my Volkswagen

Beetle, drove to Colorado, and joined my buddies to drink and ski my way back to sanity.

Within a week of intense distraction, my sense of a stable world began to rebuild. I don't know if it was the beer, my rowdy friends, or spending so much time in nature, but I breathed a massive sigh of relief as that unworldly two-week experience faded and I regained my sense of reality.

I returned to Michigan and resumed my job as a surgical orderly. But something had changed. The hangovers from my drinking binges couldn't completely erase the hangover of my otherworldly experiences. Within a few months I felt stable enough to begin venturing back into what I had experienced. I knew that something profound, and profoundly disturbing, had happened. Even though I had successfully forced myself back to reality, I had glimpsed a new world, and dreams were a big part of it. So began my exploration into the world of sleep and dream.

I started reading everything I could about dreams. I read Sigmund Freud, Carl Jung, and countless books from psychologists, scientists, mystics, and quacks.[2] They were helpful but also incomplete. I still couldn't understand what happened. One day I started reading about Buddhism and was immediately struck that "buddha" literally means "the awakened one." What does that mean? Awake as opposed to what? What did the Buddha awaken from, and what did he awaken to?

The more I studied Buddhism, the more I understood what had happened to me. These teachings were the only thing I encountered that could explain my outrageous two-week ride. Inspired by the story of the Buddha and the resonance of his teachings with my experience, I became committed to "waking up," which makes me a Buddhist in the purest sense. For the past thirty years I have continued my study and practice of this gentle tradition. When I finally came upon the Buddhist teachings on dream yoga, which is when you strive to have lucid dreams with the goal of doing specific practices within them, I knew I had come home.

Even though I consider myself a Buddhist, I'm primarily interested in the pursuit of the truth, and discovering the nature of reality. This truth may include or transcend traditional or even New Age religion, as well as science and philosophy. I'm interested in personal evolution, and I don't care what does it. So while the teachings in this book are based on the wisdom of the Buddhist tradition—and in particular, Tibetan Buddhism—they also come from psychology, science, and my own experience. No one has a patent on truth. Just as my experience joined day and night, this book will continue the theme of unity as I join the wisdom of the East with the knowledge of the West in an attempt to bring this wondrous world of the night into the crisp light of the day.

As a final thought, there is promise and peril in sharing spiritual experiences, including powerful dreams. The promise is that it can inspire and connect you to others. The peril is that it can inflate the ego, and deflate the potency of the experience. In my Buddhist tradition we are advised not to share these experiences. The renowned Tibetan master Tulku Urgyen Rinpoche ("Rinpoche" is an honorific term meaning "the precious one") said that talking about spiritual experiences is like being in a cave with a candle and giving your candle away. You're left in the dark. These experiences arise in the sanctuary of silence, and they should remain in that sanctuary.[3]

In the lucid dreaming literature there are many books where authors convey their proficiency by reporting how many lucid dreams they've had, describing how easily they can induce them, or sharing transformative dreams. I understand the need for this, and often find inspiration in their reports. Mastery in lucidity has no established credentials, so writers instill confidence in their readers by sharing their experiences. We also don't have role models in this young field, certified dream heroes we can emulate.

What do you do when modesty is the result of mastery? How do you convey that mastery without violating the modesty, or prevent slipping into a performative contradiction (that is, unwittingly falling into the trap you espouse to avoid)?[4] This is why you'll have a hard time finding masters of dream yoga. They don't talk about their experiences. As the Taoist tradition proclaims, "He who knows does not speak. He who speaks does not know."

So even though I start this book by sharing a life-changing experience, I will tread a middle way, erring on the side of omission. I will occasionally rely on the dream reports of others to convey what is possible in the night. It's a delicate dance, this tiptoe between conveying inspiration and feeding self-aggrandizement. Even humility can cloak arrogance. Suffice it to say that many of the most powerful experiences of my life continue to occur in my dreams. These dreams are often more vibrant than anything in waking reality, and they have frequently changed my life. I believe in the night.

This is a dream. I am free. I can change.

TENZIN WANGYAL RINPOCHE

Introduction

Adventures in Consciousness

THE JOURNEY WE are about to take in the course of this book is both fun and profound. Most people have no idea about the extent of possibilities that exist for this adventure in consciousness, an adventure in the darkness of the night.

We begin our journey with lucid dreaming. "Lucid dreaming" is when you realize you're dreaming, but without waking up from the dream. You're fully conscious within the dream and can do almost anything you want within it. Lucid dreaming is the ultimate in home entertainment. Your mind becomes the theater, and you are the producer, director, writer, and main actor. You can script the perfect love story or the craziest adventure. Lucid dreaming can also be used to solve problems, rehearse situations, and work through psychological issues. (For books specifically about lucid dreaming, see the suggested reading list at the end of this book.) From the trivial to the transcendent, lucid dreaming is a spectrum of experience mostly concerned with worldly matters and self-fulfillment.

Going deeper, lucid dreaming can develop into dream yoga, and become a spiritual practice. This is not to say that lucid dreaming isn't spiritual. It can be. But as a practice, and in contrast to dream yoga, lucid dreaming doesn't have as many spiritually oriented methods. "Yoga" is that which yokes, or unites. Dream yoga unites you with deeper aspects of your being; it is more concerned with self-transcendence.

Other traditions work with sleep and dreams for spiritual purposes, including Sufi and Taoist dream practice, aspects of Transcendental Meditation, and Yoga Nidra. I will focus principally on Tibetan Buddhist dream yoga because this is a specialty of this branch of Buddhism.

From the etymology of "buddha," all the way to the nocturnal meditations, this tradition has explored the nighttime mind for over twenty-five centuries. In the biographical poem the *Buddhacarita* ("Life of the Buddha"), it is said that the Buddha attained his enlightenment through four "watches of the night." In the first watch, the soon-to-be Buddha gained recollection of his past lives and knowledge of the cycle of rebirth. In the second watch, he saw that all beings go through this cycle and that karma drives the wheel of life. During the third watch, he saw the means of liberation from this cycle. And in the fourth watch, just at the break of dawn, he attained the great awakening and became the Buddha. Following his example, we will similarly "watch" the night in a new and illuminating light.

The exact origin of dream yoga is opaque in Buddhism. Some scholars trace dream yoga back to the Buddha. Namkhai Norbu, a master of the Nyingma school of Tibetan Buddhism, says it originated in the tantras (especially the Mahamaya Tantra), which are shrouded in mystery and authorship.[1] Guru Rinpoche, the founder of the Nyingma tradition who brought Buddhism from India to Tibet, taught dream yoga as part of his cycle of teachings. In the Kagyu and Gelugpa traditions, dream yoga is taught mostly in the Six Yogas of Naropa, which is perhaps the oldest certain source. Naropa gathered the Six Yogas but was not their author. Lama Thubten Yeshe says, "The Six Yogas of Naropa were not discovered by Naropa. They originated in the teachings of Lord Buddha, and were eventually transmitted to the great eleventh-century Indian yogi Tilopa, who in turn transmitted them to his disciple Naropa."[2] But the Indian master Lawapa ("master of the blanket," also known as Kambala) is the author of dream yoga as presented in the Six Yogas. He passed the teachings on to Jalandhara, who passed them to Krishnacharya, who taught them to Naropa. Tilopa, who is the founder of the Kagyu tradition, attributes dream yoga specifically to Lawapa.

My study of dream and sleep yoga comes from all these lineages (and others as well), but my practice of dream and sleep yoga is mostly from the Six Yogas of Naropa. Four of the Six Yogas will be central to our journey in this book: illusory form yoga, dream yoga, sleep yoga, and *bardo* yoga. The other two yogas are *chandali* (inner heat) yoga and *phowa* (ejection of consciousness) yoga, which are beyond the scope of this book.

We tend to think of yoga as physical, stretching the body into various postures, but there are also mental yogas that work to stretch the mind. As a mental yoga, dream yoga may leave stretch marks on your mind. But stretching, at any level, is good for growth. Just as physical yoga makes your body more flexible, dream yoga makes your mind more flexible: that is, adaptable, pliable, malleable, supple, accommodating, compliant, amenable—and open. Who wouldn't want a mind like this? Once a mind is open and pliable, you can wrap it around all sorts of new experiences.

With dream yoga, instead of using your mind as an entertainment center, you turn it into a laboratory. You experiment with dream meditations and study your mind using the medium of dreams. At this point you become a "spiritual oneironaut." Oneirology is the study of dreams, and oneironauts (pronounced "oh-NIGH-ro-nots") are those who navigate the dream world. Just like astronauts explore the outer space of the cosmos, oneironauts explore the inner space of the mind.

While dream yoga originated as a Buddhist practice, the Dalai Lama says, "It is possible [to practice dream yoga] without a great deal of preparation. Dream yoga could be practiced by non-Buddhists as well as Buddhists. If a Buddhist practices dream yoga, he or she brings a special motivation and purpose to it. In the Buddhist context the practice is aimed at the realization of emptiness [the nature of reality]. But the same practice could be done by non-Buddhists."[3] Emptiness is a core doctrine in Buddhism, and a central theme of our journey. It is also one of the most misunderstood concepts in all of Buddhism. We will return to the concept of emptiness frequently in this book and gradually unpack it.

Taking this practice further, dream yoga can develop into "sleep yoga," an advanced meditation in which awareness spreads not only into dreams but into deep dreamless sleep. Staying awake during dreamless sleep is an age-old practice in Tibetan Buddhism. With sleep yoga, your body goes into sleep mode, but your mind stays awake. You drop *consciously* into the very core of your being, the most subtle formless awareness—into who you truly are.

If you want to go even further, there's one final destination of the night. Dream yoga and sleep yoga can develop into "bardo yoga," the famous Tibetan practices that use the darkness of the night to prepare for the darkness of death. "Bardo" is a Tibetan word that means "gap, interval, transitional state, or in between," and in this case it refers to the gap between lives. If you believe in rebirth and want to know what to do after you die, bardo yoga is for you. On one level, all of dream yoga and sleep yoga is a preparation for death.

Lucid dreaming, dream yoga, sleep yoga, and bardo yoga are the evolution of the "dark practices" that comprise this book. Illusory form yoga is their daytime counterpart. These practices are designed to bring light into some of the deepest and darkest aspects of your being. In this book we'll focus mostly on lucid dreaming and dream yoga (including the daytime practice of illusory form), with some discussion of sleep yoga and a brief survey of bardo yoga for those who are interested in these more advanced practices. An entirely new world of "nightlife" awaits you in the dark, and with the techniques presented here, you will have everything you need to safely explore this deep inner space.

While I've never seen anyone get into trouble with dream yoga, as with any discipline it may not be for everyone. People with dissociation or depersonalization tendencies should consult with a mental health professional before undertaking lucid dreaming or dream yoga. Those with psychotic predispositions, or anyone suffering from a loss of a stable sense of reality, could potentially worsen those dissociative states of mind. As with any meditation, it's always good to check your motivation. If you're looking to escape from reality, the nighttime meditations are probably not for you.[4]

So who is this book for? It's for anyone interested in the thrill of waking up in their dreams, and having the time of their life in the privacy of their own mind. It's for anyone wanting to make better use of the twenty-four hours of each day, and for those wondering what happens when they sleep and dream. It's for intrepid pioneers interested in exploring the frontiers of consciousness, and the nature of mind and reality. It's for anyone interested in psychological and spiritual development, those who want to learn about the creative powers of the mind, and those who want to prepare for death. Finally, it's for those drawn to Buddhist practice, and interested in waking up in the spiritual sense.

This may seem ambitious. But remember that if you live to be ninety years old, you've spent thirty of those years sleeping, and entered the dream world around half a million times. That's a lot of time in a state of consciousness you know very little about. Don't you want to change that? Think about how much you could learn in "night school" if you had even a few of those thirty extra years.

How to Read This Book

While this book shows you how to have lucid dreams and what to do with them, it is designed to go deeper. Many fine books (listed in the suggested reading list) are available to introduce you to the world of lucid dreaming. This book is written to show you how vast and profound this world truly is, and how far it can take you. It's more of a philosophical and spiritual journey into the practices of the night, geared to support the practices themselves and the experiences that unfold from them. If you want to limit your journey to the wonders of lucid dreaming alone, you will learn how to do that. But the heart of this book is to show you that dreams can be used to remove suffering and achieve lasting happiness, which is one way to define enlightenment.

This book is therefore about waking up from the delusion that results in samsara, which is the conventional world filled with dissatisfaction and suffering (and set in contrast to nirvana, or enlightenment). As the political commentator Bill Maher says, "Anytime there's mass delusion, bad things follow." This comment applies to the full spectrum of delusion, from cults all the way down to delusions about the nature of reality. As we will see, we are all unwitting members of the cult of materialism, the mass delusion that things are fundamentally solid, lasting, and independent, the central characteristics of samsara. Our mission in this book is to point out this delusion, a fallacy that Buddhism defines as being asleep to the true nature of things, and to wake up from it. And anytime there's mass awakening or truth, good things follow.

While lucid dreaming is more of a Western phenomenon, dream yoga, sleep yoga, and bardo yoga come mostly from Tibetan Buddhism. Our journey will unite both worlds, the best of the East and West. The Indian philosopher Mahadevan said that the main difference between Eastern and Western philosophy is that the West develops its view of reality from a single state of consciousness (the waking state), while the East draws from all states of consciousness, including that of dream and sleep. It's more comprehensive.

The Tibetans have been exploring these states of consciousness for over a thousand years, with the explicit intent of using sleeping and dreaming as ways to understand life and death. This isn't merely philosophical understanding, but knowledge that is designed to remove suffering. So while dream yoga and sleep yoga (let alone bardo yoga) can seem esoteric and otherworldly, they have extremely practical applications for how to live.

Because the spectrum of nighttime practices, ranging from lucid dreaming all the way to bardo yoga, covers such a wide range of experiences, this book takes a broad-spectrum approach. This is in line with several themes that structure this book: the three levels of mind, as discussed in chapters 2, 9, and 10, and the three levels of body, as discussed in chapters 5 and 10. These three levels go from gross to subtle, outer to inner, the familiar to the unfamiliar. This threefold approach is inherent throughout the corpus of Buddhist teachings, which themselves are presented via the Three Yanas and the Three Turnings.[5]

The following material will therefore go from the familiar to the unfamiliar, from the exoteric to the esoteric, from easy to more difficult. For example, most people are familiar with the psyche and the outer body (which here will be treated as the first levels of mind and body), so this material is straightforward. However, most people are not familiar with the concepts of the "clear-light mind" and the "very subtle body" (here discussed as the third levels of mind and body), so this material may be more alien.

This book is like a tour into your innermost self. As many guide-books say, we're going to leave familiar territory and journey into foreign lands. It takes an intrepid spirit to leave the comfortable and familiar and travel into the unknown, but as any seasoned world traveler knows, the moments of hassle and discomfort are worth it. You will return from this inner journey, just as you would any outer sojourn, a better and more worldly person. You will become infinitely more cosmopolitan because you will connect not just to the people you might meet in places like Istanbul or Delhi (if you were to venture out into the world), but to all people everywhere as you venture into a shared inner domain.

This inner journey may take you temporarily out of the comfort zone of your familiar home in the gross mind and outer body, but it will eventually deliver you to your true home in the center of yourself, and the bed of mind that you share with all sentient beings. Then you might arise from this bed and come back from this inner journey to re-inhabit your outer forms, and your everyday life, with the newfound treasures you have discovered within. And perhaps, just like the masters of old, you will then offer these riches to others and invite them to do the same.

While this book generally progresses from gross to subtle, and familiar to unfamiliar, there are early sections that may stretch you, and conversely there is material toward the end where you can relax. You can either read these challenging sections, or simply skip them and go on to easier information. Many of these sections begin by alerting the reader about challenges to come, but others glide into deeper material without such a preface.

I've tried to make this book as accessible as possible, sprinkling in personal stories and anecdotes, injecting supporting quotes, and constantly showing how these sometimes esoteric teachings apply to every moment of our lives. I endeavor to pay homage to the depth of this material while providing the occasional oasis of ease. Like any good yoga, this book will stretch and then relax. And as with physical yoga, the best way to expand and grow is to feel the stretch, and let it work on you as you gently lean into it.

As a note to encourage the reader, all the chapters prior to actual dream yoga practice (chapter 14) are designed to set the stage for dream yoga. In Buddhism, it is often taught that the preliminaries are more important than the main practice. If you plow a field, remove the weeds, fertilize it properly, and do so during the correct season, the seeds you plant will flourish. If you don't, it's like dropping seeds on untilled ground in the dead of winter. Dream yoga is subtle. Without working the field of your mind in advance, it may not take root.

Finally, you will find many endnotes to further enrich the material. With these endnotes I give myself the license to write with freedom. You can refer to them during a first reading, skip them entirely, or attend to them in a second reading of the book. I'll often read the endnotes of a book collectively when I finish reading each chapter. My hope is that they will augment the main text without distracting you.

We'll start discussing the many benefits of the nighttime practices right away, and summarize them in chapter 19. If you just can't wait, or want to know why you should bother with these nocturnal meditations, then jump ahead and read chapter 19 now. The numerous benefits may surprise you.

Three Wisdom Tools

To take this journey inward, we're going to engage the three *prajnas,* or "wisdom tools," of hearing, contemplating, and meditating.[6] Hearing, or reading, about something leads to contemplating upon it, which leads to meditating on it. By reading and thinking about this material, you will be engaging the first two wisdom tools. In our voyage this is like filling the gas tank, getting a good map, and stocking up on all the necessities for a big trip. But the journey truly begins when you start to meditate, when you actually turn the ignition on and engage the yogas that take you within. This is when you'll replace the map with the territory, savor the uniqueness of this trip, and make your own discoveries as you travel into the core of your being.

The three wisdom tools are the way we ingest, digest, and metabolize the teachings until they literally become us. If we remain at the level of hearing and contemplating alone, we'll remain at the level of mere philosophy. The teachings may tickle your intellect or entertain you, but they won't fundamentally change you.

Once you chew on the material and bring it into your system through the embodied practice of meditation, the teachings can transform you because this is when you *feel* them. Otherwise the material stays safely and aseptically tucked away in your head. The three wisdom tools take information from your head and deliver it down into your heart and guts. This is where you really feel things, and where you're truly fed. This is where you transform cerebral data into somatic fiber.

We're going to try to uproot the basis of samsara, which involves transcending fear. And as the religious scholar Reza Aslan says, "Fear is impervious to data." You're not going to get at it by hearing, or even contemplating. To transform fear, you have to work at the level of feeling, which is where you touch what you're trying to transform—exactly what meditation is designed to do.

When you're around someone who has done this inner work, and has fully incorporated the teachings with deep meditation, *you* can feel it. You can tell that this is a person who practices what they preach and is someone you can trust. For me, this has always been a guide for identifying an authentic teacher. Is what they say more than just talk? Do they embody their teachings? Do they live their truth? I have had the good fortune of being around some of the most intelligent people on this planet, from famous scientists to world-renowned philosophers. I find them infinitely fascinating. But the ones who really touch me, who truly move me, who inspire me to change, are the most meditative people on this planet.

It is through the three wisdom tools that knowledge is transformed into wisdom. So the real point of this book is meditation, or yoga, the final instrument of wisdom. Take these teachings and yoke them to your life through the meditations presented in the following pages.

The Tibetan word for "meditation" is *gom*, which means "to become familiar with." It is through meditation that you will become familiar with previously unfamiliar inner states of mind and body.[7] It is with meditation that you take this miraculous tour into the cosmos within. So while there is plenty in this book to feed the casual tourist, the book comes to life when you make the journey for yourself. As the Buddha himself said of his teachings (but in the language of today), "Don't take my word on it. Find out for yourself."

> From the point of view of the Buddhist teachings, the way
> to make progress is to have a deeper understanding of
> our own mind, which amounts to understanding that the
> world and our perception of it are illusory.

DZIGAR KONGTRUL, *Buddhadharma*

1

What Is a Lucid Dream?

"LUCID DREAM" IS a term hinted at by the scholar Marquis d'Hervey de Saint-Denys (1822–1892), but which was coined by the Dutch psychiatrist Frederik van Eeden (1860–1932).[1] In the West, lucid dream accounts go back as far as Aristotle, with the first Western lucid dream report written in 415 CE by Saint Augustine. A lucid dream is when you wake up to the fact that you're dreaming, but you still remain in the dream—that is, you're dreaming and you know it.[2] The validity of lucid dreaming was scientifically proven in 1975 by the psychologist Keith Hearne at Hull University, and then independently by Stephen LaBerge in 1977 at Stanford.[3] LaBerge is arguably the father of modern lucid dreaming, and his books *Lucid Dreaming: The Power of Being Awake and Aware in Your Dreams* (1985) and *Exploring the World of Lucid Dreaming* (1990, coauthored with Howard Rheingold) are classics. Prior to these pioneering studies, the idea of "lucid dreaming" was mostly dismissed by the scientific community. How can you be awake and dreaming at the same time? LaBerge and Hearne proved that you can, and lucid dreaming gained a foothold in the West.

In that magical instant of awakening within the dream, everything changes. What just a moment ago had total control over you now comes under your control. Instead of being blown around help-lessly by the dictates of the dream, you now dictate the dream. You can do whatever you want, and no one can see you. You can fly, have sex with a movie star, or rob Fort Knox.[4]

Dreams are truth-tellers.[5] They reveal our deepest unconscious tendencies, as any psychologist or dream interpreter can attest.[6] This same maxim applies to working with dreams on a spiritual level, as we will see throughout this book. The moniker for dream yoga in the classic texts is "the measure of the path." Dream yoga will show you a great deal about who you are, and where you stand on the path.

Try this brief contemplation, and be ruthlessly honest: What would you do if you could become invisible? What might that reveal? Would you act selflessly or selfishly? Plato addressed this issue in *The Republic*, where he talks about the "Myth of the Ring of Gyges." In this myth the shepherd Gyges discovers a magical ring that gives him the power of invisibility. Plato uses this myth to talk about morality—what would you do if you were invisible and nobody could hold you accountable for your actions? Would you work to benefit others (which, in Buddhist terms, would reveal an evolved being with a purified mind), or would you fulfill your wildest fanta-sies (which would reveal a normal being with a defiled mind)? Gyges used his invisibility to fulfill his raw desires. Lucid dreaming gives you a chance to live the myth of Gyges, and to learn from it.

Lucidity is not an "all-or-nothing" affair. There is a spectrum rang-ing from barely lucid to hyper-lucid, and from the shortest flashes of lucidity to lucid dreams lasting over an hour. For example, being barely lucid might involve acknowledging on some level that you're having a dream, but not acting with full comprehension. You might still flee from perceived danger, or treat dream characters as if they were real. Hyper-lucid dreaming would be full comprehension of the dreamlike nature of your experience in the dream, recognizing that even the sense of self in the dream is being dreamt. Hyper-lucidity could also refer to colors and forms in the dream that seem more vibrant and real than anything in waking experience. You can also be non-lucid in a dream, become lucid to it, then drop into non-lucidity again.

The good news about lucid dreaming is that even though it may take practice to have such dreams regularly, it just takes one instant of recognition and you're "in." One flash of recognition transforms a non-lucid dream into a lucid one. I've been to many lucid dream seminars where people get discouraged by their inability to trigger lucidity, but then the next night it suddenly happens. That single instance is often enough to ignite a passion for lucid dreams. There's nothing quite like a lucid dream, and when you have one, it's irresistible to want more. The following chapters will show you how to have these magical dreams.

Facts and Figures

Here are some general facts about lucid dreaming: Young children tend to have lucid dreams more frequently, an occurrence that drops off around age sixteen. Younger people in general are more likely to have lucid dreams than older folks. Lucidity occurs as early as age three, but it seems most likely to happen around ages twelve to fourteen.[7] On average, lucid dreamers have three to four lucid dreams each month, with the average length of lucidity being about fourteen minutes. Some 58 to 70 percent of people will have at least one lucid dream during their life.[8]

The benefits of lucid dreaming are remarkable. Here's a sampling:

- Lucid dreaming can aid with nightmares and depression. Up to 8 percent of adults suffer from chronic nightmares. In a study at Utrecht University in the Netherlands, participants underwent lucid dreaming treatment (LDT), which included coming up with alternative endings to their nightmares. Those who were able to do so reduced the number of their nightmares.[9]

- Lucid dreams can boost your confidence, help you overcome shyness, manage grief, and give you the chance to rehearse things, like a performance or presentation. They can also prepare you for events you expect to be emotionally difficult, by giving you the chance to experience them in your dreams in advance of the actual worldly event. For example, a friend of mine was able to prepare for her mother's approaching death by having lucid dreams about that sad event and using those dreams as opportunities to practice letting go. This form of anticipatory grief can soften the blow of real grief.

• Lucid dreamers may be better at solving problems, according to recent studies. In some problem-solving situations, people need to "step back from perceived reality, reflect on it, and evaluate the perceptual evidence," write the authors of this study. How does this connect to lucidity in dreams? The same authors continue, "For the insight that leads to lucidity, people also seem able to step back from the obvious interpretation and consider a remote and, at the time, implausible option—that it is all a dream."[10] In other words, new perspective can be innovative. The biggest problem of them all is samsara, which is the confused world of conventional reality defined by dissatisfaction and suffering, and lucid dreaming has the potential to solve even that.

• Lucid dreaming has been shown to improve motor skills, which means it has the ability to help you with any physical activity, from playing the piano to athletic performance. It makes sense, because lucid dreams activate the brain in the same way as waking life. If you work on a math problem in your dream, for example, your left hemisphere is stimulated just as it would be during the day. If you sing in your dream, the right hemisphere is activated. If you do squats in a lucid dream, your physical heart rate increases. The extraordinary thing is that the effects from your nightly activity continue into the day. Training your dream body can train your physical body. For those with no time left during the day to do things, it's like adding a night shift.[11]

- Lucid dreaming can facilitate healing. One doctor published a paper about a patient with a twenty-two-year history of chronic pain who cured himself overnight with a single lucid dream. "I'm no expert on lucid dreams," says psychiatrist Mauro Zappaterra. "But the man woke up with no pain. He said it was like his brain had shut down and rebooted. A few days later, he walks in the VA pharmacy and actually returns his medication—300 tabs of levorphanol. To me that's pretty convincing evidence."[12]

Lucid dreaming is becoming the latest rage. People are using it to get an edge on their competition. Researchers are working with it to treat PTSD. Sleep scientists in Germany are using it to enhance focus and performance in athletes. Actors, inventors, artists, writers, and musicians are increasingly practicing lucid dreaming to enhance creativity. The psychologist Janine Chasseguet-Smirgel writes, "The process of creation [is] accompanied by the capacity to communicate with the most primitive layers of the unconscious"[13]—layers of the unconscious that can be accessed in your dreams.

Dreaming in general has been connected to creativity for eons, and the literature is replete with examples. The German chemist Friedrich Kekule discovered the molecular structure of benzene in a dream, James Cameron's dream of a robot-man eventually became the movie *The Terminator,* Robert Louis Stevenson came up with the plot for his novella *The Strange Case of Dr. Jekyll and Mr. Hyde* in a dream, and Paul McCartney's song "Yesterday" came to him in a dream.

The current popularity of lucid dreaming is both a blessing and a curse. We'll explore the blessings throughout this book. The curse is that dreams, as being unreal, are often not taken seriously. Cultures that honor dreams are often dismissed as primitive. "It's just a dream" is a trivializing comment, albeit one with provisional valid-ity. But if we dismiss our dreams and discharge lucid dreaming as just another virtual reality game, we will dismiss a profound oppor-tunity to explore the nature of mind and reality. The truly primitive cultures may well be those that dismiss the power of dreams, and therefore ignore the unparalleled opportunities for growth.

In this book we're going to talk about how to strengthen the world of dreaming as a way to weaken the world of daily appear-ance, so that worldly things don't have as much power over us. In technical terms, we can almost say that we'll reify, or materialize, the dream world in an effort to de-reify, or dematerialize, the waking world—until both are seen as equally real or unreal, and we awaken to the illusory nature of both. That's where freedom lies, and that's what "waking up" in the spiritual sense means.

We'll have much more to say about lucid dreams throughout the book. Right now, let's look at a map that can help us understand where we're going when we sleep and dream, and then explore how to get there.

My dreamlike form
Appeared to dreamlike beings
To show them the dreamlike path
That leads to dreamlike enlightenment.

THE BUDDHA, from the *Bhadrakalpa Sutra*

2

A Map for Practices of the Night

BEFORE WE START a journey, especially one into darkness, we need some idea of where we're going and what lies ahead. We need a good map. In Buddhism this is called "right view," which is the first factor in the Eightfold Noble Path.[1] "View" is a good term because it denotes a sense of vision and path. It's akin to philosophy or outlook, but more practical. Without a good view it's easy to get lost, detoured, or trapped in dead ends. Having no view is like crawling around on the ground like a worm. You can waste a lot of time. But with a bird's eye view, you can see exactly where you're going, and therefore get there faster.

A good map is important for the practices of the night because some people are afraid of what they might find in the depths of their mind. Some people are afraid of the dark. The mind is uncharted territory, shadowy, and sometimes scary. Nightmares hide in the dark alleys of the night, along with all sorts of ghastly unconscious elements. If you're on a spiritual path, the deeper mind is also strewn with all kinds of booby traps and obstacles that can bump you off your path. Having the right view is like aiming a floodlight into the night, which illuminates the journey and can eliminate the fear.[2]

A central theme of this book is learning how to establish a healthy relationship to fear, and to replace that fear with courage. We'll use the darkness of the night as a segue into transforming fear into fearlessness. Everything we do in life requires some guts, whether it's applying for a job, buying a house, asking someone for a date, taking a trip, opening a business, making a presentation, learning how to meditate, or starting something as different as dream yoga. Even getting out of bed on a bad day can take some nerve. As the motivational author Matthew Kelly says,

> The most dominant emotion today in our modern society is fear. We are afraid. Afraid of losing the things we have worked hard to buy, afraid of rejection and failure, afraid of certain parts of town, afraid of certain types of people, afraid of criticism, afraid of suffering and heartache, afraid of change, afraid to tell people how we really feel . . . We are even afraid to be ourselves. Some of these fears we are consciously aware of, while others exist subconsciously. But these fears can play a very large role in directing the actions of our lives . . . Fear stops more people from doing something with their lives than lack of ability, contacts, resources, or any other single variable.[3]

Courage, on the other hand, is the spark of life that propels us beyond the straitjacket of our fear. Nothing of importance is ever accomplished without courage. Look at the giants of history. Without bravery their lives would have slid into mediocrity. Kelly states that "the measure of your life will be the measure of your courage." When you die, do you want to be measured by your fear and what held you back, or by your courage and what moved you forward? Do you want to live on the sidelines as a mere spectator, or get onto the playing field of life and really live it?

While courage catalyzes, fear paralyzes. Fear, and the hesitation born from it, smothers life so that it burns on a pilot-light level. Things are safe, but semi-dead. The colloquialism "frozen in fear" takes on entirely new dimensions on the spiritual path and the meditations of the night. We're going to melt that frozen fear and replace it with calm courage, so that we can fully come to life.

On a spiritual level, fear is what keeps us from waking up. This fear is mostly our fear of the dark. <u>Darkness represents the unknown, or the unconscious</u>. We're always afraid of what we don't know or can't see. Darkness, in other words, is a code word for ignorance and the trigger for fear.[4] This darkness, or unconsciousness, has two levels: the relative and the absolute. Their distinction is important.

The Relative Level

The relative level of our unconscious mind is where repressed psychological stuff hangs out, the spiders and snakes of our darker mind. When Sigmund Freud said that dreams are the royal road to the unconscious, he was referring to this relative level. There's a reason we repress unwanted experiences into our unconscious mind. They're just too painful or frightening for consciousness. But what we refuse in conscious experience turns into the refuse (rubbish) of the relative unconscious mind. As the saying goes, "What we resist, persists." We didn't want to face this refuse when it was initially experienced, and we generally don't want to face it when it arises in our dreams, in therapy, or in meditation. But if we want to wake up and grow, face it we must.[5] Carl Jung wrote,

> The personal unconscious contains all psychic contents that are incompatible with the conscious attitude. This comprises a whole group of contents, chiefly those which appear morally, aesthetically, or intellectually inadmissible and are repressed on account of their incompatibility. A man cannot always think and feel the good, the true, and the beautiful, and in trying to keep up an ideal attitude everything that does not fit in with it is automatically repressed.[6]

These shadow contents scare us only because we don't know about them. They can arise in dreams, but they mostly generate fear when the dream is non-lucid. With proficiency in lucid dreaming, these frightening dreams become lucid to us, and lucidity leads to control.[7] So instead of running away from frightening dream experiences, and further repressing the elements that sparked the scary dream, we can face our demons with awareness—and therefore fearlessness—and purify the elements that give rise to the dream. In so doing we also purify our unconscious mind.[8] It's like lifting up a slab of flagstone in the middle of the day and having all those slimy critters slither away from the light. The only difference is that with the light of awareness, the creepy critters don't just slither away to reappear somewhere else. They disappear forever.

You're going to have scary dreams whether you engage in lucid dreaming or not. With lucidity you can remove the fear by gaining control. Surveys have shown that while many non-lucid dreams tend to be unpleasant, most lucid dreams are pleasant. It makes sense. Why would you be afraid of something you can control?

Some writers suggest that you can look for an ally in your dreams, a "pacemaker," or an internal dream guide who can accompany your descent into the unconscious. If you have a connection to Tibetan Buddhism, there are protectors that you can supplicate to help you on this inner journey. I'm certain that guardian angels and the like can also be engaged to hold your hand. While viable, these are only relative forms of protection, ones that I have never needed. The ultimate form of protection is having the right view, and seeing through any apparent threat. In the final analysis it's just your mind "in there," and that mind is basically good. If you don't reify the contents, nothing can hurt you.

The Absolute Level

The importance of a complete view of the unconscious mind becomes evident when we go beyond this relative level and arrive at the absolute ground of unconsciousness. This remarkable view, which is shared by many spiritual traditions, is a deal-maker when it comes to dream and sleep yoga. It's vital not only for the nighttime meditations, but for any spiritual practice. If the relative unconscious mind were the only destination of the nighttime yogas, it could be a deal-breaker, because of all the unwanted elements stuffed into that level of mind. Who wants to end up in a bed of spiders and snakes? The absolute view illuminates our final spiritual destination, day or night. It allows us to see through the dark relative levels and to take ultimate refuge in the light that shines within.

According to this more complete view—which you can prove for yourself with the practices in this book—the deepest level of your unconscious mind, who you really are at the ground of your being, is perfectly pure and utterly good. Down there, below what seems to be the deepest, darkest, and scariest aspect of your being, is the totally awakened state, the light of enlightenment.[9] It's what Buddhism calls "buddha nature" (your awakened nature), and it has also been termed "basic goodness." I will discuss it using a Tibetan Buddhist term, as the "clear-light mind."

This absolute level of the unconscious mind is radiant, loving, beneficent, and wise. The spiders and snakes of the relative level are replaced with sages and saints. When accessed and made conscious, this is the level of mind from which the buddhas operate. This is where your own awakened nature also resides, and is waiting for you to discover it. Through dream yoga you can yoke to this Buddha within, and wake up to who you really are.

Even though you may not know about this level yet, just having this view is enormously helpful. It changes everything. Instead of having something to fear in the darkness of the night, you now have something to look forward to. You're going to drop into the divinity of your being, into an essence that never dies, never changes, and is forever awake. Your relative unconscious mind may have some surprises for you, but if you know that's not who you really are, that below that haze is luminous purity, you can replace anxiety with anticipation.

This journey will therefore show you how to become fearless in the dark. Once again, this is not just the darkness of the night, but the darkness of the unknown aspects of your own mind, which is symbolized by the night. What happens when you travel consciously through the night, with the practices outlined in this book, is a condensation of what happens during the entire spiritual path. So this beautiful view not only informs the meditations of the night, but every practice of the path.

When you fall asleep every night, you're actually falling awake. You just don't know it yet. My task is to help you know it, and to transform this divine view into your direct experience.

Relative Defense

The relative level of your unconscious mind is like a protective shield. Its job is to protect ignorance, for it is the very embodiment of ignorance. This level is what keeps you in the dark, and therefore asleep, in both the physical and spiritual sense. To be asleep in the spiritual sense means to be unaware of your unawareness. It's the perfect blind spot—one you don't even know you have. The relative level of your unconscious mind doesn't want you to wake up to the truth, or to see the blind spots of this outer layer of unconsciousness. Because this underworld is filled with unpleasantries (it's the refuse heap after all, the landfill of rejected experience), it's very effective in keeping you away from the truth that lies below, the absolute reality that underlies all relative appearance.

The relative unconscious mind is the birthplace and bed of the ego, and it will do everything in its power to keep you from going deeper.[10] For the ego, ignorance really is bliss. It tries to keep you from the truth, because to penetrate the bed of ego is to see through its façade, and for the ego, that is equivalent to death. Ego feels as if it will evaporate if it goes below the thicket of the relative unconscious mind, so it kicks and screams to keep you away from the deeper truth of your absolute undying self. Ego is just protecting itself, but in doing so, it ensures your suffering. As we will see when we discuss the clear-light mind, ego *does* die (or is, more accurately, seen through) when we drop from the relative to the absolute levels of the unconscious mind. Thus, from ego's perspective, the defensive strategies are justified.

Knowing about the clear-light mind within is fantastic news from a spiritual perspective, but unwanted news from ego's perspective. Since we mostly operate from ego's point of view, without a bigger picture of where we're going when we drop into the absolute nature of our mind, fierce protection in the form of resistance can arise when we (ego) think about exploring the darkness of the night.

Most people just don't want to go there. They don't want to be bothered with things like dream yoga. They'd rather just sleep.

The principal means of "protection" are overt fear and covert apathy, or laziness. Fear is the lifeblood of the ego. To see through the prickly defenses of the relative unconscious mind means seeing through our fear of the dark. It's like going on a quest for the Holy Grail and learning that it's at the bottom of a deep, dark well. We look down the well and see all sorts of slithering creatures on the surface of the water. Without a map assuring you that the Grail is below the grime, there's no way you're going to dive into that well.

"Fear" is etymologically connected to "fare." Fear is the fare, or toll, that must be paid in order to grow. If we really want to wake up, we need to *follow our fear* into and through the darkest aspects of our being, for that is where the brightest light abides.

When Joseph Campbell uttered his famous maxim, "Follow your bliss," he was speaking a partial truth. It is important to follow your bliss, and it can take courage, but if that's all you do, you'll just get blissed out. From a spiritual perspective, it can be more valid to say, "Follow your fear." But similarly, if that's all you do, you'll just get freaked out. The Buddhist concept of the "middle way," or "not too tight, not too loose," is the ideal guide. Don't become an extremist and lose your way by getting either snared in bliss or scared away by fear.

In our journey into nighttime darkness, "follow your fear" takes on additional significance. Fear is the minion of ignorance—where you find ignorance, you will find fear. This is important because ignorance itself is so subtle. It's virtually invisible, another massive blind spot, something we're asleep to. In my spiritual community we talk about "*klesha* attacks," where the Sanskrit word *klesha* means "emotional upheaval." It's basically when someone loses it. It's easy to identify klesha attacks of passion, aggression, jealousy, or pride, for example, but I've never been able to say, "I'm having an ignorance attack." This is an irony, because if I see the world as solid, lasting, and independent (dualistically), I'm under attack. It means I'm under attack right now, I just don't see it. This blindness is particularly damaging because every other visible klesha, and therefore all our suffering, arises from this one, the stealth bomber of ignorance.

So you can use your fear, which is much more visible, to work with your ignorance. When you feel fear, you're getting down to it. You're approaching some level of ignorance, and therefore the opportunity to transcend it. If you're serious about waking up in this life, and don't know where to go or what to do, go to the places that scare you. But be intelligent about it. Don't go to physically dangerous places, or slip into mere thrill seeking. Use your fear of the dark to lead you to the light, not into mere entertainment.

I have used this maxim to guide much of my life. It's the reason I went into three-year retreat nearly twenty years ago. Nothing scared me more than having to face my mind so directly for so long. It turned out to be the most transformative three years of my life. It's the reason I started doing dark retreats.[11] Nothing scared me more than going into a pitch-black cabin for weeks on end to face my mind so intensely. These retreats continue to be among the most rewarding experiences of my life. It's the reason I've studied and *practiced* death so extensively (my 2013 book *Preparing to Die* was inspired by this study and practice). Nothing scared me more than the darkness of death. This study and practice has removed my fear of death. And, of course, this theme continues each night as I explore the darkness of sleep. But because I trust my map so completely, I have absolutely no fear of this inner terrain.

Oddly enough, I have always found *enduring* bliss within my fear. Following my fear has always led me to real bliss, not the transient enjoyment that often results from following my bliss alone. And strangely enough, following my bliss often leads to fear—the fear of losing my bliss. You get the point: following your bliss can result in fear; following your fear can result in bliss. This applies to our fear of the dark. If you're afraid of the darkness of your own mind as it manifests in the night, a map that shows you that bliss (the absolute unconscious mind) is what awaits you beyond the fear (the relative unconscious mind) can make all the difference, and inspire you to take the plunge.

This is also why many spiritual traditions are described as *warrior* traditions.[12] In Tibetan, warriors *(pawo)* are "those who are brave." Spiritual warriors are those who are brave enough to explore the deep inner space of their own mind. It's dark in there. And it does take courage. But it's only fearful if we don't know who we truly are, and if we remain ignorant to the fact that fear only exists at the relative levels of our unconscious mind.

I don't want to overstate this relative level, and therefore paradoxically keep people away from exploring their mind as they sleep and dream. Many people are already excited about traveling consciously into the night, and for them I say: welcome aboard! But for others a good flashlight can help.

This map of the unconscious mind will become clearer, and the journey more comfortable, when we discuss the levels of mind further in chapters 9 and 10. The more we can see where we're going, the more inspired we'll become. We'll have much more to say about transforming fear, ignorance, darkness, and sleep into fearlessness, wisdom, light, and awakening.

In summary, fear, the primordial emotion of samsara, is the active expression of ignorance. Ignorance is usually too subtle to see, but fear is something we can all relate to. This ignorance is basically unfamiliarity, not knowing who we really are. By becoming familiar with (the very definition of meditation) who we are, we transform ignorance into wisdom, darkness into light, and replace fear with fearlessness. That is our journey in this book.

The Power of the Map

Another possible concern with dream yoga is the subtle nature of the journey. Some people may feel they can't do it. But I have taught dream seminars for years, and in my experience almost everybody, with patience, can have lucid dreams and therefore practice dream yoga. Sleep yoga is a different matter, which is why we'll only discuss it relatively briefly in this book. But for those who are interested, keep in mind that as you develop stability in dream yoga, sleep yoga becomes increasingly accessible.

Even if you can't accomplish the following practices, just knowing about lucid dreaming, dream yoga, and sleep yoga will change the way you relate to sleep. But more importantly, this material will change the way you relate to life. Even if it's left at the level of the map alone, this view of reality is powerful enough to change the way you live.[13] It's a treasure map that can alter the course of your life.

Lucid dreaming, dream yoga, and sleep yoga have a common outcome: increasing awareness. While this book focuses on the nighttime practices, it's actually about bringing light into any aspect of life. Like a supernova exploding deep in the universe of your own heart, the light will eventually arrive at the surface of your life and transform it.

Anything that heightens awareness is beneficial. While the ultimate goal is to develop constant awareness and achieve the awakening of a buddha, even if the view only expands your awareness to a fraction of that totality, it will help. In doing these practices for over thirty years, heightened awareness has been the greatest benefit. I see more. Life isn't so burdensome. My world has become softer, more playful and childlike.

As we will see, awareness is one way to talk about lucidity in an expanded sense. The beginning, middle, and end of the path, or what Buddhism refers to as ground, path, and fruition, are all about nurturing awareness/lucidity, which is what we will do using the medium of our dreams. As an overview of our journey, and its practical implications, Buddhist psychotherapist Bruce Tift says,

> The whole journey is—and always was—about being
> present with [waking up to] reality. But something
> must differentiate the ground, or starting place [being
> asleep], from the fruition [awakening]. When we begin,
> the ground—our day-to-day reality [what we'll refer
> to as "appearance"]—is experienced as if it were the
> whole story. We believe it to be completely real [like a
> non-lucid dream]. Not only that, but we embellish it
> with a running commentary in our mind—"content"
> that keeps us from noticing the "context" in which
> our experience is arising. During the path phase, we
> gradually shift our perception so that we no longer focus
> solely on the content of our experience—our thoughts,
> feelings, sensations, and ideas. Instead, we begin to
> recognize [wake up to] the context in which these

experiences arise—a context that can never be captured and understood conceptually. We call this context "awareness." We still experience the content [the dream], but we are simultaneously aware that it's not the whole story; it does not completely represent reality [we've become lucid]. So you might say that the ground is our present-moment experience without awareness. The fruition is that very same experience with awareness. The path creates the conditions for this shift of perception [waking up] to arise . . . this whole approach is not about improving the content of our experience. Instead, it's about creating a shift in how we relate to the experiences we are having at any moment . . . freedom [waking up] arises from a profound disidentification with [seeing through] any content.[14]

We'll return to these themes throughout the book, and gradually unfold this summary quotation, which (with my insertions) shows us how we can wake up to our life by waking up to our dreams.

There are many times when I'm unable to trigger lucid dreams, or too lazy to even try. That's okay. The view behind these practices still affects everything I do. This will become clearer when we discuss the daytime practice of dream yoga, illusory form, which is introduced in chapter 12.

We'll also return to a deeper exploration of the map in chapter 9, when we discuss the levels of mind. After the next chapter on sleep cycles and how to use them, we will proceed directly with how to start having lucid dreams.

By and by comes the Great Awakening, and then
we shall find out that life itself is a great dream.
All the while fools think that they are awake, busily
and brightly assuming that they understand things.

CHUANG TZU, *The Tao of Abundance: Eight Ancient Principles
for Abundant Living*

3

Understanding Sleep Cycles

WE TAKE SLEEP for granted, but it's literally a lifesaver. Without
sleep you would die. There's a rare genetic disorder called "fatal familial insomnia" that usually occurs in middle age, lasts about a year,
and always ends in death. There is no cure. Much more common is
sleep apnea, which afflicts more than 22 million Americans.[1] With
this condition, a person stops breathing up to thirty times an hour
and therefore never gets enough restorative sleep. Those suffering
from sleep apnea have a significantly higher risk for heart disease,
stroke, and a host of other illnesses.[2] It's a silent killer.

Up to 75 million Americans have sleep disorders (there are over
seventy sleep disorders),[3] and over 25 percent of Americans take a
prescription medication to help them sleep.[4] In 2010, Americans
spent 30 billion dollars in the sleep-assistance industry.[5] Sixty-two
percent of adults in the United States report sleep problems several nights a week.[6] One-third of working Americans, or over 40
million people, don't get enough sleep.[7] Even if you don't suffer
from sleep apnea, sleep problems contribute to diabetes, obesity,
anxiety, depression, immune suppression, substance abuse, strokes,
heart disease, accidents, mood disorders, and death.[8] The sleep scientist William Dement says, "Sleep is one of the most important

predictors of how long you will live—as important as whether you smoke, exercise, or have high blood pressure or cholesterol."[9]

Dream yoga may or may not help with sleep disorders. It's not meant to be a medical treatment. But it can help people relate to their disorders in a new way, and provide ways to take advantage of them. If you suffer from insomnia, for example, you can use your sleeplessness to practice lucid dream induction techniques. You can take sleep obstacles and turn them into opportunities.

To sleep well you must literally do nothing. For many of us that's not easy. But doing nothing, and doing it well, is one aspect of meditation. So the preparatory meditations for dream yoga that we will introduce can help with things like insomnia. It's a nice twofer: meditation can help you "wake up" in the spiritual sense, while helping you fall asleep in the biological sense.

Why Do We Sleep?

No one knows exactly why we sleep or dream, despite many theories. We may sleep to digest learning, to integrate memories, or for memory consolidation, taking short-term memory and making it long-term. We may sleep to boost our immune system, and therefore prevent disease. Animal research has shown that sleep contributes to brain plasticity and neurogenesis, which is the formation of new neurons in the brain. Evidence also suggests that sleep cleans the brain, flushing out toxins.[10]

In Eastern medical theory, sleep balances the elements, which become disturbed during the day. In this view, there are five main elements in the world—earth, water, fire, wind, and space—and likewise there are five elements within us. With insomniacs, there is often too much "wind," which tends to kick us out of our body and into our head. When we go to sleep we unwind, or un-wind. We drop back into our body (our personal earth) and ground ourselves.[11] When we really get out of balance, we don't just get tired, we get sick. Sickness then forces us to sleep, and to balance the elements. When I'm stressed and "windy," I invariably get a cold and have to sleep. In Buddhism, wind is considered the most powerful element. The epic Kalachakra Tantra, "The King of Tantras," asserts that "wind" creates and destroys individual and collective world systems. If it can do that, it can surely keep us up at night.

In the Buddhist view, sleep is a product of ignorance. Indeed, "sleep" is another code word for ignorance. Buddhas, as "the awakened ones" or "the ones who know," literally don't sleep.[12] Their body may go into sleep mode (they lie down at night), but their minds never black out. The historical Buddha Shakyamuni, for example, allegedly went to Tushita heaven in a special dream body to teach his mother as his body slept. So when the tradition asserts that buddhas don't sleep, it doesn't mean they stay up all night doing physical activity. It means that ignorance has been completely removed, and they remain forever awake, or lucid, through all states of consciousness—waking, dreaming, and dreamless sleep.

Markers of progress on the spiritual path are tricky, but one marker may be less sleep. We have to be careful, however, because some people simply need less sleep, which may have nothing to do with spiritual realization. But the literature is replete with stories of advanced meditators needing just an hour or two each night of sleep. This may be due to less grasping during the day, and less internal conflict.[13] The normal conceptual mind is constantly grasping at everything, which is akin to lifting weights all day. It's exhausting. Think about how tired your bicep would get if it were constantly doing curls. As the mind relaxes its vicelike grip on thoughts and things, which happens with meditation, it doesn't get so tired. When we sleep, we finally get to relax and rest. But if we're relaxed and rested all the time, which is the mind of a buddha, there's no need to relax the mind at night.[14]

Why Do We Dream?

As for why we dream, many researchers believe that dreaming helps connect various levels of memory, integrating more recent events within long-term memories. Dreaming may also help us sort through what is most relevant to our well-being, and one study suggests that we dream to ease painful memories.[15] Other studies submit that sleeping and dreaming stimulate lateral thinking, which is an indirect and creative approach to problem solving.[16]

REM sleep (described below) is associated with the activation of brain areas dealing with emotions, which implies that dreams may be a form of emotional metabolism.[17] Dreams may help us digest important events. In REM-deprivation studies, where dreams are cut from life, people are quickly thrown out of physiological and emotional balance. One can infer that, from an evolutionary point of view, dreams are essential for health and well-being, even if we don't know why.

According to the Dalai Lama, and every resource I could find, there is no explanation within Buddhism for why we dream. Perhaps it's purely soteriological, or "pertaining to deliverance." Perhaps we dream, and wake up from our dreams, to show us how we can deliver ourselves from samsara.

Types of Sleep

To most effectively learn lucid dreaming, which is the platform for all the other nighttime practices, it helps to understand and take advantage of our sleep cycles. Sometimes it's best not to disturb sleep; other times we can make use of a sleep cycle to trigger lucid dreams.

There are two main kinds of sleep: non-REM, or quiet sleep, and REM, or paradoxical sleep. REM sleep is called "paradoxical sleep" because while the brain becomes more active during this stage, muscles become more relaxed. Non-REM sleep is associated with restoration, deep relaxation, and an idling brain. People who suffer from sleep apnea don't spend enough time in non-REM sleep, and therefore don't get the needed restoration. (REM sleep is the sleep stage used in lucid dreaming and dream yoga. Non-REM sleep is used in the stage associated with sleep yoga.)

REM sleep, which accounts for about 25 percent of sleep in most people, is associated with rapid eye movement (REM), muscle twitches, sleep paralysis, an active brain, and dreaming. Sleep paralysis (atonia), which is when voluntary muscles become temporarily paralyzed, usually goes unrecognized, but sometimes we can be aware of it. The awareness of sleep paralysis results from an "out of sequence" REM state. We're not supposed to be conscious of our body in REM sleep. We're supposed to be sleeping or dreaming. But that's what happens during glimpses of sleep paralysis—we're partly conscious when we're not supposed to be. It's a temporary mix of brain states that are normally separate. In recognized sleep paralysis, REM encroaches into wakefulness; in lucid dreaming, wakefulness encroaches into REM.

I tend to notice sleep paralysis during naps, when I'm partly asleep and partly awake. It feels as if I'm in a straitjacket, or as if someone is pinning me down. Before I understood what was happening, it was a panicky experience. Sleep paralysis is nature's way of preventing us from acting out our dreams. With certain disorders, such as REM sleep behavior disorder (RBD), sleep paralysis doesn't work, and folks do things like beat up their sleeping partners, completely unaware of doing so. People have been arrested and prosecuted for this bizarre form of domestic violence. When my dog is dreaming, I often see him twitching and semi-barking, and I wonder what he might be chasing in his dream. Without his temporary paralysis he would probably leap up and run into a wall. Sleepwalking and sleep talking are different, and occur in non-REM sleep when there is no paralysis.

In lucid dreaming and dream yoga, we don't engage with non-REM sleep because we're generally not dreaming during non-REM sleep and we don't want to disturb that restorative stage. The time to apply our efforts is during REM sleep, when dreams are mostly happening. Understanding the following stages helps us determine when to apply our dream-induction techniques.

Stages of Sleep

We go through five stages when we sleep. Each stage is associated with a brain-wave frequency, which is correlated with brain activity. We tend to view sleep as a simple matter of "turning off," but sleep is actually a very active state. Our brain-wave activity is more varied during the night than it is during the day.

Until recent improvements in technology refined our understanding, scientists measured four principal brain-wave states—beta, alpha, theta, and delta—as determined by an EEG, or electroencephalogram.[18] Waking consciousness is associated with beta and alpha, and sleep with theta and delta. Beta waves pulsate at a frequency of 13–40 cycles per second (or hertz) and are associated with states of concentration and stress. Alpha waves have a frequency of 8–13 hertz and are associated with more relaxed waking states. When we go to sleep, the brain downshifts from waking beta and alpha to theta (4–8 hertz), and eventually to "neutral," or the deep sleep of delta (0–4 hertz).[19]

As brain waves settle from beta into alpha, we enter a pre-sleep stage called the "hypnagogic" phase, which is a kind of gap (bardo) between waking and sleeping (from the roots *hypnos,* "god of sleep," and *agogia,* "leading to"—a lovely image). During this stage it's common to have feelings of falling, or hearing someone call your name, experiences called "hypnagogic hallucinations." The boundaries between inside and outside, self and other, blur. Hypnagogic phenomena are interesting for meditators, especially during long meditation sessions, as one dips in and out of sleep on the cushion, and therefore in and out of hypnagogic states. We'll have more to say about hypnagogic experiences later, and how to use them, for they are a way to practice "lucid sleep onset." Another common event during this pre-sleep stage is called the "myoclonic (or hypnic) jerk," which is when you suddenly jerk awake for no obvious reason.[20]

The surrealist Salvador Dalí took advantage of hypnagogic states to tap into the creative power of his unconscious mind, giving rise to many of his dreamlike paintings. Dalí and his surrealist colleagues saw dreams as central to their work. To stay in the pre- and post-dream state for as long as possible, Dalí devised a system where he held a spoon cradled over his chest that would fall onto a plate when he dozed off, waking him up. He then reset the arrangement over and over, which allowed him to drift between waking and dreaming consciousness for extended periods. Thus he extracted images from his unconscious-dreaming mind and used them to seed his conscious surrealist art. Dalí's paintings are a form of "bardo" art, drawn from the gap between waking and dreaming.

Stage 1, which lasts about five or ten minutes, is very light sleep. This is when it's still easy to wake someone up. The difference between deep relaxation and slipping into stage 1 sleep occurs gradually and subtly. If you wake someone up during this stage, they often report that they weren't really asleep. Brain waves during this stage decrease from alpha to theta. We spend about 4 to 5 percent of sleep here.

Stage 2 sleep is slightly deeper and characterized by a decrease in breathing, heart rate, and body temperature. The brain is still mostly in theta, but interspersed are two wave features that are the defining characteristics of stage 2 sleep. "Sleep spindles" are a sudden increase in wave frequency, and "K complexes" are a sudden increase in wave amplitude. This stage lasts about twenty minutes, but as with any stage the time is variable. We spend about 45 to 55 percent of total sleep here.[21] Stages 1 and 2 are considered light stages of sleep.

Stage 3 is the beginning of deep sleep, when brain waves drop into the slower delta range. It's a transitional stage between light sleep and the deep sleep of stage 4. There is no crisp distinction between stages 3 and 4 except that stage 3 is when less than 50 percent of brain waves are delta, and stage 4 is when more than 50 percent of waves are delta. We spend about 6 percent of sleep at stage 3. In 2007, the American Academy of Sleep Medicine decided to group stage 3 and stage 4 together, making four stages instead of five. In this book I will be using the pre-2007 classification because it still seems to be the one most employed.

Stage 4 is our deepest sleep and lasts about thirty minutes in the first sleep cycle. (We cycle through these five stages four to five times each night, as described below.) It's characterized by profound muscle relaxation and rhythmic breathing. This is where we're fully offline. Stage 4 is restorative sleep, when the body releases human growth hormone, undergoes cellular and biological repair, and gets the rest we need. We spend about 12 to 15 percent of total sleep at stage 4, but that percentage decreases dramatically as we age (from up to 20 percent as a young adult to 3 percent by midlife), and by age sixty-five this "slow wave" sleep can disappear altogether. Aging is therefore inversely proportional to the amount of slow wave sleep. Because the release of growth hormones also decreases, lack of deep sleep can account for many aspects of aging, including decreased sex drive, fatigue, increased body fat, loss of muscle tone and strength, thinning of the skin, memory loss, and diminished immune function.[22] Stages 3 and 4 are when it's the most difficult to wake someone up. If someone wakes up from this state, they're usually groggy, grumpy, and disoriented. Bed-wetting and sleepwalking tend to occur at the end of stage 4.[23]

After resting in deep dreamless sleep for about thirty minutes, we briefly come back up to stage 2, but instead of coming all the way back up to stage 1, we enter a new stage, REM sleep, or stage 5. In other words, stage 1 is replaced with REM sleep. After REM, we go back down through the stages again. REM sleep is when we dream the most. Brain waves come back up from delta to alpha, which means your brain returns to its usual daytime frequencies. Heart rate and respiration quicken, and voluntary muscles are paralyzed. You actually consume more oxygen during REM sleep than you do when awake, unless you're doing something aerobic. People often worry that lucid dreaming and dream yoga could make them less rested. Since most of our restorative sleep occurs in delta wave sleep, and dreams mostly occur during REM sleep when the brain isn't resting anyway, this worry is unfounded.

"Sleep architecture" represents the cyclical pattern of sleep as we move between the different stages. It gives us a picture of what sleep looks like during the night, as presented in a graph called a "hypnogram" (see figure 1).

We go through these five stages four to five times each night, in about ninety-minute cycles. After each REM period, we have brief moments of awakening, up to fifteen times a night, when we toss and turn. This creates an opportunity to bring awareness to our dreams before cycling back into stage 2 sleep.

The first REM period is short, about five to ten minutes. This is why we rarely remember dreams from the early part of the night. If we have a non-REM dream, it tends to be less intense and emotional, often just a recollection of events from the day. As the night progresses, REM periods increase and non-REM periods decrease. The first half of the night is mostly non-REM, and the second half transitions into mostly REM. Just before awakening we can be in REM sleep for forty-five minutes to an hour, which is why we mostly remember our morning dreams. This is prime-time dreamtime.

By understanding these cycles, we can tune in to the times for ramping up our efforts. Don't waste your time trying to have lucid dreams in the early part of the night. Get your restorative sleep. Wait until REM sleep is at its peak. When I do dream yoga retreats and have the luxury of taking naps during the day, I often practice lucid dream induction techniques throughout the night. This means I set my alarm to go off every ninety minutes, which is when I'm most likely to be in REM sleep. I don't recommend this as a regular practice, unless you can take naps during the day. During daily life the time to concentrate your efforts is a few hours before waking up.

This is all we need to know about the science of sleep to launch us into the nighttime practices.

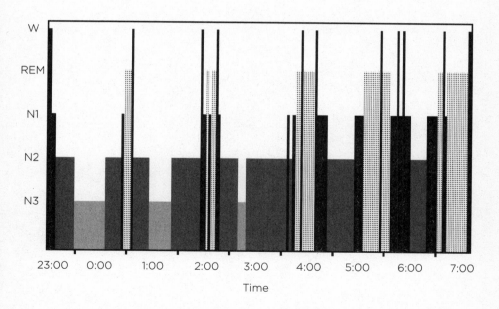

FIGURE 1   This hypnogram shows the alternating pattern between the four stages of sleep. (N = non-REM sleep; W = waking.) REM sleep is depicted by the dotted bar, which gets wider (lasts longer) as the night progresses and peaks in duration just before the person woke at 7 a.m. *Courtesy of Kristen LaMarca, PhD, and Nevin Arora, MD, of Integrative Insomnia and Sleep Health Center, San Diego*

Milarepa does not suffer, because he knows that this life is like a dream and an illusion. At the same time, he sees that sentient beings suffer precisely because they take this life to be truly existent.

KHENPO TSÜLTRIM GYAMTSO RINPOCHE,
composed extemporaneously at Dorje Denma Ling,
translated by Ari Goldfield

4
Western Lucid Dream Induction Techniques

IN THE NEXT few chapters we will explore the techniques that allow us to wake up in our dreams. The present chapter focuses on Western induction techniques, and the following chapter looks at Eastern techniques, providing a broad approach that joins the modern knowledge of the West with the ancient wisdom of the East. In my own training, I spent my first decade practicing Eastern techniques, with hit-and-miss results. When I supplemented these meditative practices with the methods from the West, my lucid dreaming took off.

Dream yoga itself hasn't changed much in hundreds of years. It was designed by beings so awake that perhaps they didn't realize that mere mortals like ourselves might need some baby steps. The classic practice texts are pithy, and therefore steep. The great contribution of modern lucid dreaming is to provide a gradual on-ramp. Lucid dreaming has much to offer for practitioners of dream yoga, and dream yoga has a great deal to contribute to lucid dreaming. Together they make fantastic sleeping partners.

In these two chapters I will introduce a variety of induction techniques. There is no need to master them all. Triggering lucidity is the point, not the technique that gets you there. We're all different. One technique may work for one person and not at all for another. The point in presenting all these techniques is that you will eventually find one that works for you. When you do, stick with that. No need to do any other unless you wish to explore more possibilities. The only danger in presenting so many methods is that you might try one for a night or two, give up, and then skip to the next. I recommend staying with a technique for at least several weeks. Give it a chance. If it's not working after that, then try another. And feel free to start with whichever particular method makes the most sense to you.

There's a story about a farmer who wanted to dig a well. He tried to find water by digging six feet in one spot, at which point he got discouraged and moved to try another spot. He dug another six feet, got nothing, and moved to another location, and then another. His lack of perseverance guaranteed failure. To get to the center of yourself with these nocturnal meditations, you have to dig deep. Potshots create potholes that will never reach far.

What makes dream yoga unique is that you become your own instructor. You're the one who knows your mind better than anyone. You're the one who knows your sleep patterns and dream quirks. You have to be honest with yourself in this practice, which is another instance of the nighttime practices as truth-tellers. You have to rely on your own wisdom, and take responsibility for your success.

See what works for you not only in the techniques but in the way you employ them. If you find it's too disruptive to practice lucid dreaming during the week, then just do it on weekends. While it's helpful at first to do a technique the way it's presented, don't be afraid to play around with it. Maybe a blending of techniques works for you, or your own method. Experiment, and have fun. If you don't enjoy lucid dreaming, you won't do it. While motivation and ambition are important, don't be hard on yourself. Go slow and easy.

The idea of the nighttime practices as truth-tellers applies to another issue. Sooner or later, these practices will reveal your passion for ignorance. There will come a point when you may say, "Screw it. I'd rather go to sleep." Many times I don't want to practice. I get lazy, or just don't care. That's when I notice my passion for ignorance and smile at it. This is a natural expression of our passion for mind-lessness, as we will see. While there may be part of us that wants to wake up, there's a big part of us that does not. For the ego, igno-rance really is bliss. We've been spiritually asleep for a long time, and waking up isn't always easy.

A central teaching in any meditation is "not too tight, not too loose." If you're too tight, or try too hard, you'll tie yourself into knots and won't fall asleep. If you don't try enough, you're too loose, and you're not practicing dream yoga. The "middle way" approach is always best. It's like tuning a guitar. Tune it too tight and the strings snap; tune it too loose and it makes a saggy sound. With balance, perseverance, and humor, you will learn how to tune your mind to make beautiful night music.

Three Key Ingredients

The three essential ingredients for lucid dreaming are (1) strong motivation, or intention, (2) good dream recall, and (3) practicing the induction techniques. If you already possess the first two, you can skip to the induction techniques below.

The first ingredient, strong motivation, is critical. Motivation, or intention, creates momentum that carries into the dream world. It's as if you are seeding the lucid dream, a technique that is basic to any level of dream induction. The word "intent" comes from roots that mean "to stretch toward" (*in-*, "toward," and *tendere*, "stretch"). Lucid dreaming or dream yoga begins by stretching the mind with intention. As we have seen, stretching is common to both mental and physical yogas. In order to wrap your mind around the dark, you have to stretch toward it. You eventually want to stretch your awareness into previously unconscious states of mind, and the warmup for that begins with your intent. Stretching in this inten-tional way therefore begins to expand your mind.

Have you ever had to get up early and not had an alarm clock? By setting a strong intention to get up at a certain time, we often wake up at that time despite not having an alarm. In the same way, we can set an internal alarm to wake us up within a dream by setting a strong intention.[1]

If you're reading this book, you've already started to set your intent. Studying the view, or philosophy, behind lucid dreaming and dream yoga strengthens it. To actually practice intention, say to yourself throughout the day, "Tonight I *will* remember my dreams. I *will* have many dreams. I *will* have good dreams. I *will* wake up within my dreams." Don't just mouth the words. Mean it. You also strengthen the intention by saying it out loud and writing it down: taking it from mental to verbal to physical. As you're lying down in bed, ramp up your intent, like a sprint to the finish line.

Other expressions of intent come from reading books, taking courses, and basically spending as much time as you can with this material. When Stephen LaBerge was doing his PhD dissertation on lucid dreaming, he was soaking in this material and had lucid dreams almost every night. My own work in writing this book has been similar. Plant lots of seeds and you'll harvest lots of plants. Do not underestimate the power of intent. The dream researchers Robert Price and David Cohen write, "Lucid dreaming appears to be an experience widely available to the highly motivated."[2]

One way to sustain motivation is to have a clear goal once you do become lucid. In lucid dreaming workshops, people often say, "My goal is to become lucid in my dreams!" When they do, they often immediately wake up and feel disappointed because the lucid dream didn't last. Why should they be disappointed when they attained their goal? They got what they asked for, so the key is to ask for more. It's therefore important to set a goal *beyond* becoming lucid, so that lucidity eventually becomes the natural state, the platform, that's required to accomplish even higher goals.

Patricia Keelin, an elite lucid dreamer, says that the more emotionally imbued the goal is, and the stronger the motivational charge, the greater the reach. For example, if you go to sleep with the passion, excitement, and anticipation that "I will wake up in my dreams because I want to fly. I want to feel the freedom of soaring through space, to see from a bird's-eye view, and to feel the wind blowing through my hair!" you've added octane to your intent. The key is to add the magical element of *feeling*, or emotional charge. So extend your intent even further into the dream world, "stretch toward" more, by infusing your motivation with passion. It's amazing how often you'll get what you really ask for.

A second essential ingredient for lucid dreaming is good dream recall. Even though we have at least six dreams each night, many people don't remember any of them. LaBerge says that until you can remember at least two dreams each night, it's better not to try the lucidity techniques.

Good dream recall begins with your attitude, which follows from motivation and setting the intent to remember your dreams.[3] Value your dreams, and then plant the seeds for better recall. If you make your dreams important, they will come to you more frequently. As the dream researcher Patricia Garfield says in her book *Creative Dreaming*, "Those who do not 'believe in' dreams or who believe them to be nonsense do not remember their dreams or have only nonsensical ones. Dreams are what you make of them . . . Dream states respond to waking attitudes."[4] Tell yourself resolutely that you *will* remember your dreams. Put your heart into it. Get plenty of sleep, and allow yourself to sleep in. Take advantage of prime-time dreamtime. The fun part of lucid dreaming is giving yourself permission to languish in bed and dip in and out of dreams.

Dream journaling, or a dream diary, really helps. Starting a dream journal highlights the intention that you're taking this seriously. You're putting your money where your mouth is. You're also progressing from mental (the intent), to the verbal (repeating the intention to remember dreams), to the physical (getting the journal). Garfield quotes the anthropologist Tanya Luhrmann, who recalled, "Many years ago, I joined a group that decided that we would write down our dreams. And my dream life changed. I seemed to dream more. I remembered more detail. I sometimes had dreams of mythic intensity."[5]

If you have a hard time remembering dreams, it helps to write down any snippet of any dream you can remember. When you wake up, ask yourself, "Was I dreaming?" Close your eyes and try to return to recapture any part of the dream. And don't move. Moving engages waking consciousness and pulls you out of the dream world. If you've already moved and think you did have a dream, return to the position you were in when you first woke up. Memories are lodged in our bodies. I have often recaptured a dream by returning to the position I was in when I had it.

Here's a daytime practice to support this. Set a timer to go off at random intervals throughout the day. When it signals, take a moment to recall your thoughts or actions from the past ten minutes. You can also adapt this type of mental backtracking to occasions when you find you've been daydreaming. This is in the family of "reciprocating practices," which means that the practice you do during the day will help you with your practice at night, and the practice you do at night will help you with your practice during the day. This type of back-and-forth, or bidirectional, practice is common in dream yoga. You're opening up a two-way street between the day and the night.

Finally, take advantage of prime-time dreaming by waking up about two hours before you normally would, staying up for fifteen minutes or so, then going back to sleep. With these tips it's easy to start remembering your dreams. With strong motivation and good dream recall, you're ready to explore the third ingredient, the induction techniques, which I'll divide into the daytime and nighttime methods.

WAKING UP AND THE REASSEMBLY OF SELF

Waking up in the middle of the night can also be illuminating in terms of how we create, or reconstitute, our sense of self. I often find that when I first wake up, especially if it's from deep dreamless sleep in the middle of the night, that I can't immediately locate myself. Sometimes literally, as in not knowing where I am, but most importantly ontologically, as in not knowing *who* I am. I'm obviously aware when I'm jolted awake, but I'm sometimes not aware of my personal identity or history.

You've probably had this unsettling experience. It takes a few revealing seconds to reconstitute the running narrative, the storyline, that ends up being "you." In my experience, sometimes the feeling is groundless and panicky, and I scramble to re-create who I am. On those occasions, I breathe a sigh of relief when I finally "find" myself. At other times it's fascinating not to locate my sense of self, and I delight in this gap of not knowing. During these more pleasant awakenings,

I watch my mind bustle about as it puts together the jigsaw puzzle—all the separate pieces of my history—that results in this ineffable feeling called "me."

This is a glimpse of egolessness, and how my ego sometimes doesn't like it. When I first wake up, there's no reference point, no me. Just pure awareness free of any narrative. If I can stay open to that groundlessness and relate to it properly, without reference to anyone (me) having this experience, it's a liberating and spacious feeling. But due to the power of habit, ego's defensive and self-generating strategies race to coalesce this open awareness into a contracted point that I then recognize as the historical me. I can literally feel this contraction in my guts. What I don't feel, because it's been happening for so long that I've grown accustomed or even anesthetized to it, is that this contraction doesn't stop. It's happening right now. I'm operating from this contracted and painful point all the time. It's a point of pinched awareness called "me," a defensive self-contraction against open space, or pure egoless awareness, that is born from my fear of egolessness.

The next time you wake up in the dead of night, or are otherwise jolted awake, try to relate to this jarring transition in consciousness in a new way. Feel the initial openness, the rapidly ensuing bewilderment, and the scramble to reassemble yourself. This kind of exploration is part of the nighttime yogas, which as a family of practices are ways to relate to any nighttime experience with a meditative and inquisitive attitude. You can learn a great deal about yourself as you fall (apart) into sleep, and come back (together) to waking consciousness.

Daytime Western Induction Techniques

A host of daytime methods provide the on-ramp for the nighttime techniques. These daily practices also help you mix dream yoga into your life, integrating these normally disparate states of consciousness.

State Checks

One useful daytime induction practice is to conduct regular "state checks." A state check means you're going to question the status of your reality by asking yourself throughout the day, "Is this a dream? Am I dreaming?" as a way of developing a critical attitude toward your reality.[6] It may seem silly to ask yourself these questions, because our usual response is, "Of course I'm awake!" But how do you know for sure?

A non-critical or unquestioning attitude causes us to miss the fact that we're dreaming when we're dreaming. We don't realize that we're dreaming because we take the dream to be real, when in fact it is not. That's the very definition of non-lucidity—"mis-taking" dreams to be real. Because we don't question the status of our reality during the day, we don't question the status of our reality at night. As you familiarize yourself with the practice of conducting state checks, the habit carries over into your dreams. When you apply it, you will suddenly discover that you *are* dreaming. That one flash of recognition is all you need to wake up in your dreams.

Conducting a state check is easy. On the back of a business card write, "Is this a dream?" Look at it periodically during the day, then take it out of your line of vision, then look at it again. If you're awake, the card will look the same the second time you look at it. But if you're dreaming, something about the card will change. If the card comes back the second time saying something else, or is in a different font, size, or color, you can be pretty sure you're dreaming. You can do the same thing with a digital watch. Look at it, look away, then look again. Is it the same on second glance?

My favorite state check is also the easiest. Simply jump up periodically during the day. If you come back down, you're probably awake. But if you keep going up, or come back down and fall through the ground, you're dreaming. I have used this countless times to trigger lucidity. Sometimes I'll jump up and just keep going; other times I'll start to come down, tuck my legs in as if I'm about to land on my knees, then bounce back up. These are things I can't do in waking reality, so I'm clued in to the fact that I must be dreaming. It's fun and it works. It's like I'm skipping my way into lucidity.[7]

THE MYTH OF KNOWLEDGE

Conducting state checks points to a deeper issue, what the historian Daniel Boorstin calls "the illusion of knowledge." "The greatest enemy of knowledge is not ignorance, it is the illusion of knowledge," he writes. The world's great discoverers have always needed "to battle against the current 'facts' and dogmas of the learned."[8] The illusion, or myth, of knowledge is one of our greatest obstacles because it's so insidious. It's a massive blind spot, or in our terms, an "asleep spot." The myth of knowledge is when you're certain you know something, but you actually don't. It's when you think something is a given, or axiomatic, but you're wrong. Emotionally, it's when you bang your fist on the table and proclaim, "That's just the way it is!" But as Mark Twain put it, "It ain't what you don't know that gets you into trouble. It's what you know for sure that just ain't so."

In the world of lucid dreaming, the myth of knowledge is when you think you're awake, but you're actually dreaming. Being stuck in a non-lucid dream is falling victim to this myth. It can be a jolt to awaken from a dream that you thought was so real. In Buddhism, the myth of knowledge is a central theme, and the awakening even more of a jolt. It's when you think you're awake, but you're actually asleep, in the spiritual sense. We're all victims of this myth. That you're awake right now just ain't so. That things exist the way you think they do just ain't so. Understanding the myth of knowledge is important on the path of waking up. As the philosopher of science Sir Karl Popper said, "It is through the falsification of our suppositions that we actually get in touch with 'reality.'"[9]

When we conduct state checks, we're taking the advice of the bumper sticker that exhorts us to "Question Authority." We're questioning the authority that what we're experiencing is real. Our journey in this book, ultimately, is to point out the illusion of knowledge and wake up from it. The futurist Alvin Toffler said, "The illiterate of the twenty-first century will not be those who cannot read and write, but those who cannot learn, unlearn, and relearn."[10] Our job here, as in life, is to unlearn and relearn. We need to strip away the myth that what we're experiencing right now is real, and to relearn that it's actually just a dream. Or as Johann Wolfgang von Goethe put it, "None are more hopelessly enslaved than those who falsely believe they are free."

Dreamsigns

Another daytime technique that ties into state checks is to work with dreamsigns. Just like with state checks, you start by working with dreamsigns during the day and then extend the practice into the night. It's both a daytime and nighttime practice, another reciprocating method. Working with dreamsigns means becoming sensitized to out-of-the-ordinary (dreamlike) events that occur during the day, and to use those strange events as triggers to conduct state checks. A primary catalyst for triggering lucidity is noticing the dreamlike nature of your experience. This is in the category of what LaBerge calls a "dream-induced lucid dream," which means you're using the content of the dream to spark lucidity. We often wake up to the fact that we're dreaming when we say to ourselves, "Wow, that's really weird . . . I must be dreaming." The strangeness clues us in. So during the day, if a bird hits your window, or a book falls off the shelf, jump up or otherwise ask yourself, "Is this a dream?" Anytime anything weird happens, ask yourself, "Is this a dream?"

When we're actually dreaming, we experience many anomalies, such as abrupt transitions of location, strange discontinuities, or bizarre occurrences. We might be flying, seeing pink elephants, or coming across any number of surreal events. If we take these in stride, as we usually do, we remain non-lucid. But if we condition ourselves to question reality when strange things happen, we condition ourselves to wake up within our dreams.

There are many kinds of dreamsigns. First are "weak" dreamsigns. These are highly improbable, but not impossible, events that occur in dreams. Seeing a strange dog walk into your dream house is weird, but not unheard of. "Strong" dreamsigns are things that can only happen in a dream, like when a chair turns into a boat or you find yourself flying. "Personal" dreamsigns are the most useful. These are common activities, situations, people, or objects that occur in your dreams, especially in recurrent dreams. This is where you take advantage of recurrent dreams. Record these activities, situations, people, or objects in your dream journal and become familiar with them. When they recur in your dreams, use your familiarization to trigger lucidity. For example, if you have a recurrent dream about your dead uncle, the only way he can appear to you as still alive is in a dream. Use his presence as a sign that you're dreaming.[11]

"Dream themes" are connected to dreamsigns, and can also help you trigger lucidity. The idea is to become familiar with your repetitive dream themes: the environments, narratives, characters, objects, and actions that occur regularly. Do this by reviewing your dream journal for repeated themes. If you have recurrent dreams about being chased, for example, or being late for a plane, use that theme to help you wake up to the fact that you're dreaming. "Wait a second . . . I've been chased like this before . . . I must be dreaming."

DREAMSIGNS AND DEATH

Working with dreamsigns also helps us prepare for death. Tibetan Buddhists believe that one of the biggest problems we have after death is not realizing we're dead. In bardo yoga, it is taught that there are classic death signs that can clue you in to the fact that you're dead. Once you wake up to the fact that you're dead, you can use the many techniques of bardo yoga to help you during this challenging time.

The classic signs to look for to verify that you're dead include (1) you cast no shadow, (2) you look into a mirror or other reflecting surface and see no reflection, (3) you walk on sand or snow and leave no footprints, (4) your body makes no sound, (5) people don't respond to you, (6) you can move unimpeded through matter, (7) you manifest miraculous power, such as the ability to fly, read minds, or travel very quickly, (8) you cannot see the sun or moon.[12] These are also some of the same signs that can help you recognize that you're dreaming. Create the habit of checking for these signs now, and that habit will carry into dream and death. Remind yourself to look for your shadow, or to check for a reflection. Am I dead, dreaming, or alive and awake right now?

I regularly work with these death signs. When I'm outside on a sunny day I'll check to see if I'm casting a shadow. I'll look for footprints when I walk in the snow. It may seem strange, but it helps me develop the habit of questioning the status of my reality.

Prospective Memory

A general exercise to induce lucid dreaming is the practice of "prospective memory." Prospective ("of or in the future") memory is remembering to do something in the future. It's almost an oxymoron, because memory is associated with the past and prospective is associated with the future. When you're trying to remember to wake up in a dream, which is a future event, you're working with prospective memory, which can be strengthened with some exercises.[13]

Once you get the gist of prospective memory exercises, the variations are infinite. The practice is to remember to do a state check whenever a specific event occurs. The event can be anything. For example, you could tell yourself that every time you see a cat, you will remember to do a state check. Or every time you hear a plane, a siren, or a dog bark, you will remember to do a state check. As your prospective memory develops, so will your ability to remember to wake up in your dreams.

I recommend setting one different trigger event per day. Tell yourself that every time you get a text message today you'll remember to do a state check. For the following day, every time you go to the bathroom, you'll do a state check. Memory is a mental muscle you can exercise, and one that can lift you into lucidity.

STATE CHECKS AND PRIMING
The Power of the Prime

Conducting state checks, or developing a critically reflective attitude, helps us interrupt the power of what psychologists call "priming." Priming is just what it sounds like. It's the mostly unconscious setup that predisposes us to see things a certain way. Priming is a fancy way to talk about expectation. If we start a sequence like 1, 2, 3, 4, 5, we are primed to expect that the next number will be 6. Our desires and expectations prime us to see what we want to see. We see the world the way we do—as solid, lasting, and independent—because we've been primed to do so by our parents, teachers, and virtually everyone alive. It's this continued reinforcement that continues into the dream state and primes us to see the dream as solid, lasting, and independent, and therefore non-lucid.

Priming is based on repetition, which is the essence of predisposition. We're predisposed to non-lucidity at night because since early childhood we have been trained to see the world in a non-lucid way during the day. Daily dreamsigns and state checks use conscious priming to trigger alertness and awareness, lucidity instead of non-lucidity, and they do so by planting these new patterns for lucidity into the unconscious mind. We're setting ourselves up to see the dream as a dream.[14]

Nighttime Western Induction Techniques

When you lie down to go to sleep, give one final push with your intention to wake up in your dreams. With as much heart as you can muster say, "Tonight I *will* have many dreams. I *will* have good dreams. I *will* remember my dreams. I *will* become lucid in my dreams." How many times has your state of mind colored your sleep and dreams? If you go to sleep stressed or preoccupied with a particular state of mind, it often seeds your dreams. We dream at night what we think of during the day. In dream yoga we want to seed the thoughts, delivered with the force of our intention, to wake up within our dreams.

The "seeding" of our thoughts and intentions is the equivalent of what Buddhists call "karmic traces." Tenzin Wangyal, in *The Tibetan Yogas of Dream and Sleep* (1998), says, "The karmic traces are like photographs we take of each experience. In the darkroom of sleep we develop the film." Do you want to have certain dreams, or wake up in your dreams? Then take the proper photographs during the day.

Mnemonic Induction

LaBerge developed a particularly effective technique that he calls the "mnemonic induction of lucid dreams." A mnemonic is a memory aid, and LaBerge got to the point with this technique where he could have lucid dreams at will. Mnemonic induction of lucid dreams employs prospective memory and is used after you wake from a dream at night and before you fall back asleep. There are four steps to this technique:

1) During the early morning, or when you awaken spontaneously from a dream, go over the dream several times until you have memorized it.

2) Then, while lying in bed and returning to sleep, say to yourself, "Next time I'm dreaming, I want to remember to recognize I'm dreaming."

3) Visualize yourself as being back in the dream just rehearsed; only this time, see yourself realizing that you are, in fact, dreaming.

4) Repeat steps 2 and 3 until you feel your intention is clearly fixed or you fall asleep.[15]

Electronic Aids

In 1985, LaBerge started designing a lucid dreaming induction device in the form of a comfortable sleep mask, a type of dream goggle. When sensors in the mask detect sufficient eye movement to indicate the REM stage of sleep, a cue is delivered via flashing lights, or sound, or both, to prompt the dreamer to become lucid. The cues enter your dream and become incorporated into it, helping trigger lucidity. It's similar to what happens when it's cold in your bedroom and you find yourself dreaming about snow or ice. Outside affects inside.

I've used several versions of these lucid dream induction devices with good results.[16] A typical dream where the light cue triggers lucidity might be me driving in a car and noticing that the vehicle in front of me is pumping its brake lights. Or I'm standing under a streetlight that starts to flash. I'll suddenly remember to associate the flashing light in my dream with the flashing light in the goggle, and I'm instantly lucid. Some of these goggles can be adjusted to your style of REM sleep, and therefore customized for optimal use. With some personal experimentation, the device is fine-tuned to your particular dream patterns.

Scientists at the Goethe University Frankfurt in Germany were recently able to trigger lucid dreams in subjects by applying a mild electric current to their scalps. Researchers found that electrical stimulation in the 40 hertz (gamma) range applied to the frontal lobe "induces self-reflective awareness in dreams"—that is, lucidity.[17] The lead investigator, Ursula Voss, says, "We can really quite easily change consciousness in dreams." She recruited twenty-seven adults who had never experienced a lucid dream. Two minutes after reaching REM, the subjects received a weak electrical current (2 to 100 hertz) to the frontal lobe area for thirty seconds. The sweet spot was 40 hertz, which triggered their brains to produce brain waves at the same frequency, and induced lucidity 77 percent of the time.[18] When this technique is refined, it could be a revolution in lucid dream induction.

Galantamine

Galantamine is an effective substance for increasing dream clarity, and therefore dream recall.[19] In its prescription-strength form, galantamine was approved by the FDA in 2001 for the treatment of Alzheimer's disease; it is sold under the names Razadyne, Reminyl, and Nivalin. In its over-the-counter form you can find it as Galantamind. It's been used in Eastern Europe and Russia since the 1950s for the treatment of various neurological disorders. Galantamine is an alkaloid extracted from the snowdrop daffodil and spider lily, which are in the Amaryllidaceae (amaryllis) family of flowering plants. It was reportedly used thirty-two hundred years ago by the Greek hero Odysseus, the hero of memory and the enemy of forgetfulness.

Many have used galantamine with great success. But some of my lucid dream colleagues report no luck, or even restless sleep as the result of taking it. As with so many induction methods, results may vary.

Galantamine works by inhibiting the breakdown of the neurotransmitter acetylcholine, which is important in generating and maintaining REM sleep.[20] Acetylcholine also supports memory. By keeping more of this neurotransmitter active in your brain, you tend to have clearer and more stable dreams. The standard dosage for lucid dreamers is 4 to 8 milligrams about six hours *after* you go to sleep, which means most people get up and take it around two hours before they normally wake up, then go back to sleep. This is perfect, because it also works with prime-time dreamtime. Try 4 milligrams and see what happens. If there are no results, increase the dosage to 8 milligrams.

Galantamine is often mixed with choline bitartrate, creating the perfect dream cocktail. I have never experienced side effects, but in its prescription strength, the side effects of galantamine include nausea, vomiting, dizziness, diarrhea, headache, decreased appetite, and decreased weight. It's not to be used in pregnant or lactating women, those dealing with depression, or those sensitive to galantamine, choline, or pantothenic acid. In its over-the-counter form, galantamine is dispensed in an unregulated industry, which means you never know what you're getting. One has to trust the manufacturer, and there are studies showing that nonregulated supplements are sometimes not what they profess to be. But in my experience, I do notice a difference in my dreams when I take confirmed doses, and no difference when I've taken a placebo.

I only use galantamine for an occasional boost and do not recommend regular use. It's better to rely on other methods, especially the meditative tools described later. But galantamine does have its place in lucid dreaming. As with any supplement, use it but don't abuse it.

Dream Induction Tips and Tricks

If you're really inspired, set your alarm to go off every ninety min-utes during the night, which is when you're most likely to be in REM sleep. Once you're awake, practice mnemonic induction of lucid dreams if you've awoken from a dream, or reset your intention to become lucid. Perhaps the single best tip is to set your alarm to go off about two hours before you would normally wake up, stay up for around thirty minutes, then go back to sleep. This method remains very effective for me, and it doesn't disrupt my sleep. You can increase the likelihood of lucidity twentyfold with this step alone. A number of dream researchers assert that joining mnemonic induction with this "wake up and back to bed" method is *the* most effective of all induction techniques. Conjoin this method with 4 to 8 milligrams of galantamine that you take when you get up, and get ready to rocket into REM with full lucidity.

Leaving a dim light on, and keeping the room cool, also helps. It keeps sleep literally and figuratively lighter. You're using an outer light to invoke inner lucidity. To practice good sleep hygiene, which is always helpful for dream yoga, eat light at night, don't drink a lot of alcohol, and remove any electronic gadgetry (TV, smart phones, computers, and so forth) from your bedroom. Also avoid using your electronic devices before going to sleep.[21]

Experiment. Find out what works for you. Remember that lucid-ity is what's important, not the technique that gets you there.

> We need a dream-world in order to discover the
> features of the real world we think we inhabit (and
> which may actually be just another dream-world).

PAUL FEYERABEND, *Against Method*

5

Eastern Lucid Dream Induction Techniques

IF YOU FIND that the Western techniques from the last chapter work, then stick with those. But there are many people who benefit from the traditional Eastern methods. Since lucid dream induction is not a one-size-fits-all practice, it's helpful to have options. I've worked with both sets of methods with good success, and therefore encourage you to explore these ancient wisdom tools.

Many of the methods in this chapter come from Vajrayana Buddhism, which is largely a Tibetan tradition. Vajrayana ("diamond vehicle") is the last of the three main schools of Buddhism, the other two being the Mahayana ("great vehicle") and Hinayana ("narrow vehicle"). The Vajrayana methods are meditative techniques that can be learned, practiced, and developed. If you don't have success with them initially, as your practice matures so will your success.

The Subtle Body

In Vajrayana Buddhism, the body is as important as the mind, and practitioners work with the body in order to work with the mind (as they do in Taoist dream yoga as well). In particular, dream yoga uses the subtle body to engage subtle aspects of mind. Dream yoga takes us deeply into ourselves mentally *and* physically. It therefore helps to learn about the inner subtle body—of where we're going within our body when we sleep and dream.[1] It's important to know that not everything physical is material. For example, fields and forces are physical but not material, and so is the subtle body. It's just as real as physical fields and forces, and exerts the same level of influence on our lives.

> Buddhism uses the mind to work with the body (via the mental yogas, or meditations), and it uses the body to work with the mind (via the inner, or subtle body, yogas). This bidirectional approach is characteristic of Vajrayana Buddhism, which is also called the "vehicle of skillful means." One way or the other (bidirectionally), because both are intimately connected, body and mind are engaged in the process of transformation.

We noted earlier that there are three levels of mind; these go from gross outer, to inner subtle, to innermost very subtle (what we will refer to later as "psyche," "substrate," and "clear-light mind," respectively). Correspondingly, there are levels of body that support these levels of mind. Our focus for the moment will be on the inner subtle body; we will discuss the very subtle body at more length when we explore the practice of sleep yoga. As a brief summary: waking consciousness is associated with the level of the gross outer body, dreams with the subtle body, and dreamless sleep with the innermost very subtle body.

The intermediate level of the inner subtle body is targeted in Chinese medicine, Indian Ayurveda, and other Eastern medical systems (via techniques such as acupuncture, acupressure, and moxibustion) for physical health. It's also targeted in many spiritual traditions (via techniques such as the inner yogas) for spiritual awakening. And just as there are outer yogas that work with the outer gross body, there are inner yogas that work with the inner subtle body. The dream induction techniques from Tibetan Buddhism engage these inner yogas.

The subtle body is a bridge between mind (the formless) and body (fully manifest form). With the inner yogas as they're engaged in the dream yoga induction techniques, we're using this subtle body to work with the subtle mind of our dreams. The subtle body has a sophisticated anatomy and physiology; our discussion here will address the four main constituents—referred to as the channels, winds, drops, and wheels. These are called *nadi, prana, bindu,* and *chakra* in Sanskrit, and *tsa, lung, tigle,* and *khorwa* in Tibetan. Each of these four inner aspects has outer-body correlates that can help us understand them.

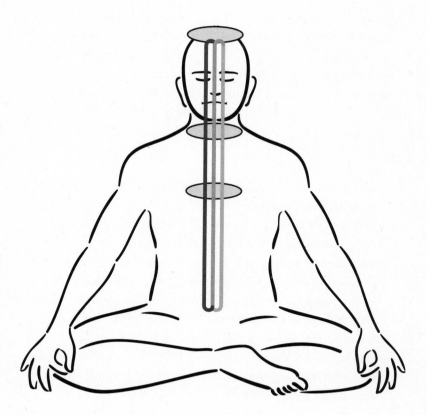

FIGURE 2 **The subtle body.** The winds *(prana, lung)* flow through the left, central, and right channels *(nadi, tsa).* The head, throat, and heart wheels *(chakras, khorwa)* are depicted in this illustration.

PROFOUND INNER REALITY

Although the subtle body isn't a material body like the outer gross body, that doesn't make it less real. In a sense it's more real, because it's the foundation for the outer body. In the Tibetan Buddhist view, the outer is an expression of the inner. The best way to explore the subtle body, and discover the four main constituents for yourself, is through the inner yogas. That's when you can prove to yourself that the channels, winds, drops, and wheels are real, because you *feel* them, and feeling is even more convincing than seeing. You can feel the winds, or prana, moving through your channels, and the bindus gathering at the chakras.

When I started doing the inner yogas and felt my subtle body for the first time, it was one of the great discoveries of my life.[2] A new dimension of being was revealed. This is when I developed conviction in what the Tibetans call the "profound inner reality." Body and mind are not the same, but they're also not different—a discovery that's achieved with the inner yogas.

1. *Channels.* The channels are the easiest elements of the subtle body to understand. Depending on which system you use, there are around 72,000 channels in our subtle body. These are like arteries, veins, or even nerves. For our purposes we only need to know about three: the central channel (*avadhuti* in Sanskrit, *uma* in Tibetan), the right channel (*pingala/rasana*), and the left channel (*ida/lalana*). The central channel runs from the top of the head to the base of the spine. The left and right channels begin at the nostrils, curve up to meet the central channel near the top of the head, then run parallel to it to a distance about four finger widths below the navel, where they merge with the central channel.[3]

2. *Winds.* Within the channels flow the subtle winds, or prana, also known as chi, life force energy, psycho-physical energy,

subtle bioenergy, even Holy Spirit in esoteric Christianity. The outer body correlate is most obviously respiration, but other parallels would include the flow of blood or the conduction of nerve impulses. The wind that flows through the right channel is called the "sun poison prana," which is a masculine, extroverted, "in the world," and very active energy. The wind that flows through the left channel is called the "moon nectar prana," which is more feminine, introverted, and receptive. The wind that flows through the central channel is called "wisdom wind," and it only "breathes" when the two outer channels, which carry confused or dualistic wind, stop breathing. This occurs in very deep meditation or death.

Pay attention to your breath when you meditate (or go to sleep) and you will notice how your respiration slows down and can even stop. There's an intimate connection between the movement of breath and the movement of thought. When all thoughts cease in deep meditation (or death), so does all the outer (breath) and inner (prana) wind that brings about that movement.

3. *Drops.* The third aspect of the subtle body are the drops (bindus), sometimes called "mind pearls." These can be the hardest to understand. Outer body correlates would include sperm and ovum, neurotransmitters, hormones, or anything that represents the concentration of life force energy. In spiritual practice, the drops are often visualized as shimmering beads of light, the size of a sesame seed. The simplest definition of bindu comes from Chögyam Trungpa Rinpoche (the renowned twentieth-century teacher of Tibetan Buddhism in the West), who referred to the drops as "consciousness." Think of them as drops of consciousness.[4]

4. *Wheels.* The final aspect of the subtle body is also the most famous—the wheels, or chakras. Chakras are energy distribution centers. Depending on the system, there are usually five or seven chakras situated along the central channel: base of the spine, genitals, solar plexus, heart, throat,

forehead, and top of the head. Outer body correlates are the endocrine centers, which are, respectively, the adrenal glands, the testes or ovaries, and the pancreas, thymus, thyroid, pituitary, and pineal glands.

The way these four constituents work together, and how this all ties into the inner yogas for lucid dream induction, is that the bindus, or drops, move through the channels, carried by the winds, and gather at the chakras to create different states of consciousness. When we're awake, the drops (which remember *are* consciousness) are gathered at the head chakra. When we fall into deep dreamless sleep, the drops fall from the head and gather at the heart. When we dream, the drops come up from the heart and gather at the throat.

One way that the inner yogas work with this natural process is through the power of visualization, which gently manipulates the process to induce lucid dreams. The idea here is that where the mind goes in visualization, the pranas go. Where the pranas go, the bindus go. And where the bindus go, so goes consciousness. We'll see how this works shortly.

MUSIC AND MANTRAS
Sound and the Subtle Body

If you don't do inner yoga, you can still get a feel for the subtle body when you're touched by sound or music. Sound is deeply connected to the subtle body. They exist at similar "frequencies," and the subtle body can be influenced by sound through processes similar to sympathetic vibrations or entrainment. For example, when you place two pianos side by side, lift the dampers off one piano, and hit a note on the other, the piano with the dampers lifted off will resonate (sympathetically) to the vibrations of the other piano. Sound, and mantra, affects the subtle body in a similar way. The next time you're really touched by music, it's your subtle body that's being touched.

Mantra, which is obviously connected to sound, also works on the subtle body. Mantras work in a number of ways, but in terms of the subtle body they serve to "straighten out" the channels through which prana flows. If you could somehow take an X-ray of the subtle body of a meditation master, you would find perfectly straight and supple channels, free of any blockage. Imagine something like smooth tubes of transparent saran wrap. If you saw an X-ray of the subtle body of a confused sentient being, you would find crinkled, stiff, and crooked channels, with lots of knots. Imagine something like wrinkled tubes of stiff wax paper. Mantras iron out the channels, which then allow the winds to flow without deflection or obstruction, which results in a clear and straight mind.

Inner Yoga Induction: Getting Started

As a prelude to any nighttime technique, there are two things you can do to settle your mind and prepare for lucid sleep. First calm your mind with ten minutes or so of meditation (described in chapter 6). Second, you can do a brief prana purification exercise, which removes the stale winds and energizes the subtle body. If you're familiar with *pranayama,* do that for a few minutes. Otherwise, take three slow and deep cleansing breaths. As you inhale, imagine pure life force energy flooding your subtle body. As you exhale, imagine that all the stagnant winds are blown out. You can do a final vigorous push at the end of your exhalation, as a respiratory exclamation point, with the sense that every last wisp of stale air is being expelled.[5]

Now, to begin the first inner yoga induction technique, lie down on your right side. Tuck your feet in slightly and rest your left hand along the top of your left leg. If possible, block off your right nostril. This is easily done by holding your right hand in a fist and closing your right nostril with your right thumb (see figure 3).[6]

This position (*mudra* in Sanskrit) is called the "sleeping lion posture," and it's the famous posture that the Buddha took when he died. You'll see statues and photographs of this mudra throughout Asia (see figure 4 on page 65).

Why do you want to do this? According to the inner yogas, you want to sleep and die in an introverted, or "feminine," mode.

Sleeping and dying are not the times to be extroverted. Things are going offline, not online. By lying down on your right side and blocking off your right nostril, you're invoking the closure of the more outgoing sun poison prana. In the world of dream yoga, this prana is "bad breath." It tends to keep us awake. Assuming the sleeping lion posture invites the winds to switch to the left channel, which is more conducive to "conscious sleep," or the ability to drop into sleep with some measure of awareness.[7]

If you pay close attention to your breathing, you may notice that every ninety minutes or so the winds switch from the left to the right channels. Have you ever noticed how one nostril or the other will be constricted or closed, for no apparent physical reason (like being plugged), and then gradually open? That opening and closing is due to the winds alternating their flow between the right and left channels.

This sleeping lion technique also helps with insomnia. If I'm dealing with periodic insomnia, I often notice that when I wake up in the middle of the night my left nostril is closed, and I'm breathing through my right nostril. I'll roll over onto my right side, assume the sleeping lion posture, and often fall back asleep. Some people have a natural disposition for this type of inner yoga technique, as well as the others presented below, while others do not. Trust your experience and do what works.

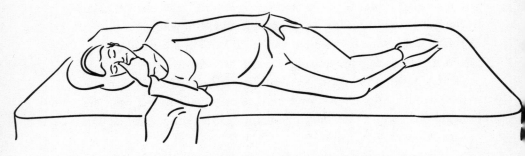

FIGURE 3   Inner yoga position for sleeping, with the right nostril closed off.

Throat Visualization

A second dream yoga induction technique, using the inner yogas, is as follows: When you lie down to go to sleep, bring your mind to your throat, which is where consciousness gathers when you dream. Visualize a red pearl or red AH there.[8] (See which image works best for you.) Each chakra is associated with a particular frequency, which can be expressed by a color and a sound. For the throat chakra, the color is red and the sound is AH.

> The mind holds on to things as it descends into sleep. If you don't use these visualizations, the mind will grab something else, like a discursive thought. More often than not, that thought is not conductive to lucidity. Just look at your mind and see for yourself. Where does your mind drift when you lie down to sleep?

In this visualization, you are pulling consciousness (the drops) from waking consciousness to dreaming consciousness, and you're doing so consciously. With this inner yoga technique you can become so adept at moving consciousness from one chakra to the next that you can go from waking to dreaming within seconds.

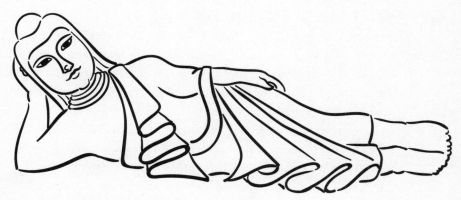

FIGURE 4   The Buddha in the sleeping lion pose.

One moment you're awake, the next moment you're in a lucid dream. (The Russian philosopher P. D. Ouspensky famously practiced and wrote about this art of voluntarily entering a lucid dream from a waking state.)

In his lucid-dreaming guidebook, *Are You Dreaming?*, Daniel Love says that a lucid dream is essentially the meeting of two seemingly contradictory states of mind: dreaming and consciousness. To induce lucidity we can either add dreams to consciousness (as with a waking-induced lucid dream) or consciousness to dreams (a dream-induced lucid dream). So what we have are techniques for *achieving* lucidity—those that help the dreamer realize they're dreaming—and the techniques for *sustaining* lucidity—those that help the dreamer to stay conscious (lucid) while falling asleep. Either way the point is to mix consciousness and dreams.

Such sudden shifts in states of consciousness may seem unbelievable, but we "fall asleep" non-lucidly every time we're swept away into a daydream or slip from mindfulness to mindlessness. One moment we're fully present; in the next we're lost in some fantasy. The shifts between waking and dreaming also happen when we dip in and out of sleep during early morning hours, or as we're falling asleep, topics we'll return to when we talk about hypnagogic and hypnopompic (from *hypnos* "sleep" and *pompe* "leading away") states.

As you gently hold the visualization at your throat, don't allow yourself to get distracted. The practice is to keep your mind at your throat for as long as you can before finally letting go and dropping into sleep. If you can do that without having anything interrupt your visualization, you stand a good chance of becoming lucid. As with every induction technique, below this is the ever-present intention, "Tonight I *will* recognize my dreams to be dreams," which perfumes your sleep and dreams.

Remember that where the mind goes, the winds go; where the winds go, the bindus go; and where the bindus go, so goes consciousness. When we *fall* asleep, it's because the bindus (consciousness) do indeed fall from the head, and they do so because the winds that keep them up there un-wind. Being all wound *up* is an interesting colloquialism in this regard.

Transitional Karma and Sleep Hygiene

With the throat visualization, as with many other nighttime induction techniques, we're working with laws of "transitional karma"—and using karma, or cause and effect, to our advantage. There are four forces of karma at work during any moment of transition—moment to moment, day to day, and life to life. In order of influence, these forces are heavy karma, proximate karma, habitual karma, and random karma. Heavy karma is the force from our most powerful good or bad deeds, or impactful states of mind. Proximate karma refers to the state of mind that is present at any moment of transition. Habitual karma is the force of our ordinary habits. Random karma arises if the other three aren't dominant.

In trying to induce lucid dreams, we're working with these laws. Habitual karma is at work when we ask ourselves throughout the day, "Is this a dream?" In other words, conducting state checks. We're creating the habit of questioning reality. If we do this frequently, we're adding weight to this habit, which then matures into heavy karma. This is what happened to LaBerge when he was heavy into the topic of lucid dreaming during his PhD dissertation at Stanford. With so much weight behind his actions during the day, it's karmically no surprise he was triggering lucid dreams at night. Author Gretchen Rubin says, "Habits are the invisible architecture of daily life. If we change our habits, we change our lives."[9]

Random karma is always in the background, and becomes less random (more deliberate) the more our intention is directed to the goal of waking up in our dreams.

Proximate karma is the one that we use the most in the nighttime induction techniques, and it's the one where we have the most control. If we can learn how to control our mind as we drop into sleep, we can transition into lucidity. Chögyam Trungpa Rinpoche talked about "first thought best thought," a phrase that was given to him by the poet Allen Ginsburg. "First thought best thought" refers to the freshness of each moment, before the "second thought" of concept barges in to color the moment. In the world of dream yoga we work with "last thought best thought," or proximate karma. This refers to how the last thought on our mind before we transition into sleep has a big impact on how we sleep. For example, if we go to sleep stressed out, this proximate state of mind will often induce stress-related dreams.

Taking a concept from bardo yoga: the last thought or feeling you have before dropping asleep tends to "reincarnate" as the first thought or feeling in your next state of consciousness.[10] If you can gently hold on to a thought, feeling, or intention before falling asleep, that thought, feeling, or intention will tend to arise in your dreams. It's basic karma, or cause and effect.

Good sleep hygiene in the spiritual sense is about going to sleep with a clean state of mind so that you can have good clean sleep and dreams. If you went for a long, sweaty run, would you go to bed without taking a shower? Similarly, don't take your dirty, discursive mind to bed. So in addition to the Western-oriented sleep hygiene tips mentioned in chapter 4, you want to settle your mind in meditation before you go to sleep, and transition cleanly into the dream yoga induction techniques as you lie down. The meaning of sleep hygiene in the inner yogas refers to purely holding your mind on the throat visualization and not allowing any random thoughts to sully your visualization. If I'm too tired or lazy to practice dream yoga, I at least try to go to sleep using these spiritual principles of good sleep hygiene. It's like taking a warm mental bath before bed.

THE VIRTUOUS SLEEPING MIND

The law of proximate karma applies to sleep in general, even if you're not doing dream yoga. Chökyi Nyima Rinpoche says,

> Just before falling asleep there's always a final thought. We can try to make that last thought a noble, benevolent thought. If we can do that, the quality of that thought can permeate our entire sleeping state . . . We can then say, from a spiritual point of view, that our sleep becomes a virtuous sleep . . . If your last thought is selfish, or even hostile, then falling asleep with that in mind saturates the sleeping state with unwholesome emotions. This is a simple idea, but it is an important one. Without too much difficulty . . . we can ensure

that a significant portion of our lives becomes saturated with goodness.[11]

Geshe Tashi Tsering adds,

> According to the Abhidharma texts, sleep is seen as virtuous, non-virtuous, or neutral depending on the immediately preceding consciousness—the mind just prior to sleep. That mind makes a huge difference to the mind of sleep. If the mind before sleep is virtuous, such as the thought that we will sleep not just to rest but to refresh the body in order to have energy to help ourselves and others, then our sleeping mind will more likely be virtuous. Similarly, if we fall asleep with a mind wholly bent on liberation, that is a wonderful way to ensure that our entire sleeping time is very positive, no matter how long we sleep.[12]

Sitting Lion Posture

Another dream induction technique from the Hindu Kriya Yoga tradition involves the *simha* pose, or the sitting lion posture. In this technique you sit on your haunches like a lion and put your hands on your lap in the "fist of non-aggression," tucking your thumbs into your palm and grasping them with your other fingers. Then tip your head back, exposing your throat, and roar three or more times like a lion. As you roar, open your fists and spread your fingers out as if you're sending prana from your fingertips. The roaring stimulates your throat chakra. When I first tried this, I had a lucid dream that night. See if it works for you.

Magic Induction Techniques

What we will here call "magical" techniques could fit into either Eastern or Western methods. A first technique is working with devotion, or prayer. If devotion is part of your path, as it is in *bhakti* yoga of Hinduism, or guru yoga in Buddhism, then use your devotion to help you wake up in your dreams. If you're a Christian, Jewish, or Muslim believer with a strong connection to the power of prayer, then use that. If you believe in higher powers or supernatural assistance, then cry out to whatever sacred form you relate to for help with your dreams.

The idea is to invoke forces outside of you and to create the sacred mood that's conducive to lucidity. In dream yoga, creating the proper environment for practice is as important as the main practice. If the right atmosphere is there, lucidity just happens.

Here's how it works. In the spiritual world, mind is in the "public domain," which means that higher energies can tune in to you. Teachers from the Nyingma tradition such as Sogyal Rinpoche and Guru Rinpoche say that it's a property of the awakened ones—from any tradition—to respond instantly when someone cries out from the bottom of their heart.[13] These entities or energies can then help you wake up in your dreams. I have a brief liturgy, which I call the "Four Dharmas of Dreams," that I often recite as I go to sleep, in which the power of blessing works as an induction technique:[14]

> Grant your blessings so that my sleep may be one with
> the dharma.
> Grant your blessings so that dharma may be practiced
> in my dreams.
> Grant your blessings so that dreams may clarify confusion.
> Grant your blessings so that confusion is transformed
> in dreamless sleep.

A second magical induction technique works with compassion. Khenpo Tsültrim Gyamtso Rinpoche, one of the greatest living Kagyu masters, says that it's hard to rush the spiritual path. Things have to unfold in their own way. But he also says there is one thing that can accelerate spiritual awakening: the heartfelt motivation to wake up in order to help others. In Buddhism this is the role of *bodhichitta*, or the awakened heart-mind, and the central aspiration of the *bodhisattva*, or one who puts the benefit of others before their own. Several of my dharma friends have gone to sleep with the strong intent to have a healing dream for a loved one who was suffering, and successfully incubated lucid healing dreams from the force of that compassionate intent.

The great master Guru Rinpoche said, "When you go to bed in the evening, cultivate the Spirit of Awakening, thinking, 'For the sake of all sentient beings throughout space, I shall practice the illusion-like samadhi, and I shall achieve perfect buddhahood. For that purpose I shall train in dreaming.'"[15]

If this liturgy doesn't work for you, make up your own. As I lie in bed, I'll often put my hands over my heart in a prayer mudra and say something like, "May the buddhas and bodhisattvas come to me this evening and help me wake up in my dreams. May I wake up in my dreams so that I can better lead others to awakening." The actual liturgy is not that important. What's important is the heart-felt feeling of compassion and devotion. The feeling and intent is what carries over into sleep and dream, not the words that elicit that feeling or intent.

Some teachers say it's good to imagine resting your head on the lap of the Buddha, Christ, or your spiritual teacher, as you fall asleep. If you have a connection to devotion, prayer, or compassion, then use your imagination, and your heart, to invoke those feelings.

Creative Napping: A Blend of East and West

Naps are a great way to work with lucid dreams, particularly waking-induced lucid dreams. It's easy to go from stage 1 sleep into REM quickly during a nap, so waking-induced lucid dreams are more likely. When I'm doing a dream yoga retreat, I'll mix day and night by waking up often during the night to take advantage of my ninety-minute cycles, and then catch up on any missed sleep by taking naps during the day. Napping is also a great way to work with the pre- and post-dream states, hypnagogic and hypnopompic respectively—those bardo-like states between waking, sleeping, and dreaming when the mind is dipping in and out of consciousness. Hypnagogic and hypnopompic states are not quite here (awake) and not quite there (sleeping or dreaming). If we bring mindfulness and awareness into these dips, it's a marvelous way to explore levels of consciousness, and to watch how one state affects the other.

Hypnagogic states may seem like a mish-mash of experiences, but researchers have distinguished at least four main stages: bursts of color and light, drifting nature scenes and faces, thought-image amalgamations, and hypnagogic dreamlets.[16] With this map of the stages, you can better practice "lucid sleep onset," and orient yourself with these road signs as you travel in and out of sleep with awareness.

Napping took on an entirely new dimension for me during my three-year meditation retreat. This traditional Buddhist retreat requires that participants sleep sitting up, in a kind of meditation box. Imagine a three-sided wooden box large enough to sit in, with an open top and front. It may sound medieval, but it's a potent literal container for extended meditation. After some initial resistance to feeling boxed in, I came to love my little cubicle, which I called "ego's coffin."

Part of the reason for sleeping in a sitting posture is that it's conducive to a lighter sleep, and therefore favorable for the nighttime meditations. During the first month of my retreat, I really struggled. I tried to be the perfect retreatant, and despite my fatigue I pushed to stay awake during my long daily sessions in the box. One day, in a moment of utter exhaustion, I pulled my robe over my head (I was a temporary monk during the retreat), leaned back in my sitting posture, and took my first power nap. Thirty minutes later I woke up refreshed and returned to my meditation.

So began my love affair with the nap. Rather than toughing it out, I listened to my internal rhythms and allowed these short breaks. Instead of taking away from my retreat, napping added clarity and energy to my practice. It got to the point where I could drop from waking to sleeping within seconds. This isn't unusual. If you're tired enough, you drop like a rock. I'm not recommending that people sleep sitting up, even though for the serious student it's an interesting experiment. I am saying that naps are a wonderful way to work with the nighttime practices during the day and to explore bardo-like states of consciousness.

It's helpful to view the transition between waking and sleeping consciousness as being like a thin membrane. When I'm awake I'm above the membrane, and when I dip into sleep or dream I'm below it, like dropping below the surface of a lake. One practice is to take a thought or image from "above" (from waking consciousness), gently hold it with mindfulness, and then transplant the thought or image below the membrane of sleep. You can then watch the thought "inflate" into an entire lucid dream—a waking-induced lucid dream—right before your very dream eyes. You're observing how thought becomes your (dream) reality. Tarthang Tulku says, "While delicately observing the mind, lead it gently into the dream state, as though you were leading a child by the hand." This is also a good demonstration of proximate karma—how the last thought on your mind in waking consciousness becomes the first "thought" (dream) in your next state of consciousness.

This is a subtle and deep meditation. If I'm not napping, I usually do this practice in the morning when I'm dipping in and out of sleep. When I finally get up and look at my daily world, I ask myself if it's any different from these dreams. I know that my thoughts literally do not create waking reality as they do in my dreams. But I also realize that thoughts have tremendous power, and that they color my waking reality.

Mindscape/Landscape

In Buddhist cosmology, there are six major realms of existence. According to the Kalachakra Tantra, each realm is created by the collective karma of the beings who inhabit it. We are collectively the creators and experiencers of this human realm, not the victims of it. If we're victims of anything, it's of our own karma, our own bad habits. The Kalachakra scholar Vesna Wallace writes "the destiny of the inanimate cosmos, which is due to the actions [karma] of sentient beings, is also the destiny of the sentient beings who inhabit that cosmos."[17] Tenzin Wangyal writes, "Like dreams, the realms are manifestations of karmic traces, but in the instance of the realms, the karmic traces are collective rather than individual . . . Although the realms appear to be distinct and solid, as our world seems to us, they are actually dreamy and insubstantial."[18]

By watching how I create an entire dream world out of a single karmic trace, or thought, I get a hint of how this same process takes place at the universal level. For me, this inner process takes place in mini-dreams, or "dreamlets." I often can't sustain these waking induced lucid dreams, but the brevity doesn't lessen the profundity. When the lucid dreamlet ends, I pop above the membrane of sleep and back into the fuzzy hypnopompic state. Then I go mindfully trolling for another thought or image, one that I can take with me as I dip back into the dream world to seed a new lucid dream. Napping has turned into a playful exploration of my mind, and an intimate demonstration of the power of mind to create a world. Mindful napping has also shown me that the same kind of creative process occurs when I drift from mindfulness into mindlessness during the day. One moment I'm awake to what's happening and fully present for my experience, but in the next I slip into mindlessness and fall into a daydream. I've crossed the "line," or "membrane," into a form of unconsciousness. The only real difference between these two forms of "napping" is that during the actual nap my thoughts can seed an entire personal reality (a dream), while during the day my thoughts are constrained by external sensory input.

Naps can boost the brain's learning capacity and help with the consolidation of memory. They reboot the brain, refresh the mind, and can actually make you smarter.[19] A University of Colorado study found that children who missed their afternoon naps showed less joy and interest, more anxiety, and poorer problem-solving abilities than other children.[20] Studies have also shown that short naps can improve awareness and productivity, along with heightened creativity, emotional and procedural memory, and cognitive clarity.[21] These scientific and spiritual assertions can change the way we relate to napping.[22]

On the subject of napping and creativity, the cognitive scientist Roger Shepard writes, "Many scientists and creative thinkers have noted that the mind's best work is sometimes done without conscious direction, during receptive states of reverie, idle meditation, dreaming, or transition between sleep and wakefulness."[23] Researchers at Georgetown University discovered that during naps, the right hemisphere of the brain, which is associated with creativity, is very active, while the left hemisphere, which is more analytic, is relatively quiet.[24] The left hemisphere, which tends to dominate the right, specializes in numbers and language processing. It's almost as if when the chattering and reasoning left hemisphere shuts up, the creative right hemisphere opens up. Lucidity training is therefore a form of creativity training.

The creative mind is set free in lucid dreams. You can do so many things you just can't do in waking reality. This freedom can be the basis of innovation, "downloading" dream insights into waking life. The dream researcher Judith Malamud writes, "[Lucidity] encourages the kind of wide-ranging, uninhibited, recombinatory mental activity that is characteristic of the creative process."[25] Making otherworldly connections that are not inhibited by worldly restraints is an absolute playground for creativity.

Just as dream content is not thought to be different from the dreamer who creates it, so also appearances are not different from mind. They *are* the very mind as it emanates.

TASHI NAMGYAL, *Pointing Out the Great Way: The Stages of Meditation in the Mahamudra Tradition*

6

A Fundamental Meditation
Mindfulness

ONE BIG DIFFERENCE between lucid dreaming and dream yoga is that typically speaking there are no meditations involved with lucid dreaming. There's no real yoga. So with the meditation in this chapter, we're stepping directly into the world of dream yoga. The core meditation for dream yoga is also the most accessible. It's the practice of mindfulness. Even if you elect to never practice in your dreams, the mindfulness meditation introduced here will help you have more lucid dreams.[1] Meditation will also help you remember your dreams, and make them more clear and stable. But before we describe how to do mindfulness meditation let's unfold the view behind it.

The Nature of Mindfulness

Mindfulness is the art of keeping your mind on the present moment. It's set in contrast to mindlessness, which is when your mind drifts away from what's happening. Mindlessness is virtually synonymous with distraction, and mindfulness is a synonym for non-distraction.

Three Stages of Mindfulness

Khenpo Tsültrim Gyamtso Rinpoche describes three forms of mindfulness. The first is deliberate or effortful mindfulness. With practice, this level matures into effortless mindfulness. Effortless mindfulness has two aspects, exoteric (or outer) and esoteric (or inner). On the exoteric level, mindfulness gets easier and eventually effortless. You find yourself being more and more present. The esoteric aspect is that effortless mindfulness is associated with awareness of the true nature of mind. We'll see why this is important shortly.

With sustained practice, effortless mindfulness matures into spontaneous mindfulness. On the exoteric level this is when you're mindful all the time. You're never distracted. On the esoteric level, this quality of mindfulness is never distracted from the true nature of mind.

We start with effortful mindfulness, which is a relatively coarse level of mindfulness that dissolves as we fall asleep. But with practice, this level refines into effortless and then spontaneous mindfulness, which do not dissolve at sleep. This means that these more advanced levels are qualities of mind that you can hold on to when you go to sleep, and that keep you aware of what's happening with your mind (phenomenologically).

Imagine a fireman's pole, the ones they would jump onto and slide down as they raced to their trucks. The oneironaut's pole is similar, but with a twist. It's conical in shape: wide at the top then thinning out at the bottom. This is what veteran onerionauts slide down as they descend into conscious sleep. Effortful mindfulness is the "widest," and it's what we start with as we lie down to go to sleep. Spontaneous mindfulness is the "narrowest," and it's what we end with as we drop into sleep. The tapered pole of these three stages of mindfulness gives us something we can hang on to as we slide from the world of form into formless sleep. In other words, deliberate mindfulness starts with bringing awareness to some form, and evolves until we become aware of formless awareness itself.

These three stages of mindfulness also have an encouraging practical application for meditation in general. When we first start to practice mindfulness, it takes effort. We're starting to turn against the enormous tide of mindlessness. If we just go along with the usual stream of mindlessness, which most people unwittingly do, we don't feel its enormous pull. We're going with the flow. But the minute we sit down and begin to practice mindfulness meditation, the torrent of mindlessness is finally felt. We start to twitch and eventually go stir crazy as we wrestle with the force of a lifetime of distraction.

But the more we practice, the easier it gets. Instead of constantly cutting the groove of mindlessness, we begin to fall into the groove of mindfulness. Our attention naturally starts to flow in that healthy direction. This is when effortful mindfulness matures into effortless mindfulness. So most of the effort in meditation comes up front. Having this view can encourage us to sustain the practice.

It may seem like we're training the mind, redirecting the flow of our attention from mindlessness into mindfulness. This is pro- visionally true. But on a deeper level, mindfulness is the natural state of the mind. If we just left the mind alone, it would always be mindful. Leaving it alone properly is the art of meditation. This is what it means to say that effortless and spontaneous mindfulness are mindful of the true nature of mind. The mind of a buddha is never distracted. It's always fully present, or awake, to what is happening right here and now. This means that the only thing we have to do to realize effortless and spontaneous mindfulness is simply relax. Just relax into the true nature of your mind, the clear-light mind, and you will be forever present—and awake.

All our effort in meditation culminates in the ability to relax. At the highest stages of the path you don't have to do a thing. You finally become a true human being, instead of an insatiable "human doing."

Mindfulness and Lucidity

To fully understand the power of mindfulness, we need to expand our understanding of lucidity, of what it means to be awake and present for what's happening—during the day or night. In an expanded sense, lucidity is virtually identical to mindfulness. Mindfulness is therefore a way to practice lucidity throughout the day. It's a way to wake up to what's happening right now. Be awake now and you will be awake during sleep and dream. What is found then is found now. In other words, mindlessness is a moment-to-moment expression of being asleep, and mindfulness is a moment-to-moment expression of being awake.[2] The Sufis proclaim that anything outside the present moment is a dream. In a song of realization *(doha)* called "Awakening at Dawn from the Sleep of Ignorance," written by the nineteenth-century Tibetan master Chokgyur Lingpa, there's a verse that says,

> Right now the beings of the three realms
> In mindlessness they all are asleep.
> Awake, they roam in their blinded states.[3]

Scientists talk about "inattentional blindness," which is when you fail to notice something that is fully visible because your attention has been directed elsewhere. Inattentional blindness is a more intense form of distraction, or mindlessness, that can literally kill. How many times have you been distracted by something, and then bumped, or even crashed, into an object? Studies of inattentional blindness reveal that visual perception is more than just photons hitting your eyes and activating your brain. To really see, you must pay attention.[4]

It's easy to extrapolate from these studies and say that mental perception is more than thoughts or images hitting your mind's eye and activating your brain. To really see, and therefore become lucid to your inner mindscape, you must pay attention. So attention, and its training, is at the heart of lucidity. And mindfulness meditation is the heart of this training.

This is where we need to remember that sleep is a product of ignorance. This isn't normal ignorance, like not knowing about a topic, but a primordial ignorance that is unaware of the nature of mind and reality. This is the ignorance that the Buddha awakened from, looked back upon from his awakened perspective, and then saw everybody still entrapped within. Everyone in the world was asleep.

So how can we work with this fundamental ignorance? How can we, like the Buddha, wake up from it? By counteracting its moment-to-moment expression, which is distraction. In other words, we can wake up by practicing mindfulness meditation.

As samsaric beings, or "sleepwalkers," we return repeatedly to any level of sleep, whether it's nighttime sleep or daily distraction, because it recharges the samsaric mind. Distraction, as the expression of ignorance, is the sustenance of samsara. When we get lost in the sleep of ignorance—lost in thought, distraction, or dreams—our samsaric lives are fed. We've hit the refresh button on confusion.

With mindfulness meditation we're working with ignorance—that is, "sleep"—as it manifests in its most common and immediate form, which is distraction. The point is this: *the distractions in daily life and the unconsciousness of sleep are two faces of the same ignorance.* It's the same thing happening at two levels. Unrecognized (discursive) thought is just the way we go to sleep moment-to-moment. Estimates put the number of these thoughts at around seventy thousand per day.[5]

As we have seen, buddhas don't sleep during the night *nor* do they sleep during the day. They're never distracted. They never forget. So forgetfulness is another way to address this important topic. In this regard, mindlessness (with an emphasis on the "less") is actually a form of primordial forgetfulness. We constantly forget to be present. Mindfulness (with an emphasis on the "full") is the expression, or practice, of remembering.

In many ways, the essence of spiritual practice is remembrance: remembering to come back to the present moment (through the practice of mindfulness), remembering to be kind and compassionate (through practices like *lojong* and bodhichitta), remembering that you're already a buddha (through practices like deity yoga, or the formless meditations like Mahamudra or Dzogchen).[6] The basis of samsara is this: we just forgot. That's the fundamental difference between a sentient being and a buddha. Sentient beings have forgotten that they're buddhas; buddhas never forget. It's a Zen-like conclusion—all this effort to learn, when all we really have to do is remember.

The Tibetan word for mindfulness is *drenpa,* which means "to recollect, remember." The word "memory" itself goes back to the Latin *memor,* which means "mindful." It makes sense. If forgetfulness is our problem, remembrance is our solution. And the practice of remembrance, of waking up, starts with remembering to come back to the present moment. It starts with mindfulness. This simple practice therefore has monumental repercussions. The spirit of re-membering starts with mindfulness, but ends with Buddhahood.

PRACTICING REMEMBRANCE

Forgetfulness (mindlessness) dismembers, memory (mindfulness) remembers. During the Last Supper, Christ broke the bread and said to his disciples, "This is my body, which is for you. Do this in remembrance of me." The forgetfulness that we manifest moment-to-moment is just a daily iteration of the primordial amnesia that occurs when we forget our true nature, our clear-light mind, and stray from this Christ consciousness within. The return to Christ, or the Buddha within, begins when we return to the present moment. We start to heal the primordial dismemberment, the fracturing away of the psyche from the clear-light mind that results in duality, every time we come back to nowness.

Nonduality, which is a synonym for enlightenment, is an abstract notion. We don't realize that nonduality is something we can *practice*. Every time you come back to your breath in mindfulness practice, or to the present moment in daily life, you are practicing enlightenment, and healing the primordial dismemberment that continues to reverberate in the mini-dismemberments that we call mindlessness. You're taking a step on the spiritual path heading back to the Buddha or Christ within you every time you stop stepping away from Christ or the Buddha and start stepping back to the present moment. You'll find the Buddha hiding within this very moment. And mindfulness will introduce you to him.

Just like tiny drops of water can eventually become an ocean, tiny moments of remembrance can eventually heal this primal dismemberment. The practice of moment-to-moment nonduality eventually results in nonduality. We may think that enlightenment exists somewhere in the vague future, out "there and then," but the key to actualizing it is right here and now.

Nonduality seems so distant only because we keep walking away from it. Every time we break away (dismember) from the present moment with our mindlessness, we're taking another step away from who we truly are, and what we really want. We unwittingly keep distancing ourselves. *We're stuck in samsara because we keep practicing it.* We're stuck in duality because we continue to exercise it.

Sogyal Rinpoche said, "To end distraction is to end samsara." The *Tibetan Book of the Dead* says, "Do not be distracted. This is the dividing line where buddhas and sentient beings are separated. It is said: In an instant they are separated, in an instant complete enlightenment." So by practicing non-distraction, we're going to wake up and end samsara.[7] This is exactly the same distraction that makes us non-lucid to our dreams. The following mindfulness meditation is therefore nothing more than the formal practice of lucidity.

Mindfulness Instruction

It's best to learn mindfulness meditation from an instructor, but you can teach yourself the basics from a book.[8] In this section I will provide the essentials. Don't worry about getting it perfect, just get it going. Meditation will develop as you spend time with it.

There are three phases to the instruction: body, breath, and mind. These three phases interpenetrate and therefore support each other. Together they create a stable tripod that reinforces lucidity.

Body

The first phase is about posture, or how to align your body. It is taught that simply by taking the proper posture, sooner or later you will find yourself meditating. An attentive posture invokes an attentive quality of mind. The posture itself is supported by an attitude (or mental posture) of dignity, nobility, even regality; so right away we see how these phases support each other.

Sit in the middle of a meditation cushion, or a chair. If you're sitting on a chair, don't lean against the back. Cross your legs if you're on a cushion, or plant your feet squarely on the ground if you're on a chair. Feel your connection to the stability of the earth. Rest your hands on top of your thighs and keep your back firm, but not stiff. A stable back represents the quality of fearlessness, but it's balanced with an open and receptive front, which represents gentleness. Fearless and gentleness are two key ingredients in good meditation, and your posture literally embodies that. Pull your shoulders back and expose your heart, which is perhaps the central instruction with posture. All the other physical aspects of posture hinge around opening your heart.

Align your head above your spine, which usually means tucking it back in. We're often "heading" out in the wrong direction, and this inclination is represented in bad posture. Rest your tongue on the back of your upper teeth, and part your lips as if you are whispering "ah." Later we'll discuss how to extend this practice into a lying down posture, which is when you close your eyes, but for now it's best to practice lucidity with your eyes open. Keep your gaze down at a point about six feet in front of you, but don't focus on anything. Let your visual field be open and receptive, like your mind and heart.

The stillness of your posture creates a new contrast medium that allows you to see, and therefore become lucid to, the contents of your mind. When you're always moving, it's harder to see the movement of your mind, which is what thoughts fundamentally are. Physical movement is like camouflage. It decreases the contrast that would otherwise allow you to detect the movement of your mind. Sit still and your thoughts are suddenly flushed out of hiding. This is why many meditators complain that meditation seems to increase thoughts. It doesn't. It simply makes them more visible.

WAKING DOWN

Philosopher Drew Leder writes, "Almost all spiritual traditions use posture and gesture as a means whereby we enter into relation with the divine. This body's roots reach down into the soil of an organismic vitality where the conscious mind cannot follow."[9] Our body is a direct link to reality, which the psyche, the most superficial aspect of mind, cannot take you to. Relating to the body is not merely simple minded, it's "trans-minded." It leads you beyond the conceptual mind and to the truth within.

Deception cannot follow you into your body. At a relative level, this doctrine is the basis for lie detectors, which detect subtle changes in the unconscious body while the conscious mind is chattering away. Consciously you can lie, unconsciously you cannot. Your body, like your dreams, is a truth-teller. You (the psyche) may be speaking your truth, but your body speaks another.[10] And remember that the practices of the night are about going deep into the mind, which means going deep into the body. This is why the body phase of meditation is so important. In many ways it's both the ground and the fruition of the path.

"Waking up" is a synonym for enlightenment, but it's just as valid to talk about "waking down" into the wisdom and truth of the body. Phase 1 of the technique invites that awakening. The great Longchenpa said, "Supreme primordial wisdom abides in the body." Sri Aurobindo echoed this: "The work of transformation is about the descent of spirit into the flesh. Embodiment more than transcendence."

Breath

Once good posture is established, bring your attention to the natural movement of your breath. Don't visualize it or think about it. Feel it. Let your awareness ride the medium of your breath. Notice how your breath feels coming in and out of your nostrils, or notice the gentle rising and falling of your abdomen. That's it for phase 2. With these two phases you're sitting and breathing, but you're doing so with lucid presence.

Mind

For phase 3, whenever anything distracts you—a thought, emotion, image, regret, anticipation—mentally say to yourself "thinking," and return to your breath (in the Tibetan view, "thought" includes emotion or any other content of the mind). The label "thinking" is gentle but precise, like popping a bubble with a feather. It's just an act of recognition that you've strayed. It's not a reprimand. Thoughts aren't bad, and you are not trying to get rid of them. You're simply recognizing how thoughts steal your awareness, and make you non-lucid to what's really happening. When the meditative traditions talk about freedom, they're not talking about freedom *from* thought, but freedom *within* thought. Thoughts are never the enemy.

I recommend at least ten minutes of mindfulness meditation every day. If you can do the practice for twenty minutes or more, that's great. But quality is more important than quantity. It's good to practice first thing in the morning, before your day gets away from you. For lucid dreamers, it's also good to practice just before going to sleep. This gathers and settles the mind, which prepares it nicely for lucid dreaming. It's great for spiritual sleep hygiene.

To summarize the technique: First, take an upright and dignified sitting posture. Second, bring your mind to the natural movement of your breath. Third, when anything distracts you, label it "thinking" and return to your breath.

Waking Up

When we say "thinking" in meditation, we're actually saying "wake up." We're waking up to the fact that we've strayed from our body and breath. "Thinking" is simultaneously a recognition of non-lucidity, our detection that we've drifted off into a mini non-lucid daydream, and it is the practice of lucidity, or waking up from that drift. Once again, if we become lucid to the contents of our mind now, we will begin to do so when we dream. It's exactly the same process. We get hooked into non-lucid dreams in the same way we get hooked into thoughts. It's just non-lucidity happening at two different levels.

Some scientists say that we're aware of less than 1 percent of what goes on in our mind at any given moment.[11] In other words, we're non-lucid to 99 percent of what's happening inside. It's no wonder we're non-lucid to our dreams! See for yourself. How often are you fully present? How often you are lost in distraction?

With practice, advanced "lucidity practitioners" can reverse these numbers. Instead of being lucid to just 1 percent of what's going on in our mind, we can become 99 percent lucid to our mind. Lucid dreams then become a natural and common occurrence. (When someone is 100 percent lucid, they are a fully awakened one, a buddha.)

To stress this point another way, every time we unconsciously follow a random thought, we're practicing non-lucidity. So whether we know it or not, we're always practicing. We're always becoming better, or increasingly familiar with (gom), either mindfulness or mindlessness, lucidity or non-lucidity. This is why we're so good at being mindless. We practice it all the time. And this is why we're non-lucid to our dreams.

There are many other benefits of mindfulness for lucid dreaming. For example, once you're lucid in a dream, the stability of your lucidity is nothing more than the stability of your mind. Not only does mindfulness meditation spark more lucid dreams, it also brings about increased stability and clarity of those dreams. Therefore, once again, dreams are truth-tellers. As your mind becomes more stable, clear, and less fragmented in meditation, your dreams become more stable, clear, and less fragmented. They're also more easily remembered. The stability and clarity of your dreams is nothing more than the stability and clarity of attention itself.

These tenets of lucidity have played out in my experience. When I go into retreat, and all worldly distractions are removed, my mind slowly transitions from mindlessness into mindfulness. Because I'm practicing mindfulness all day, I gradually find myself more aware of my dreams. Eventually my non-lucid dreams are replaced with lucid ones, and finally they become more clear and stable. Instead of the colloquialism "What goes up must come down," for the dream yogi it is "What goes down (during the day) must come up (at night)."

So you want to be lucid at night? Meditate during the day.

This is thy hour O soul,
Thy free flight into the wordless,
Away from books, away from art,
The day erased, the lesson done,
Thee fully forth emerging, silent, gazing,
Pondering the themes thou lovest best:
Night, sleep, death and the stars.

WALT WHITMAN, "A Clear Midnight," from *Leaves of Grass*

7

The Lion's Gaze

THE JOURNEY OF meditation altogether, and the night-time practices in particular, points to one of the central tenets in Buddhism that lies at the core of this book. It's implicit in everything we've discussed, and will discuss. Before we move on to the advanced meditations, let's make it explicit. This tenet is also the secret to unconditional happiness. If it's understood, it leads to that happiness; if it's not understood, it leads to endless dissatisfaction and suffering. It's so foundational that even the word for "Buddhist" in Tibetan alludes to this underlying principle.

In or Out

In Tibetan, the word for "Buddhist" is *nangpa,* which means "insider." Buddhists are those who realize that happiness is an inside job. They know that meaning and joy come from within. This is another way to talk about Buddhism as a non-theistic tradition. There's no need to look for salvation outside or in the future, as the theistic traditions maintain. Look within, right now, and you will find what you seek. As Yogi Berra said, "You can observe a lot just by watching," especially if it's in the right direction.

I once saw a cartoon that summarized this playfully. In the cartoon there's a sweet Christian monk holding up a big placard proclaiming, "Christ is coming!" Standing in the background is a reserved Buddhist monk with a small sign that says, "Buddha here now."

This "insider" theme is central to the nocturnal meditations, and to sleep in general, because when we go to sleep we're being forced inside. Everything that would seduce us out into the world is turned off, so in we go. For the untrained eye, it's dark inside. Not much to see. But for the trained eye, which is the meditative eye that has adapted to (become familiar with) the dark, there's an entire world tucked away in here. Extraordinary vistas, and wondrous mindscapes within, await the skilled eye. Meditation and the nighttime practices can illuminate this inner world, transform the darkness into light, and help us see everything—day or night—in a shining new light.

When you first step outside into the night, you can't see a thing. But if you're patient and keep your eyes open, eventually all sorts of things start to appear. Your vision accommodates to the dark, and you see things you didn't see before. In exactly the same way, when you first turn your mind's eye within as you start to practice the nighttime yogas, you can't see a thing. Especially in deep dreamless sleep, which is at first totally black. But if you're patient and keep this inner eye open, an opening that's initiated with daily meditation, eventually all sorts of things start to appear. In particular, the deeper levels of mind, the substrate and then the clear-light mind (discussed in detail in chapter 9), begin to stand out. Turning your gaze within, and seeing things you've never seen before, is the essence of meditation in general, and the nocturnal practices in particular.

Conversely, the word for "non-Buddhist" in Tibetan is *chipa*, which means "outsider"—that is, those who look outside of themselves for meaning and happiness. As the country music song recorded by Johnny Lee says, "They're lookin' for love"—and everything else they want—"in all the wrong places."[1] "Outsiders" are always heading in the wrong direction, lost in worldly distractions. In Christian theology, the Greek word for sin is *hamartia*, which means "to miss the mark." We're constantly missing the mark because the target of happiness is 180 degrees off. Once again we've got it completely backward. We keep aiming outside, then wonder why something is missing, why life seems off the mark.[2]

Until we enter a meditative path (and if we're not careful, even while on the path), most of us are outsiders. We feel that external things will make us happy, so we spend our lives chasing things, people, or circumstances, like the proverbial rainbow. To look out is to move out. Most importantly, we spend our lives chasing our thoughts, as meditation quickly reveals. This pursuit of thoughts and things is the basis of materialism and consumerism, and therefore all our suffering.[3] The philosophy professor Peter Kreeft writes, "Suicide, the most in-your-face index of unhappiness, is directly proportional to wealth. The richer you are, the richer your family is, and the richer your country is, the more likely it is that you will find life so good that you will choose to blow your brains out."[4]

Material richness is often directly proportional to spiritual poverty, because all those expensive toys result in expensive distraction that bankrupts your soul; what you're getting isn't what you really want. Remember that to end distraction is to end samsara, and conversely, to amp distraction—to amp being seduced out—is to amp samsara.

The "outsider" trajectory took on force with the advent of artificial light, which coaxes us out and away from ourselves at a time when nature is inviting us in. In his 2003 book *Dawning of Clear Light: A Western Approach to Tibetan Dark Retreat Meditation,* Martin Lowenthal writes,

> Our desire to eliminate darkness takes both material and spiritual forms. The harnessing of electricity and the invention of the light bulb have not only extended our days and transformed our rhythms of work, *they have deepened our preoccupation with external images* [emphasis added], especially with the coming of television and computers . . . We pay for this exclusive orientation toward light with fear of the dark, a flight from mortality, and superficial lives relegated to experiencing only the surface of reality. [We pay the price of heightened distraction.] This denial and fear of darkness lead to addictions that keep us from experiencing . . . depth.[5]

I'm writing this on December 21, the darkest day of the year. For many people, this time of year is the most depressing, because the blanket of darkness becomes oppressive.[6] SAD, or seasonal affective disorder, runs rampant. Alcoholism, and other forms of distraction (like the wild consumerism around Christmas), increase during the dark season as we wrestle with the suffocating nature of darkness, and the way it almost forces us into ourselves. It's not the darkness that we really dread, but having to face ourselves without the distractions of external light. Chasing external light has a shadow side as it keeps us heading out and away from our inner selves. "Outsiders" love artificial light, because it facilitates the impulse to head out. And they resist darkness, because it tends to interrupt that trajectory.

Renunciation

In Buddhist thought, discovering the futility of finding happiness outside, the folly of chasing external light and external satisfaction, is called "renunciation," and it's a crucial element on the path to awakening. Nighttime yoga does not require that you become a Buddhist, of course, but it does require that you shift your focus.[7]

True renunciation is often accompanied by some type of life crisis, which can happen at any age. The crisis occurs when you have what you think you need to be happy, but you're still not satisfied. It occurs when you ask, "Is this all there is?" which in our terms translates as "Is appearance all there is? Is there something behind these superficial things?"

You've got the mate, the job, the car, the house, and you're still not happy. The crisis is actually a grand opportunity. You're finally *waking up* to the fact that outside things cannot make you happy, and that skin-deep appearances are unsatisfactory. You've climbed to the top of the ladder only to discover it's up against the wrong wall.[8]

Meditation and the nighttime yogas show us that this external trajectory, and hence our suffering, all starts when we follow our thoughts out. We buy into external things, literally and figuratively, in exactly the same way we buy into our thoughts and emotions.

In the context of dream yoga, "outsiders" are those who are seduced into the projections of the mind and get lost in the dream. "Dream" at this level refers to any projection of the mind that we get overly involved with, and therefore lose our lucidity in. One definition of non-lucid, in this context, means getting excessively involved in the projections of our mind, mis-taking those projections to be solid and real. So "dream" at this level refers to any thought, emotion, or fantasy that sucks us in, and that we take to be real. We buy it, and therefore become non-lucid. In other words, *we lose the essence in the display*. We lose the empty essence of the mind in the luminous display of the mind. We've lost our mind. Or at least an integral part of it.

As the poet Rumi is quoted as saying, "What comes into being gets lost in being and drunkenly forgets its way home." Our job is to sober up and find our way home. So what we need to do is wake up *from* the luminous projections of the mind (the thoughts and emotions that we take to be so real) and wake up *to* the emptiness. We want to *find* the essence in the display.[9] The result is discovering that everything is illusory—just like a dream.[10]

"Illusory" has a specific meaning in Buddhism. To say that something is illusory means that how it appears simply isn't true. Appearance is not in harmony with reality. "Outsiders" are those who get lost in appearance and end up living a lie; "insiders" discover the reality behind mere appearance and wake up to the truth. From a psychological perspective, Carl Jung put it beautifully when he said, "Your vision will become clear when you look into your heart. Who looks outside dreams. Who looks within awakens."[11] Philosophically, Plato (in *The Symposium*) put it this way: "The mind's eye begins to see clearly when the outer eyes grow dim."

"Outsiders" are those who are overly involved in, and therefore non-lucid to, the contents of their mind and the contents of the world. They falsely identify with the things in their world and the thoughts in their mind, which are both the display of their own mental projections. The great master Jamyang Khyentse Chökyi Lodrö said, "The root of all phenomena is your mind. If unexamined, it rushes after experiences, ingenious in the games of deception. If you look right into it, it is free of any ground or origin." "Insiders" are those who see through, or "cut through," those same thoughts and things and wake up to the actual nature of everything. They accurately identify themselves as the empty projector, not the reified projections.

The modern Tibetan master Nyoshul Khen Rinpoche says,

> The nature of everything is illusory and ephemeral.
> Those with dualistic perception regard suffering as happiness
> Like those who lick honey from the edge of a razor blade.
> How pitiful, those who cling strongly to concrete reality!
> Turn your attention within, my heart-friends![12]

Tulku Urgyen Rinpoche said, "Samsara is mind turned out, lost in its projections. Nirvana is mind turned in, recognizing its true nature." If there is a summary quotation for our spiritual journey, this is it. The dreaming mind is turned (tuned) out, lost in its projections. The awakened mind is turned (tuned) in, waking up to its true nature.

Developing the Lion's Gaze

One analogy in Tibetan Buddhism is that of "the lion's gaze."[13] The lion is the king of the jungle, fearless and uncontested. His gaze is set in contrast to the gaze of a dog. The teaching is that if you throw a stick out and away from a dog, the dog will chase after the stick. But if you throw a stick out and away from a lion, the lion will chase you. The lion's gaze is set upon the thrower, not the thrown. We all have the gaze of a dog, forever chasing the sticks thrown out by our own minds. We're constantly running after the thoughts and emotions that are endlessly tossed up from within.

I have a dog and often take it to a dog park. It's fun to watch the pups chasing after balls and sticks thrown by their owners. Are we any different? Just look at your mind. Whenever anything pops up, we go after it. We buy into it. That's getting seduced into the projections of our own mind. That's getting lost in the display. *That's* non-lucidity. And that's the basis of our suffering.

In order to find the essence of things as they are, we have to look within. Just as the lion is fearless in the jungle, it takes a fearless gaze to look deeply within the jungle of our own mind. It takes courage to look into the dark, and even more guts to step into it. This is why we started with a proper view, or gaze—the lion's gaze. If we know that at the other end of the darkness of our unconscious mind is eternal light, we will go fearlessly into that good night because we realize we're heading toward dawn.

The only way to reason with an illusion is to stop believing it.

BRITTANY BRONSON, *New York Times Sunday Review*

8

Advanced Meditations and Visualizations

WITH THE IMPORTANCE of inner work established, let's look at some advanced induction techniques that turn, and tune, us inward.

A Twenty-One-Breath Settling Meditation

To further bring lucidity into the night, and to encourage the turn within, we can progress from sitting meditation to more advanced meditative aspects of dream yoga induction, such as lying down meditation. Even though sitting is the most common way to practice, there are other ways to meditate in the traditional texts: standing, walking, and lying down.

While the sitting posture introduced earlier is important, we don't want to limit the meditative mind to one position—literally and figuratively. Restricting meditation is a common trap, especially with beginners. If we only practice sitting meditation, we'll leave our meditation behind when we leave our seat. In some spiritual communities it's common to exhort members to "hold your seat" in daily life, especially when things get rocky. One of the best ways to practice "holding your seat" is to get off of it during formal sessions and hold your meditative mind as you do so, which is what this exhortation truly means. Part of our journey with the nighttime practices is to stretch the meditative mind, and hence awareness, into all the postures of life. Working with different positions nurtures that stretch.

As a meditation instructor I often see how quickly students "lose their seat" when they stand up after a session and engage the world. Their meditation is fragile, and overly dependent on one position. In my own early experience, I was humbled to discover how hard it was to meditate when I lay down or when I got sick. My practice mind went out the window as I went to bed. But ever since I started practicing meditation while lying down, I have found it increasingly easy to extend my meditation into sleep and sickness, and slowly into everything I do.

It's fine to develop meditation on the cushion, which acts like an incubator, but problematic to only associate meditation with sitting. We can't live our life in an incubator. To survive in the world, our meditation has to grow up. We want to develop industrial-strength meditation, an adult meditative mind that can extend deep into the night, and even survive death. In order to do that, we practice in different postures.

In chapter 5 we discussed the sleeping lion posture. If that position works for you, then you can practice the following meditation in that posture. But it's often easier to do so lying on your back. Once again, do what works.

Lie down and place your hands on your belly. This helps ground awareness in the natural movement of your breath. It also helps the mind unwind, because awareness of your belly brings the inner winds down from your head and into your body. Close your eyes and feel your belly.

Because lying down is associated with sleep, our mind tends to be too loose when we take this posture. It's easy to lapse into a sloppy and mindless state. To counteract this tendency, start this meditation a bit tighter by counting twenty-one breaths. One inhalation and exhalation count as a breath. You may notice that your breathing, and therefore counting, gets slower as you progress. As we've seen, there's an intimate connection between the movement of your mind (thoughts) and the movement of your breath. After counting twenty-one breaths, stop counting and just feel your breath. Transition to mindfulness of breath alone.

As a final refinement, transition from mindfulness of breath into a direct mindfulness of mind. In other words, after a few minutes of following your breath, transition your awareness from your breath to your thoughts. But this time instead of labeling your thoughts "thinking," do something progressively more subtle. When you recognize a thought (that you would have previously labeled "thinking"), follow that thought back to its source. From where does that thought arise? Where does a thought go when it dies? You may not know what that source is yet, but follow the thought back in and see where it takes you. Instead of letting the thought take you out and away like it usually does, gently grab its hand and let it take you down and in. Go from an "outsider" to an "insider." It's like trying to follow a ray of the sun back to the sun.

With this refinement, instead of thoughts distracting you from your meditation, they *become* your meditation. This is a subtle practice, so don't tie yourself into knots trying too hard. It has to be gentle and precise, and it takes practice. You're approaching the thinnest end of the oneironaut's mindfulness pole and cultivating a very refined awareness. But if it can be done, the very thought that would otherwise send you out into the world now leads you directly to your clear-light mind.

Two things can happen if you follow this thought back in. The first is what we already talked about in "napping meditation," where we use hypnagogic states to trigger lucidity. In other words, you can watch the thought dip below the membrane of waking consciousness and inflate into an instant lucid dream. The second thing is that you can witness that thought, which is a subtle form, dissolve into complete formlessness. Watch it melt into no-thingness, or emptiness, like a snowflake hitting a hot rock. The first option can be used to work with dream yoga, and the second one with sleep yoga. With sleep yoga, it's like dropping down our pole into the vast inner space of dreamless sleep. Even if you can't do it, just the effort will point you in the right direction for the practice of the nighttime yogas, and help you maintain awareness as you fall asleep.

EMPTINESS

Emptiness is an underlying theme of our journey. Emptiness is one of the most important, and misunderstood, topics in Buddhism. Emptiness is not nothingness (which is nihilistic), but no-thingness. "Openness" is perhaps a better word because it removes the nihilistic tinge. If you look closely at anything, you will see that it arises in dependence on other things, so emptiness refers to the lack of (empty of) inherent existence. Everything is relative to everything else, which is why scholar Robert Thurman refers to emptiness as "the universal theory of relativity." No man is an island. Nothing stands alone. Emptiness replaces an "egological," or "thing-oriented," view with an "ecological," or "systems-oriented," view.

Emptiness challenges the very idea of "thingness." With the proper view of emptiness, the *appearance* of a thing—an entity that is solid, lasting, and independent—is replaced with the *reality* of relationship. In other words, in reality there is *only* relationship, which is another way to talk about emptiness. There is no such thing as a thing. In popular parlance, there are no nouns in reality, only verbs. Emptiness is important because when we get lost in appearance (just like getting lost in a non-lucid dream), we suffer. "Waking up" is largely about waking up to the empty nature of whatever arises, which liberates us from the trap of mere appearance, the bad dream of samsara.

Lotus Visualization

Visualization practice is a marvelous preparation for lucid dreaming. It's just like it sounds. If I say, "Visualize an apple," you can easily bring an image of an apple to mind. It's that simple. We can use the power of visualization, which is just a form of controlled imagination, as a tool for triggering lucidity. In Vajrayana Buddhism, visualization is part of a family of meditations called "generation stage practice," where "generation" and "visualization" are virtually synonymous. You generate a visualization as a way to work with the creative powers of the mind.[1] If this kind of meditation resonates with you, you may discover that as your visualization gets stronger, which means your ability to visualize gets more clear and stable, so do your dreams. You're exercising the same mental muscle. Dreaming and imagining depend on the same areas of the brain.[2]

I've been doing generation stage meditations for twenty-five years, and have noticed a relationship between my proficiency in visualization and my ability to have lucid dreams. Whether this is due to the mindfulness associated with visualization practice, or visualization itself, something is improving. In perhaps a similar vein, the preeminent dream researcher Jane Gackenbach has shown that "hardcore" gamers—defined as those who play video games for more than two hours, several times a week, and have done so since before the third grade—were more likely than their peers to experience lucid dreams. If you're in an artificial reality for hours every day, it makes sense that you might recognize an artificial reality at night.[3]

Try this experiment. Imagine, or visualize, your favorite fantasy. Really get into it; see it as clearly as possible. Get your other senses involved. "Feel," or even "hear," what you're visualizing. Is there any substantive difference between getting absorbed in a visualization and getting caught up in a dream? In one sense, a daydream is an involuntary and non-lucid visualization, and a visualization is a voluntary and lucid daydream.

The difference between a daydream, a nighttime dream, and a visualization is the intentionality and focus. With a daydream or nighttime dream, your imagination ("visualization") runs wild. There's no yoga here. The undisciplined mind takes off and gets lost in itself. Generation stage practice is a yoga, so it takes effort. You're working to control the creative powers of your mind, not indulge them.

There are a number of ways to begin visualization practice. You can hold an apple, or any object, and really look at it. Then close your eyes and bring that apple to mind as clearly as possible. Visualize every detail. With generation stage practice, in addition to exercising your visualization muscle, you're also exercising your mindfulness. So visualization is a double-barreled meditation for inducing lucidity.

We touched on visualization practice in a previous chapter when we talked about visualizing a red pearl, or AH, at your throat. What you want to do now is lie down on your back, do the twenty-one-breath meditation to settle your mind, then visualize either the red pearl or the AH at your throat. If you're so inclined, take the sleeping lion posture and do this. See what works.

Once you feel comfortable with this level of visualization, move on to the next phase, which is to visualize a four-petaled red lotus at your throat (see figure 5). With visualization in general, it's easier to start with a larger image in your mind, and then make it smaller. Start with a lotus the size of figure 5, then shrink it down to the size

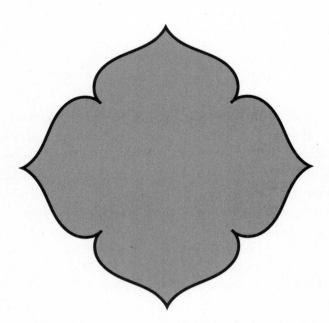

FIGURE 5   **Red lotus.** Visualize the image of a lotus in vivid red as you transition from waking to sleeping consciousness.

of a silver dollar, a quarter, or even a dime. Really good generation stage meditators can focus their minds so intently, and for so long, that they can visualize every detail of a deity (some say hundreds of deities) in a dot the size of a sesame seed. Let this inspire you, not intimidate you. With enough practice, you could do the same.

I recommend one preliminary step before attempting the lotus visualization. Take a red crayon, pen, or marker and trace the lotus on a piece of paper. Start at the top and slowly circumscribe the lotus, going in a clockwise direction. Focus intently on what you're doing. Use your mindfulness and see if you can make one "lap" around the lotus without being distracted. Try to outline it without gapping out. It's both a test and a practice of your mindfulness. This will help you when you start to visualize the lotus at your throat. If one "lap" without a break is easy, then try two, three, or even more. This will help your visualization and get it into your system. It helps you get a *feel* for the practice.

Many generation stage practitioners think that visualization is exclusively a mental exercise, but it's just as much a somatic one. Visualization comes to life when you feel it. There's no such word, but you get the point: visualization is "feelingization." Tracing the lotus on a piece of paper strengthens this aspect of generation stage practice.[4] Remember that we're dropping from our head into our body when we fall into sleep. By tracing the lotus, it's almost as if we're preparing to hand the baton of mindfulness from our (conscious) head into our (unconscious) body. In other words, as we start to lose the visualized image of the lotus when we fall into sleep, our somatic memory of the felt sense of the lotus takes over. This acts as a subtle bridge from waking to sleeping consciousness, and allows us to sustain our mindfulness as we fall asleep.

Start by physically tracing out the lotus a few dozen times. Go slowly and feel your way into it. You want to plant the feeling of the red lotus into your body so that the somatic aspect of visualization takes over when the thinking (imagining) aspect fades. In dream and sleep yoga, we're trying to sustain our awareness as we go from awareness of form (consciousness, head) to formless awareness (unconsciousness, heart-body). This isn't easy. Without preparation it won't happen. Working with these subtle practices now will help you relax into them when you fall asleep. Practice turns into performance when you hit the sack.

After you've gotten a feel for the lotus by tracing it out on paper, the next step is to close your eyes and trace it out in the space in front of you. You can use your finger as a pen, and move it around the visualized lotus as you circumscribe it mentally. You're starting to transition from form (the pen and paper) into the formless.

The next step is to practice visualizing the lotus at your throat. Do this in formal sitting meditation first as a way to etch the visualization in your mind and throat. It also stamps your motivation. You're taking this seriously, and are willing to work with it in formal practice. After taking your sitting posture, close your eyes and begin to trace out the lotus in your throat. Be slow and deliberate as you circumscribe the form. As a test, and a further practice, see if you can keep the "pen" of your mind down on the "paper" of your throat without making any gaps in the outline as you go around. In other words, see if you can trace the lotus without being distracted. Once again, dream yoga is the "measure of the path." Play with how fast or slow you go around, and how that affects your mindfulness. If you have to go quickly to keep the "pen" from coming off the "page" (from being distracted), that's okay. It's a practice after all.

Bringing this level of structure to your mindfulness can help you sustain your focus by challenging you a little. It may seem too tight at first, mostly because the untrained mind is usually so loose. If you're too loose when you start any bedtime meditation, you'll just flop into sleep in your normal non-lucid way. We start tight to control the mind, then gradually loosen the visualization as we loosen our hold on the world of form.

Descent Visualizations

As a further refinement of the lotus visualization—which so far has taken us from seeing the lotus, to visualizing it, to feeling it—now try to *become* the lotus. Start by putting your heart into your throat, so to speak. Give the lotus some depth by visualizing it in three dimensions, like the petals of a real flower. Then make it quiver or flutter, like it's alive. Zap some electricity into it. If you leave it at a cartoon level, you'll have cartoon-level effects. Wake it up, so it can wake you up.

Once you get a sense of merging with the lotus, the next step is to take it to bed. Lie down and start with the twenty-one-breath settling meditation, then bring your awareness to your throat for the lotus visualization. Trace it out with your mind's eye. Notice how gaps in the tracing occur as you dip in and out of sleep. Gradually release the intensity of the focus and allow yourself to drift into sleep. Because you have the visualized tracing as a kind of ruler, or measure, you can more clearly notice your descent into sleep. This noticing is your lucidity at work. If you've gained some mastery with the three phases of mindfulness, you can watch how effortful mindfulness (tracing it with your mind's eye) transitions into effortless mindfulness (the tracing dissolves, but you're still aware of what's happening).

For those who have a relationship to Buddhism, there's one more visualization you might try. Visualize a blue AH, yellow NU, red TA, and green RA on the four petals, and a white OM at the center. You can do this in English or Tibetan (see figure 6). The colors aren't

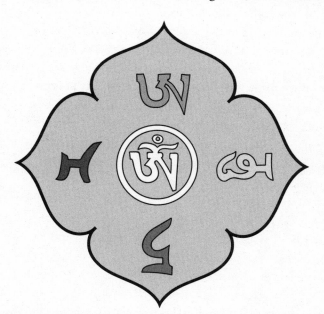

FIGURE 6 **Red lotus with Tibetan seed syllables.** Visualize a blue AH on the top petal, a yellow NU on the right petal, a red TA on the bottom petal, and a green RA on the left petal. The OM at the center is white.

random; they have a subtle effect on consciousness. You may recognize these as the five "seed syllables" of the five *dhyani* (meditation) buddhas; they will infuse the visualization with the qualities of devotion and empowerment.[5] It's a nice way to let the buddhas tuck you in to sleep.

Start this visualization the same way you did for the red lotus that was sketched without these seed syllables. In other words, draw out the lotus on a piece of paper, then draw in the letters of the syllables. It's best if you can do the letters in their respective colors, but you can also let your imagination color them in later. Once you get a feel for it, trace this out with your mind's eye in the space in front of you, then transition into visualizing this in your throat. Now take it all to bed.

When you lie down to go to sleep, and after you do your twenty-one-breath settling meditation, bring your awareness to the blue AH. Trace out the AH over and over, in English or Tibetan. When you start to get drowsy, switch over to the yellow NU. Trace it out until your mind gets heavier. This is very individual, so you have to be your own guide. Maybe stay on the NU until you start to notice some gaps in your mental tracing of the letter. At that fuzzy point, switch to the red TA, and trace it until you start dipping in and out of sleep. When there are plenty of gaps in your tracing, and you're really starting to lose it, move to the green RA on the left. At this point you're barely conscious. In the very last moments before blacking out, switch to the white OM in the center and allow yourself to slide into sleep. It's almost like you're going down the drain of consciousness and into the pipe of the unconscious mind. But this pipe is special, because it's been insulated with the essence of the five buddhas.

If I happen to drift away from a letter, I'll come back to either the last petal I was at before zoning out or to the petal where I feel I should be. I don't start at the beginning and work my way back down, though that approach might work for you. For example, if I'm at the left petal with the green RA before zoning out and I come back "up," I'll place my attention back onto the green RA and see if I can slide down to the white OM. Discover what works for you.

Because this practice is subtle, when you first start the descent visualization it's often clumsy. It takes time to get a feel for it. I wrestled with the Tibetan letters initially. Then I wasn't sure where to place the visualization at my throat, or how big it should be. There was also the challenge of when to switch from one petal to the next. I often zonked out before getting to the OM, or even the RA. This is when my passion for ignorance really came out! But with practice, and a determined but light-handed approach, it started to gel. Instead of just plopping into mindless sleep, I was able to walk myself mindfully into the dark. So be patient. Realize that you're working with subtle meditations that are designed to match the subtlety of sleep and dream.

This descent visualization is not only different from person to person, it will be different from night to night. If you're really sleepy, the entire ride around the lotus can happen in a few minutes, or even seconds. If you're not that tired, it could take half an hour or more. Don't worry about perfectly dividing your descent into five tidy and evenly timed stages. Don't get too hung up on details. That's too tight. You might spend most of your time on the first petal, then proceed rapidly through the other three. The idea is that as we spiral down into sleep, awareness spirals down into the clear-light mind. It's important to remember, however, that it can only be the clear-light mind if we're able to recognize it. Otherwise it remains ignorance, or the usual blackout, as we'll see when we discuss sleep yoga.

What we're doing is replacing our firemans pole with a spiral staircase. This invites a more articulate descent, and therefore an ability to descend lucidly. Otherwise, it's all just mish-mash as we fall asleep. Through the power of association, you can get so proficient in this that you can step yourself down into sleep consciously.[6] It's almost a form of self-hypnosis, and another example of a "waking-induced lucid dream" technique. These techniques are partly intended to show you how much is possible even before you enter sleep and dream.

Remember that where the mind goes (with your visualization) the pranas go; where the pranas go, the bindus go; and where the bindus go, consciousness goes. With these visualizations, you're consciously directing your awareness from your head into your throat, from waking into dreaming consciousness. In terms of the inner yogas, you can imagine that the four petals are all hanging off of the central channel, and that when you drop into the OM at the center of the lotus, you're dropping into the central channel. The central channel is associated with nonduality and wisdom. Duality cannot perceive nonduality; consciousness cannot see wisdom. That's why most of us black out when we fall asleep (more on this in the chapter on sleep yoga).

> The mind naturally holds on to things as it descends into sleep. If it doesn't have something like these visualizations, it will latch onto discursive thoughts and you will fall into sleep non-lucidly. Before the advent of electric dimmers, we turned on lights with the flick of switch. The light was either on or off. These visualizations act as a dimmer for consciousness. Instead of just flicking the light of consciousness off, we can slowly dim our awareness and retain a few "photons" as we slide into sleep. Then when dreams arise, the dimmer comes back up and we illuminate our dreams with this refined lucidity of mind.

People often ask what vantage point to take during the visualization. It's usually assumed that you're looking down at the throat visualization from somewhere behind the eyes, which is where we think the mind's eye resides.[7] It's fine to start the throat visualization from this perspective, because that's where the bindus (consciousness) are during waking consciousness. So begin by looking down on the lotus and tracing it out. As you get drowsy and begin the progression clockwise around the lotus, you may notice that your perspective starts to change. When I do it, my perspective descends. If bindu is consciousness, and the bindus drop toward the heart as you fall into sleep, your visualization of the lotus could also drop.[8]

If you're able to do it perfectly, by the time you work your way around the lotus and move to the center of it, you're no longer visualizing the lotus from anywhere above. You've fallen into it and *become* the lotus.

Pep Talk

Bedtime, as the archetype of ignorance in the spiritual sense, is a sanctuary for the ego. This is where ego puts up its most defensive "do not disturb" sign, and goes to hide out and recharge.[9] As spiritual practitioners, many of us are half-heartedly committed to waking up. Our renunciation is feeble. We're willing to let meditation work on us during the day, but even then it's only on our terms. We might practice thirty minutes a day, and only when it's convenient. But nighttime is my time. You can rouse me during the day, but don't try to rouse me at night.

When I did my first month-long meditation retreat nearly thirty years ago, I discovered how much I treasured the darkness of ignorance, and how far I was willing to let in the light. During this retreat I practiced basic mindfulness twelve hours a day, which was very difficult for me. I felt like a wild stallion tethered to a hitching post. My favorite part of the day was when I was finally able to plop into bed. This was when I could breathe a big sigh of relief and just indulge my discursive mind. All day long I kept bringing my mind back to my breath, but at night I let it run wild. It was like spending the night at the movies.

Because I was a serious student, and definitely too tight during the day, the contrast between daytime effort and nighttime indulgence was dramatic. I didn't just feast on my discursive mind at night, I gorged on it. It was almost rebellious, like a kid getting away with something while the parents are away.

After the second week of the retreat, my evening extravagance was rudely interrupted. Because I was creating so much momentum with my meditation during the day, it started to spread into the night. Instead of being able to indulge my rebellious mind at night, I unintentionally found myself being more and more mindful. Rather than celebrating the fruits of my efforts during the day, and rejoicing in how meditation was spreading into my life, I nearly panicked when mindfulness penetrated my nighttime sanctuary. I tried to work with this meditative invasion for a few evenings, but after several sleepless nights of wrestling with my mind, I decided that meditation wasn't for me and resolved to leave the retreat. I preferred to be ignorant.

I packed my bags, but in a gesture of courtesy decided to talk to my meditation instructor before leaving. He was very skillful, and gave me the space to leave. But he also suggested a few things I could try to better relate to what was happening, and encouraged me to give them a chance. Because of his confidence and reassurance, I was able to implement his suggestions and finish the retreat.

This was my first experience, years before I began dream yoga, of how I didn't want meditation to work on me while I slept. It showed me how much I lusted for mindlessness and craved ignorance. For the ego, ignorance really is bliss. I've obviously tempered that stance and now invite meditation to work on me while I sleep. But it took patience, perseverance, and a great deal of humor.

If you only want to practice during the day, the spiritual path is full of skillful means to wake you up. If the nighttime yogas are too obtrusive, you could limit your efforts to the daytime practice of illusory form, described in subsequent chapters. But if you want to take complete advantage of this precious life and the full spectrum of skillful means, then the nighttime meditations can help. Once again, dream yoga is a truth-teller. It will show you how far you're willing to go to wake up. Shechen Kongtrul Rinpoche, one of the main teachers of Chögyam Trungpa Rinpoche, once told his student, "Someday you're going to go [to the West]. You might just find that they're a lot more interested in staying asleep than in waking up."[10]

When we get on the spiritual path and do practices like dream and sleep yoga, we need to understand that these methods are inconvenient. How much light do you really want to bring to the darkest corners of your life? Are you willing to let that light expose you? How protective are you of your shadows?[11] In the service of comfort, how important is deception? These are not meant to be punishing inquisitions, but rather invitations that can show you where you stand on the path, and where you want to be.

The Tibetan word for renunciation is *nge jung,* which means "definite emergence." It's rare. Most of us are just "partially emerged." We haven't given up hope for samsara. Partial emergence is where we begin on the path, and it's an important step toward withdrawing from our addiction to comfort and spiritual sleep. But we should also recognize that it is partial and that there's more to go.

After decades of doing these nighttime practices, there are still times when I just want to enjoy sleep or indulge my dreams. If I'm in a lucid dream, I'll sometimes use the first part of the dream to indulge the freedom, then switch to a practice mode. I want to enjoy my dreamtime, otherwise I won't enjoy my dream yoga.

Find your balance on the tightrope of the nighttime yogas. If you're too tight or too loose, you'll fall off. The biggest tripping point is discouragement and our passion for ignorance. Knowing this can help you identify these obstacles, keep you balanced, and therefore keep you going.

If you release what is within you, what you release will save you. If you do not release what is within you, what you do not release will destroy you.

GNOSTIC GOSPEL OF SAINT THOMAS, *The Gnostic Gospels*

What lies behind us and what lies before us are small matters compared to what lies within us.

RALPH WALDO EMERSON

9

Illuminating the Deeper Mind

IF YOU'VE COME this far on your journey into the night, you are ready to have a better understanding of the levels of your mind, from outer to inner. The journey into darkness each night is a journey toward the inner mind, and we can illuminate this darkness by understanding these deeper levels. If we understand that we're heading into radiant light—not dark—when we fall into sleep, we can use that "black light" to inspire us into spiritual awakening. So let's develop the dream map we introduced in chapter 2.

Sleep is a descent from surface consciousness into the two levels of unconsciousness: the dream level and the dreamless sleep level. The model we will use to frame this descent is not a Western view of the mind but rather a blend of Western thought with Buddhist views. These levels have been explored and mapped by meditators for centuries. With the nighttime yogas, or with the appropriate daytime meditations, you can experience them for yourself.

From a Buddhist perspective, the simplest description of mind uses a three-tiered model.[1] All our dreams come from these three levels: the psyche, or the outermost superficial conscious mind; the clear-light mind, or the innermost deepest unconscious mind; and the substrate, which is an intermediate unconscious level that constitutes everything in between.

The Psyche

The psyche—that is, the surface or conscious level of mind—is the shallowest level, and the one from which we normally operate. You only have to look at your everyday experience to see this exterior level. It's this most dualistic mind that skims across the surface of life and that is defined by a sharp distinction between inside (self) and outside (other).

Most of us spend our entire conscious lives at this surface level. It's the easiest one to identify with. That's the problem. The psyche is who we think we are, so we're very attached to it. We're unaware of (asleep to) our deeper self, and therefore we float on the surface of mind, never savoring the depths that await us below. Hence we suffer, because this outermost level is akin to the surface chop in an ocean. Life here is like a piece of cork bobbing up and down on rough waters, high one day and low the next. By floating on this surface we are, ironically, drowning in ignorance.

This level is defined by grasping, which is the basis of the psyche and what keeps it afloat. Isn't this what most of us do? We grasp after thoughts and things as if our life depended on it—for on one level, it does. It's habitual and automatic. We feel that if we stopped grasping, the psyche, which is virtually synonymous with ego, would disappear. With nothing to hold on to, the psyche would dissolve into the deeper levels of mind from which it arose—which is exactly what happens every night when we fall asleep.

This grasping also results in our belief that the psyche is all there is. A primordial form of identity theft occurs when the psyche grasps onto itself as the only level of mind. The psyche steals awareness from our deeper and truer levels of identity, and consolidates it at this superficial level. It's a kleptomaniac, clutching everything in the inner and outer world, all the while saying "me" and "mine" like a spoiled two-year-old.

To relocate our true and spiritually mature Self, we have to "lose" or release our false self, the psyche. We have to stop grasping and grow up. To stop grasping and "lose your mind" may seem like a tragic state of affairs for the psyche, but not if you know what's potentially to be found. It's only your superficial mind that is lost (released), and your true identity that is therefore found. Lose your psyche to find your soul. It's a "lost and found" that can happen every single night.

Lie in bed, watch all your thoughts pop up (the psyche initially stands out when you lie down), and then watch them dissolve as you dissolve into sleep. If you didn't *let go* of the superficial mind you would never *fall* asleep. Hold on and you stay up; let go and you drop down.[2] Grasping after the contents of this level not only creates suffering during the day, it creates the suffering of insomnia at night.

To access the deeper levels of our being, we need to release the superficial levels. This is standard spiritual instruction that takes on new meaning in the meditations of the night. But because we're not familiar with these deeper levels, we don't recognize them as we sleep and dream. We don't wake up to our true nature. We, as the psyche, black out.

As Freud famously suggested, the psyche is like the tip of an iceberg. It may be all you see, but below the surface lies the vast bulk of the berg—which in Buddhist terms consists of the massive "substrate mind" and the infinite "clear-light mind." In the field of cognitive neuroscience, research confirms that human mental activity is constantly and thoroughly influenced by processes outside our conscious awareness.[3] Our journey is to bring these processes into awareness.

The Substrate

From the gross and familiar outer mind we move to the more subtle and unfamiliar inner levels, to domains that we're tucked into when we slip into sleep. The psyche emanates from a deeper intermediate level, which is referred to by a number of different names: *alaya vijnana* in Sanskrit, eighth consciousness or "storehouse consciousness" in Yogachara Buddhism, or the relative unconscious mind, to name just a few. The psyche is the surface or conscious aspect of what we think of as "ego," and the substrate is the deeper or unconscious aspect of ego. Substrate + psyche = ego. While the psyche is our outer and onstage life, the substrate is our inner and backstage life.

I like the term "substrate mind" because it implies "something that underlies or serves as the basis or foundation."[4] Not only does this definition suggest something that lies below, but it plays on the word "lie." The psyche is the biggest lie of them all because it's the lie of appearance. The psyche is the part of us that gets pulled into seeing and believing things the way they seem to be, and therefore misses the deeper truth of how things actually are. That "looks can be deceiving" is a central tenet of this book. In a non-lucid dream, what *appears* looks like reality, but it's not. Lucidity, day or night, is about waking up from that deceptive look. We're not only pathological liars in a philosophical sense (because we're living the lies generated by the psyche), we're pathological believers. We believe in the truth of appearance, the propaganda of the psyche, which is the mother of all lies.[5] We're suckers for the superficial.

There's a big difference between *appearance* and *reality*. Reality is the truth. That's what we're after on the spiritual path, as well as with the nighttime yogas. Appearance is what covers and obscures reality.[6] At the end of the path, we don't actually attain enlightenment. We simply cease to be deluded—by appearances.

It's like being at the movies. You can be totally sucked into a film and suddenly wake up to the fact that what you're lost in is just the play of light on a screen. This tiny shift in perspective has monumental repercussions. You're instantly liberated from the drama. Sam Harris writes of this common analogy, "Your perception is unchanged, but the spell is broken. Most of us spend every waking moment lost in the movie of our lives. Until we see that an alternative to this enchantment exists, we are entirely at the mercy of appearances."[7]

In Buddhism, thought is often referred to as the mere movement of the mind, and it constitutes the world of inner appearances. If this movement is overt, as in a powerful stream of thoughts or an emotional tidal wave, it sweeps us away. If the movement is covert, as in the constant undertow of subconscious thought, it sucks us into constant distraction or daydreams. If the movement is unconscious, as in a non-lucid dream, we get drawn in and lost in that current. Inner or outer; overt, covert, or unconscious; we spend our lives lost in the movies.

The point is that we think appearances, inner or outer, will make us happy, but this is a delusion, a mere substitute satisfaction. Only reality can truly satisfy.

His Holiness the Seventeenth Karmapa says,

> [Modern products] are custom-made to suit our greed
> and grasping. They are exactly tailored to deceive us with
> their appearances. As I see it, however, the bigger problem
> is the gullibility of our mind. This is what really leaves
> us vulnerable to the deceptive allure of things. In other
> words, we ourselves are the bigger problem. Sometimes
> we are like small children; when it comes to assessing our
> own needs, we often show no sign of maturity. Just think
> about it: When a little child cries, the easy way to stop
> him is to give him a toy. We dangle it in front of him and
> wave it around to catch his attention until he reaches out
> to grab it. When we finally hand over the toy, he quiets
> down. Our goal was just to stop his crying. We did not
> try to address the child's underlying needs. We gave him
> something else to desire, and tricked him into falling silent
> for the time being.[8]

The psyche is the childish nature of our mind, constantly seduced into the glitter of mere appearance. It grasps after things because it believes in them. And it tricks us into taking appearances to be real. We cry for our adult toys, temporarily fall silent when we get them, then scream for more when we get bored with what we have.[9] This is the modus operandi of the immature psyche. It's only when we discover the futility of the psyche and its substitutes that we'll truly quiet down, and through that silence find ultimate satisfaction in the level we will here call the clear-light mind.

So we live a life divided, asleep to our truer self. The great divide is between onstage appearance and backstage reality, between the outer psyche and the inner levels of the substrate and clear-light mind. We're walled off from our true self, with no transparency to the light within. That wall temporarily crumbles every night when we fall asleep, but without an understanding of what is revealed behind this iron curtain, we miss the nightly reunion with our deeper self.

The substrate mind has the largest bandwidth of the three levels and is the hardest to pin down. It's deeper than the psychological unconscious (which in chapter 2 we called the "relative unconscious mind") that is accessed through psychoanalysis and other forms of therapy. The psychological unconscious can be seen as the uppermost levels of the substrate mind, which itself is more of a spiritual unconscious.

While it's getting closer to the truth (that is, closer to the clear-light mind below the substrate), the substrate is still deception, but much more subtle. It's the fundamental lie that gives birth to all the secondary lies of the psyche. It's the fundamental lie because this is the level where duality is born. The substrate is the basic fault, in every sense of that word. It's the fault, or split, that fractures reality into self and other, and it's what we can therefore blame (fault) as the source of all our suffering. It's also a fault as in "error or mistake."[10] This basic fault, fracture, or failure is what is healed on the spiritual path altogether, and in the nighttime yogas in particular.[11]

The substrate mind is that which projects all the appearances of the relative world. It's the bedrock of the ego (or psyche), and it's a bed we drop into every night when we fall asleep. The substrate is the cradle of samsara. It's a deeper and therefore much more insidious level of deception, precisely because it is so unconscious. We don't know that we don't know. That's a real blind spot—the ignorance, the sleep, of which we are unaware. This substrate mind is constantly whispering lies to us so silently that we don't consciously hear it. That's what makes it so dangerous.

Until we access the substrate *consciously*—for instance, with deep meditation or dream yoga—it remains unconscious. When we work with the substrate mind, we're working with the tectonic plates of experience. What happens "down there" affects everything that happens "up here," as any depth psychologist or spiritual teacher knows. Personal earthquakes arise when these deeper plates move. These psychic ruptures can be catastrophic for the superficial psyche, which depends on deception and the illusion of stability for its existence, and is easily shaken when the truth bursts its bubble of lies. But these quakes are lifesaving for your spirit, for they indicate that the clear-light mind at the core of your being is starting to break through.

This sort of seismic quake is what happened to me during the experience I shared in the prologue. My view of the world shifted, and the house of cards that had been my life came crashing down.

Like a physical earthquake, things are never the same when the psyche is so shaken up. These life-altering events can arise spontaneously or they can be cultivated through spiritual practice, where the catastrophe is more controlled.

Because the bandwidth is so wide for this intermediate level, it's helpful to know that the further we descend into it, the more spiritual it gets. It's not all repressed garbage down there. Our psychological refuse lies at the upper levels of this bandwidth. But the bottom of the substrate blends into the clear-light mind, which is where all the good news resides.

One of the central messages of lucid dreaming, once again, is that appearances can be deceiving (that is, the appearances of a dream seem so real). When this message is taken into daily life, it can point out new options, alter established patterns of behavior, and help us find innovative ways to work with difficult situations. This has obvious practical implications. But a deeper spiritual implication is that lucidity can help us work with the most difficult situation of all, which is samsara altogether. It can help us solve the problem of confused conventional existence.

The Clear-Light Mind

Both the substrate and the psyche emanate from the deepest, and fundamentally ineffable, level of mind that in this book we refer to as the clear-light mind. When the Buddha attained his enlightenment, he woke up *from* the psyche and substrate and *to* the clear-light mind. This level has a number of names—ground of being, buddha nature, basic goodness, dharmakaya, rigpa, changeless nature, and so forth—but "clear-light mind" is perfect in the context of the nighttime yogas because it suggests the brilliant luminosity that is constantly shining at the core of our being. This is the light of the awakened mind that never turns off. Knowing about this mind, even at the level of the map, is like a beacon that directs you toward safe spiritual harbor.

The light of the clear-light mind does not refer to physical light. It refers to the capacity of the mind to perceive its contents, and to know. During the day, we see things when they're illuminated by the light of the sun. But we also see things when we dream. What illuminates these dream images, or any mental image? It's the light, or luminosity, of the mind. The Dalai Lama writes, "As the primary feature of light is to illuminate, so consciousness is said to illuminate its objects. Just as in light there is no categorical distinction between the illumination and that which illuminates, so in consciousness there is no real difference between the process of knowing or cognition and that which knows or cognizes. In consciousness, as in light, there is a quality of illumination."[12]

While the internal light of the mind shares some similarities with external light, there are some critical differences. For one thing, when we talk about the clear-light mind, we're talking about nonduality. We leave duality behind when we drop below the psyche and the substrate. This is where it gets tricky, because the conceptual mind, which is trying to understand the clear-light mind, is by nature dualistic. And duality can never understand nonduality. (Trying to do so often results in paradox.) We'll have more to say about this when we discuss sleep yoga, which is all about exploring this foundational mind. For now, the point is to realize that the light of the mind is not physical light.

While the clear-light mind cannot be pinned down and definitively located anywhere (because it is immanent everywhere), it has a provisional location at our heart center. A seventh-century BCE text, the *Brhad-aranyaka Upanishad*—the oldest of the Upanishads and considered the most important—teaches that the self *(atman)* is the inner light that resides within the heart, surrounded by the subtle inner breath. The Buddhist correlate is the "indestructible bindu" that resides at the heart, which is another term for the very subtle body, and something we'll discuss in our chapters on sleep yoga.

When you fall into the deepest level of sleep, you're falling into the light of the clear-light mind, whether you know it or not. This level of mind is utterly faultless, in every sense of that word. There are no fractures here, no mistakes, failures, fallibilities, or fallacies. This is the nondual wisdom mind, all good, perfectly pure, and replete with all the qualities of enlightenment. It is the enlightened mind. While the psyche and the substrate are both the relative mind, the clear-light mind is the absolute. People often talk about "altered states of consciousness." From the perspective of the clear-light mind, anything other than it is an altered state.

This is the ultimate bed of reality that gives rise to both samsara and nirvana.[13] There is nothing beyond or below this level. It transcends, or "subscends," time and space. It does not enter the world of time and space, and is therefore formless and changeless. Infinity and eternity are feeble attempts to describe that which is pre-spacial and pre-temporal.

At this level it's no longer even "your" mind, but the universal awakened mind common to all beings, so it's "the" clear-light mind, not "your" clear-light mind. As the *Brhad-aranyaka Upanishad* states, "Here a father is not a father, a mother is not a mother . . . a thief is not a thief, a murderer not a murderer." You have released your false self, and temporarily dropped the different masks you wear at the level of the psyche. But you have found your true Self, the unmasked and "faceless" mind within. You've come face-to-face with who you really are.

> Certain meditations are called "cutting through" practices (*trekchö* in Tibetan). What they cut *through* is false appearances—the delusions of the psyche and the substrate mind—and what they cut *to* is the clear-light mind.[14] Dream yoga, sleep yoga, and illusory form are in the family of these "cutting through" meditations.

The enlightened ones operate from the level of clear-light mind and never leave it. They "look up" at those caught in the snare of the psyche and have compassion for the suffering that ensues from that trap. Buddhas can still function at the level of the dualistic psyche, and they do so in order to communicate with beings like us, but they have "subscended" this small mind.

When the traditions talk about "liberation," they're talking about being liberated from exclusive identification with the psyche. The liberated ones have awakened to the full spectrum of their identity, but take ultimate refuge in their clear-light mind. So the primordial identity theft that occurs at the level of the psyche is finally recovered at the level of the clear-light mind. This is who you really are.

> The Catholic mystic Thomas Merton wrote, "What can we gain by sailing to the moon if we are not able to cross the abyss that separates us from ourselves? This is the most important of all voyages of discovery, and without it, all the rest are not only useless, but disastrous." The abyss that separates us from ourselves is the psyche and substrate, and the voyage to the center of our self can be made with the vehicle of dream yoga.[15]

The clear-light mind is therefore Big Mind, the all-inclusive mind that not only emanates all the levels of the relative mind but also holds its emanations. In other words, the clear-light mind holds your universe in its compassionate embrace, like a divine mother cradling her beloved child. The substrate mind and the psyche are the children, the radiance or shine, of the clear-light mind, and they are therefore never separate from it. Things only *appear* to be separate at the relative levels of mind, and from the perspective of those who remain asleep.

We can dip into the clear-light mind whenever we fall between the cracks of discursive thought, which operates at the level of the superficial psyche. This means that we can touch into the clear-light mind not only in deep dreamless sleep, but between each and every thought. It's always available. But without spiritual training, it's rarely recognized. Because our conscious mind (the psyche) is almost always directed out and away from the clear-light mind, we constantly miss it. This disconnect is the source of our suffering.

The clear-light mind is where intuition and extraordinary knowing comes from: things like ESP, clairvoyance, and clairaudience. Intuition comes from being "in tune with" the clear-light mind, which means being in tune with everyone else at this pre-thought level. Because the clear-light mind transcends space and time, all kinds of extraordinary knowing occurs when we tune in to it.

Compassion also comes from the clear-light mind, because it's the level of unity. While things like intuition and psychic ability are interesting aspects of extraordinary knowing, true extraordinary knowing is knowing that you are not separate from me. Your suffering then becomes mine, and "I" want to get rid of it. This, of course, is why the awakened ones are also the compassionate ones. When they look at others, they don't see others. They see "themselves."

It's for this reason that they can offer such extraordinary advice: they've seen through themselves, and so they can now see through you. Everything becomes transparent for one who sees the world through the clear-light mind. This mind clarifies and illuminates everything. A buddha knows you better than you know yourself, because while you may not see your substrate and clear-light mind, they do.[16]

I experienced this penetrating insight during my first interview with Khenpo Tsültrim Gyamtso Rinpoche. It was because of this event that I asked him to be my teacher. Before my interview, I carefully collected my questions and reviewed them. When I was admitted into his chambers, all my questions suddenly evaporated. My mind went blank. It wasn't from nerves, because I was calm when I walked in. But simply being in his absolute presence erased my relative questions. (Many years later, I heard Garchen Rinpoche share similar stories of students having their relative mind erased in the presence of a spiritual master.)

Rinpoche looked at me with great kindness. When I met his gaze, I was stunned. It's impossible to describe, but looking into his eyes was like looking into infinite space. I wasn't looking into the eyes of a human being. I was looking into the cosmos. There was a chilling sense that no one was there behind those eyes.[17] (It was only years later that I finally understood that I was gazing into the clear-light mind. And nobody, no ego, lives at that level.)

When the translator asked me if I had a question, I was able to gather myself enough to ask one. As the translator relayed the question, Rinpoche looked at me in the most amazing way. He had a whimsical look on his face, almost the look of a jokester, someone who knows the punch line of a joke you are about to get. I felt an unshakeable certainty that he was seeing right through me (it's so hard to talk about anything related to the clear-light mind, because it transcends language or concept). It felt like he was reading my karmic DNA, or somehow penetrating to the essence of my being. I was completely exposed, but also totally loved.

Words escape me even decades later, but with time has come understanding. While he heard my superficial question, he was really listening to my innermost being. He didn't get distracted by my surface presentation, by my psyche and its silly questions, but addressed the deepest aspects of my soul. Rinpoche heard questions I didn't even know I had. He knew me better than I knew myself, which is why I felt I could surrender to his wisdom. Sogyal Rinpoche speaks about this deeper part of us:

> Two people have been living in you all your life. One is the ego, garrulous, demanding, hysterical, calculating; the other is the hidden spiritual being, whose still voice of wisdom you have only rarely heard or attended to. As you listen more and more to the teachings, contemplate them, and integrate them into your life, your inner voice . . . is awakened and strengthened, and you begin to distinguish between its guidance and the various clamorous and enthralling voices of ego. The memory of your real nature, with all its splendor and confidence, begins to return to you. You will find, in fact, that you have uncovered in yourself your own *wise guide,* and . . . you will start to distinguish between its truth and the various deceptions of the ego.[18]

This is the voice that Rinpoche heard within me, and then pointed out.

Through the practice of dream yoga, we fundamentally "change our mind." We change our mind, and therefore our identity, from the psyche to the clear light. We tune in to the wise guide—or the "wise guy"—within. It's a change that changes everything.[19] Paraphrasing Steven Levine, we're not physical beings (the psyche) with spiritual experiences (glimpses of the clear-light mind). We're spiritual beings (the clear-light mind) with physical experiences (temporarily lost in the psyche).

For most of us, until we enter a spiritual path, we don't really have a choice but to identify with the psyche. It's our conscious experience after all. What else can we identify with? Spiritual practice introduces us to the deeper and more liberating aspects of our being, which allows us to dis-identify from who we think we are, and progressively identify with who we really are. Our essential purpose in life is to become the best version of ourselves. The clear-light mind is that version.

The Calling of the Clear-Light Mind

Does the clear-light mind lie passively waiting for us, like a lonely mother longing for the return of her lost child, or does it exert an active influence on our conscious lives? We've seen how the relative unconscious mind exerts a massive influence on our lives. What about the absolute unconscious mind?[20] Sogyal Rinpoche writes,

> Our buddha nature [clear-light mind] has an active
> aspect, which is our "inner teacher." From the very
> moment we became obscured, this "inner teacher"
> has worked tirelessly . . . trying to bring us back to
> the radiance and spaciousness of our true being . . .
> ceaselessly working for our evolution—using all kinds
> of skillful means and all types of situations to teach
> and awaken us and to guide us back to the truth.[21]

Even though it is highly filtered and distorted by the strata of the substrate and psyche, once we become attuned to it, we can see the subliminal workings of the clear-light mind operative in everything we do. By understanding its influence, we can begin to separate substitute gratifications (driven by our substrate and psyche) from authentic gratification (driven by our clear-light mind). We switch our allegiance from appearance to reality, outside to inside. This is a monumental switch, because it places us firmly on the spiritual path, heading in the right direction.

For example, the clear-light mind expresses itself in our longing for happiness. We all want to be happy. If we examine this longing closely, it's fundamentally the longing for unity, or nonduality. Unhappiness is the result of duality, and manifests as the feeling that something is missing or incomplete. We're not exactly sure what's missing, but something is off. If we only identify with the psyche, something *is* missing. Our identity is incomplete, so our longing is accurate. But the sense of what satisfies that longing is not.

For most of us, what satisfies this longing is the acquisition of form, or outer appearance. There's an "other," usually a person or object, that we want to unite with or otherwise possess. At the moment of unity, when we acquire the object or person, there's a brief *relative* experience of nonduality. We're temporarily happy when we get what we want. Hence is born the universal itch of consumerism, which itself arises from the illusion of materialism (that there really is an "other" out there), which is a product of our belief in the psyche and its limitless forms. When we procure one of those forms, we scratch this primal itch. We feel full. But we're actually just getting fat. We're "eating" the wrong thing, so the hunger always returns.

As we've seen, at heart we're not fundamentally longing for appearance. We're longing for reality. We just don't know it. So we spend our lives pursuing substitute gratifications at the level of form, or appearance, gobbling up everything with the thought that the next thing will make us happy. But things will never satisfy. Substitutes are substitutes. We'll never be happy if we pursue outer forms. We're homesick for the absolute, but this yearning is expressing itself in these relative, and therefore unsatisfactory, ways.

In our terms, what we really pine for is the clear-light mind. Our true self is the natural unity that we seek, and that truly satisfies. This longing for the absolute percolates up through the levels, like a beacon from a distant lighthouse in the fog, to be distorted, and therefore expressed, in relative ways as our lust for external form. This longing, and its distortion, fundamentally drives everything we do on the surface of our lives.

Author Richard Louv writes about "nature deficit disorder," and asserts that human beings, especially children, are spending less time in nature and therefore succumbing to a host of problems. With so many distractions, the "great outdoors" isn't so great anymore. But nature still calls, even if we don't hear it. Not listening to that primal call creates a deficit in our being.

Even more foundational, and therefore more problematic, is "nature of mind deficit disorder." This disorder gives rise to the problem of samsara altogether. All of our problems are secondary expressions of this fundamental deficit in our being. The mystics and dreamers of the past were intrepid explorers of this "great indoors," and invite us to do the same if we really want to be happy.

In the Mahayana schools of Buddhism, a synonym for the clear-light mind is the "great mother," *Prajnaparamita.* She is great because she gives birth to all of samsara and nirvana. She's the mom we truly long for. Prajnaparamita is the primal mother who is silently calling out to us from within to come home. She beckons us with her comforting silence, a silence that calls out in the stillness of the night. She's also known as "the mother of all the buddhas," for when we return to her lap and dissolve into her primordial embrace (becoming one with her), we wake up to our true nature and are reborn as an awakened one. She is therefore the mother of our enlightened mind.

The fact that you're even interested in things like meditation or dream yoga means that you've heard the call and have started the journey home.

We are such stuff as dreams are made on,
and our little life is rounded with a sleep.

SHAKESPEARE, *The Tempest*

10
The Mind's Fuzzy Boundaries

AS THE FOUNDATION for the upper levels of the relative mind,
the clear-light mind can infuse (and penetrate) both the psyche and
substrate: the relative is an expression of the absolute and therefore
reducible to it. And both aspects of the relative mind can work on
each other. But it's not a totally two-way street all the way down. In
other words, while the upper two levels of mind can be profoundly
affected by the clear-light mind, the clear-light mind itself is never
affected by what happens at either the psyche or substrate. It remains
untouched. That's why it's called the "changeless nature." Anything
in the relative world of space and time can't touch that which transcends space and time. The relative levels obscure the absolute, which
results in us being unaware of it, but they can't faze it.

Communication Between the Relative Levels

What we do at the conscious level (psyche) impacts the unconscious
level (substrate), and what we do at the unconscious level impacts
the conscious level. For our purposes here, this is important because
it means that what we think can impact our dreams—a process we'll
use to change our non-lucid dreams into lucid ones—and what we

dream can impact our thoughts—a process we'll use to change our non-lucid *lives* into lucid ones. With dream yoga, we change our minds, and therefore our lives, using the medium of our dreams.

Dream yoga affects this transformation in two ways. First, dream yoga changes the structure of the relative unconscious mind so that it has a beneficial impact on our conscious mind. Second, it gradually removes (purifies) the relative unconscious mind altogether, so that the clear-light mind can shine without obstruction.[1]

For now we'll discuss the first benefit. Dream yoga transforms the unconscious mind directly, which then *uploads* imprints into the conscious mind, gradually transforming it.[2] In this way, dream yoga works in the opposite direction from most spiritual practice, which *downloads* imprints from the conscious mind into our unconsciousness.

In spiritual jargon, we talk about "planting seeds" through our daily meditations and good deeds. Our daily practice (or habits) plants good "karmic seeds" in the substrate, which will ripen in good future experience. In dream yoga we do this more directly, by more consciously (lucidly) working with our unconscious mind. Instead of just planting seeds, it's almost like we're transplanting flowers. Because it's more direct, this means that transformation can take place more quickly. Our practice ripens and flowers into life faster. This is encouraging, because dream yoga can be subtle and difficult. It's subtle and difficult because it's so direct. But persistence pays rapid dividends with this practice, and understanding this aspect of the view behind dream yoga can instill this persistence.

So dream yoga and its daytime practice of illusory form—discussed in more detail in later chapters—takes full advantage of the natural two-way street between the conscious and relative unconscious mind. "Illusory form" is a practice that involves continually reminding yourself that everything you perceive is illusory, or not what it appears to be. As a daily practice, illusory form works to stop bad traffic from flowing down (we stop imprinting our unconscious mind with the false data of seeing this world as solid, lasting, and independent); and dream yoga, as a nighttime practice, works to direct more good traffic to come up (among other things, we start imprinting our conscious mind with the truth that this world is like a dream). Dream yoga works to plant good habits at the dream level that then impact our waking life; illusory form works to remove bad habits at the waking level that then impacts our dreams.

Simply put, what we do "down there" has a beneficial effect on what happens "up here," and what we do "up here" has a beneficial effect on what happens "down there." Hence dream yoga and illusory form are reciprocating, or bi-directional, practices, and create a positive feedback loop. Backstage always controls onstage. Our unconscious mind really runs the show. But if we come to know that mind, we can work much more directly, honestly, and openly with the director to make this daily show a good one.[3]

Permeability

There are two ways to look at lucid dreams. One is that lucid dreaming is unnatural, but becomes more natural through training. This view is logical and encouraging: practice lucid dreaming and you'll have lucid dreams. But if lucid dreams only arose in those who practiced, we would expect lucidity to be limited to this practice population. There are many people who have spontaneous lucid dreams with no practice, which supports an alternate view.

This second view, which is less common but even more encouraging, is that lucid dreaming is an inherent capacity.[4] It's a logical consequence of asserting the clear-light mind as the natural ground of the mind. The clear-light mind, by definition, is always lucid, and you can tap into glimmers of that lucidity with spontaneous lucid dreams. Joining this view with the first view, the closer you get to the clear-light mind with spiritual practice, the more lucid you'll become. The glimpses turn into a steady gaze.

One lucid-dream researcher, Paul Tholey, regards our usual non-lucid dreams as a form of consciousness disorder; he suggests that lucidity is in fact the natural order. Along the same lines, the philosopher Evan Thompson, in his study *Waking, Dreaming, Being: Self and Consciousness in Neuroscience, Meditation, and Philosophy*, recounts an interview with a young woman who reported that when she

first heard about lucid dreaming, she was surprised to learn
that there was any other kind. All her dreams were lucid.

The first view maintains proper *effort* as the primary ingredient for
lucidity; the second view maintains proper *relaxation* as the key
ingredient.[5] If lucidity is our natural state, we only have to relax into
it. We can reconcile these disparate views by saying that the first is
the relative view while the second is more absolute. Our journey
will emphasize the relative, because it's more approachable, but the
absolute view is our natural state and is our focus for the moment.

> We're "human doings" more than we're human beings,
> always on the go and doing something. It's difficult for us
> to relax, which at the spiritual level means relaxing into
> who we truly are, the clear-light mind. If we could just *be*,
> lucidity would spontaneously dawn.

If lucidity is innate, why don't we have more lucid dreams? Why
do we have such a lack of permeability to this innate lucidity, our
clear-light mind? It's because the clouds are too thick. The density
of the relative unconscious mind obscures this capacity. From a psychological point of view, Jung discovered that people who were able
to resolve (purify) issues at the level of their personal unconscious
became more permeable to the deeper integrating, and spiritual
aspects, of their being. From a spiritual point of view, purification
of the refuse of the relative unconscious mind reveals the lucidity of
the absolute unconscious.

The biggest barrier to permeability, and therefore lucidity, is our
exclusive identification with the psyche and its outer forms. We're
not transparent, and therefore not porous, to our deeper self because
we don't believe there is one. The psychologist William James said
that reality is what we attend to. Attend only to your outer psyche
and it becomes your reality and a barrier to your deeper self. Attend
to your inner clear-light mind and it will become your reality and

the gateway to enlightenment. By changing your attention from outer to inner, you can free yourself from the constricted psyche and open to deeper and truer levels of identification. The onset of lucidity is a consequence of that openness.

Spiritual practice dislodges this exclusive identification with the psyche and its outer forms, as does the grace of personal crises. One psychotherapist writes, "Though painful and unstable, [periods of crises] may provide the only opportunities for the life-giving source within us to permeate the barriers we have erected. This infusion . . . is a gift which is bestowed when the conscious self has been shaken, or to some degree is less fortified."[6] The true gift is that you don't have to wait for a crisis to break through the fortifications of the psyche and the substrate. Spiritual practices, including the nighttime yogas, do it much more gracefully. It's a controlled crisis, because you can do it on your terms.

By allowing the coarse outer levels of our being to melt (which results in a vulnerability that is often perceived as a crisis for the grasping psyche), we open ourselves to vast increases in lucidity. This is why it's so important to have a complete map of the mind and an understanding of who we actually are. If we remain frozen at the surface and only identify with that, we may never have lucid or transformative dreams.

To put it an irreducible way: on an absolute level you don't actually need any of the induction techniques. You only need to relax.

Dream Destination: The Clear-Light Mind

Spiritual practice—whether it's the sudden enlightenment of the "cutting through" meditations or the more gentle approaches of gradual enlightenment—is about removing the obscurations of the relative mind (psyche and substrate) and dis-covering the absolute clear-light mind. The more we remove these obscurations, the thinner the psyche and substrate become. When these veils are thinned out enough, the light of the clear-light mind breaks through like the sun shining through a break in the clouds.

This light, which is the light of pure awareness, may be felt as an increased level of insight, intuition, coincidence, or spiritual experience. You might start having special dreams and feelings, like the ones I shared in the months leading up to my two-week breakthrough. When you start to look within—through contemplation, meditation, or the nighttime yogas—you're drilling holes through the relative levels of your mind and accessing vast natural resources within. You're making your psyche and substrate more porous.

Once you see this light, and who you really are at the bottom of your being, you will come to see *everything* in a new light. You will no longer identify with the surface levels of your identity. You're no longer fooled. When you take refuge in your clear-light mind, you still have access to the psyche—you just don't identify with it. You use the psyche, as the limited tool that it is, to work with others who are still attached to that false sense of identity. But you don't let it use you. You reside at a level that is far more divine.

BEYOND CUTTING THROUGH

Although cutting through confusion and waking up to who you are completes the path of wisdom, the journey continues as you now express that wisdom as compassion. In Buddhism this is called "twofold" benefit, which refers to the ultimate benefit for self and for others, and marks complete enlightenment. The ultimate benefit for yourself is realizing there isn't one—the discovery of egolessness/emptiness, or selflessness. That's wisdom. It's about seeing through the façade of mere appearance (the psyche/ego) and discovering your clear-light mind. But if this is all you realize, as noble as it is, it's still a partial enlightenment, a "onefold" benefit.

Complete realization has to include others. So the ultimate benefit for others is helping them wake up to this same truth. To help them stop hiding from themselves, and to become transparent to their own clear-light mind, the ever-present Buddha within. This is the path of compassion, which is how wisdom, or emptiness, expresses itself. The discovery of selflessness leads to acts of selflessness. Compassion completes the path, which of course means that the path is never truly complete, because there will always be more beings to help.

This deepest of the three levels of mind, the clear-light mind, is our final destination in dream yoga (or in any type of daytime meditation practice). If we can recognize it, we really do have something to look forward to in the silence of the night—and the end of life. This is where we go every night when we fall asleep, and this is where we go when we die. If we can recognize and then sustain the recognition, this is what we can bring with us to illuminate every action during the day. But because most of us do not recognize our clear-light mind, we leave it behind as we ascend back to waking consciousness. We ironically leave the light (of nondual wisdom) and enter the dark (of dualistic ignorance). We forget where we've been, and continue to sleepwalk through life. The purpose of the nighttime practices is to help us remember, as we saw in chapter 6 (and will revisit at the end of this book).

If we can understand the clear-light mind as our destination, we also understand that we're actually the most awake, the most enlightened, in deep dreamless sleep. When we "wake up" in the morning, we're actually falling asleep, in the spiritual sense. Our superficial psyche is the most confused, dualistic, and un-illumined part of our being. We've got it completely backward!

The Indian sage Ramana Maharshi summarized this jolting truth by claiming, "That which does not exist in deep dreamless sleep is not real." The Sufi master Hazrat Inayat Khan said, "We do not realize that, when we are awake, we are covering ourselves from another world which, in fact, is more real . . . The difference between the sleeping and waking is when we cover ourselves from what is more real, we say, 'I am awake' and, when we cover ourselves from what is unreal and illusion, we say we are asleep."[7]

That we have it completely backward is the irony that the Buddha awakened to.[8] He saw the painful joke that we play on ourselves. He saw that the ascent from the clear-light mind into the psyche each morning is an ascent from wisdom to confusion, nonduality to duality, nirvana to samsara, light to dark. Seeing this for ourselves is the point of our dream yoga journey.

Hide and Seek

Dream yoga has the potential to reveal every aspect of ourselves, personal and transpersonal. The relative (personal) aspects are revealed in dreams anyway, as any dream interpreter can attest. This is often shadow material, and it must be brought to light if we want to be free.

Below that, once again, is the absolute (transpersonal) aspect of ourselves, our clear-light mind. Even though spiritual practitioners clamor for that awakened state, some are also afraid of it. We (ego) are afraid of the thermonuclear power of the awakened mind. Small mind is intimidated by Big Mind. Because of this conflicted relationship to the core of our being—our spirit wants it, but our ego fears it—we play this cosmic game of hide and seek. As we have seen, we throw ourselves out into form, get lost in it, and then try to find our way out (via the spiritual path). We get lost in our projections, overly involved in the creative forms of the mind, and falsely come to identify with thoughts and things. Form embezzles awareness.

The practice of dream yoga, however, makes us transparent to ourselves, revealing every hidden part of us, and therefore we can finally relax. We can relax because *if there's nothing left to hide, there's nothing left to seek.* The path to awakening comes to an end. Remove the obstacle of seeking, and you've arrived.

The nighttime yogas are particularly effective in developing this transparency, because the ground of ego (the substrate) hides out in the dark. The nocturnal meditations expose this hiding place, and therefore cut through the primary veil that obscures the clear-light mind. The "cutting through" meditations therefore allow us to *see through* internal and external obscurations.

Because it goes so against our Western grain, this central point cannot be overstated: what we're really seeking lies within at the level of the projector, not the projection. When we discover that, external seeking comes to an end, and so does samsara.[9]

> Dreams are real while they last. Can we say more of life?

HAVELOCK ELLIS, quoted in *Lucid Dreaming: A Concise Guide to Awakening in Your Dreams and in Your Life*

11

A Taxonomy of Dreams

IN DREAM YOGA, three general classes of dreams can be correlated with the three levels of mind—psyche, substrate, and clear-light mind—we have been exploring. These correlations can help us to distinguish between dreams we should pay attention to and ones we can ignore.[1]

Karmic, Non-Karmic, and Clear-Light Dreams

In dream yoga, most of our dreams can be considered karmic, or "samsaric," dreams, and these carry no real meaning—the meaning derived from them is the meaning we bring to them. These dreams arise from the superficial psyche, or the upper bandwidth of the substrate, which means they're unstable. They're images of rambling thoughts, and like those thoughts, they can be ignored. Think of them as neurological noise.

This doesn't mean, however, that we can't use these dreams to trigger lucidity. Any dream can become lucid and therefore used for dream yoga. But without lucidity, these dreams are just mental static. In Buddhist jargon they arise due to karmic traces from our daily lives, hence their title as "karmic dreams." Even if we have dreams of spiritual teachers or teachings, these still tend to be karmic dreams, just better ones.

As we stabilize our mind in meditation and bring greater awareness to our lives, this stability and awareness naturally extends into the dream state and we begin to experience a second category of dreams: "non-karmic dreams." Whereas karmic dreams are usually "small dreams"—fragmented and meaningless—non-karmic dreams are often Big Dreams. They can change your life.

There are two major types of non-karmic dreams, the first of which we can call "dreams of clarity." Dreams of clarity can arise at any time for anyone, but without spiritual training (such as dream yoga) they tend to be rare. What the poet Kabir said of death also applies to dream: "What is found now is found then."[2] If your mind is unclear and unstable during the day, you will experience unclear and unstable dreams at night (karmic dreams). If your mind is clear and stable during the day, you will experience clear and stable dreams (dreams of clarity) at night.

Dreams of clarity come from well below the psyche, in the deeper bandwidths of the substrate. These dreams therefore present information from deeper levels of the mind and from more positive karmic traces ("non-karmic," for this type of dream, means no negative karma is involved). The mind here is not always bound by space and time, and the dreamer can meet with other beings or with deeper aspects of their own mind arising in the form of beings.[3] In my experience, they tend to arise just before awakening, or at the crack of dawn. Unlike samsaric dreams, these do deliver teachings and messages. They are like "letters to ourselves," which is how Freud referred to information brought up from our dreams.

They also feel different. Traleg Rinpoche explained that these special dreams have three qualities that help us separate them from meaningless dreams. First is their compelling nature. They're gripping and persuasive, even forceful. Second is their content. The material in the dream has weight and applicability. Third is their form—that is, how the dream actually appears, how it came to you, and the usually positive nature of the dream.

I have used these dreams as guides for nearly forty years.[4] In my dream journal I have a special section for dreams of clarity. I date and analyze them, and often come back to study their insights. Accounts are legion of history's great thinkers, from both East and West, receiving teachings in such "big dreams." The nineteenth-century Tibetan master Dudjom Lingpa told of "teachings given to me in the dream state by my guru, the noble and supreme Avalokiteshvara," and said that "I met my guru Longchenpa in a dream where he gave this pointing-out instruction."[5] The French philosopher René Descartes said that a three-part dream delivered the foundations of the science he was to create, and he proclaimed that this was the most important experience of his life.

Because the mind is not bound by space and time at the deepest levels of the substrate, it's possible that experiences of *déjà vu* (from French, "already seen") come from the level of non-karmic dreams. When you have that eerie feeling that you've seen something before, maybe it was from a forgotten dream of clarity.[6]

Finally, we have a third and deepest class of dreams, which is when dreams arise nondualistically from the clear-light mind. This advanced kind of dream tends to occur when someone is engaged in subtle practices like sleep yoga. In a "clear-light dream," the dreamer remains in the clear-light mind, and there is no sense of a subject (you) perceiving an object (the dream). The dream is reflexively aware. It just knows itself. Even the description of these divine dreams is hard to understand from a dualistic perspective.

Clear-light dreams occur when thoughts arise in your daily meditation united with nondual awareness—that is, you can see the arising of thought as inseparable from the clear-light mind; you see the inseparability of samsara and nirvana.[7]

Most of us feel that thoughts interrupt our meditation, that they distract us. But at a certain point thoughts *become* meditation, and therefore never distract. We never get lost in thought. Thoughts (and eventually dreams) are finally seen to be what they really are: the luminous nondual expression of the clear-light mind. That's also when thoughts, as well as things, arise as illusory forms. At this level, thoughts (and dreams) become an ornament of the mind, not an obstruction to it.

Dreams of clarity arise from a deep and relatively pure aspect of mind, and from positive karma, but (unlike clear-light dreams) they still arise in duality. As a final distinction: both samsaric dreams and dreams of clarity can be either lucid or non-lucid, but clear-light dreams are always lucid. When you have a clear-light dream you always know it, because this advanced experience arises within the recognition of the clear-light mind, which is always awake (lucid).

When do these different types of dreams tend to occur in the course of a night? Dreams in the early part of the night are short and conditioned by recent events. They usually arise from just below the psyche. Dreams in the middle part of the night can also arise from just below the psyche, or from tapping into older memories and karmic traces, which come from the deeper bandwidth of the substrate. The final dreams at the end of the night are often the most interesting and revealing, and tend to tap into the substrate, or even deeper into the clear-light mind.

Some Other Types of Dreams

Dreams have been categorized into as many types as there are dream researchers. Psychological studies, for instance, refer to impactful dreams, anxiety dreams, existential dreams, alienation dreams, transcendent dreams, extraordinary dreams, and normative dreams.[8] Psychologically, once the repressive and controlling conscious mind (psyche) is relaxed or removed, all kinds of unconscious elements bubble up into awareness. Dreams reveal those bubbles: the good, the bad, and the ugly aspects of ourselves. This, of course, is why therapists beginning with Freud have emphasized the therapeutic benefit of working with dreams. They are an opportunity to integrate the fractured and refused aspects of ourselves.

In order to be a complete human being, let alone a buddha, we need to both grow up and wake up. We need to develop psychologically (growing up) and spiritually (waking up). The psychologist John Welwood coined this important distinction, and the philosopher Ken Wilber writes about it as the difference between vertical (growing up) and horizontal (waking up) enlightenment. In sweeping terms, the West specializes in growing up through *stages* of consciousness; the East specializes in waking up through *states* of consciousness. These are complementary, not combative, approaches to human development.[9]

In this book, however, we will mostly forgo discussion of the psychological aspects of dreaming in order to go deeper.[10] We want to drop below the tip of the iceberg, and get beneath the psyche. (One way to summarize the difference between psychology and spirituality in terms of dreams is to say that psychology keeps the dream of life from turning into a nightmare; spirituality wakes you up from the dream.[11]) On a more esoteric level, we can speak of archetypal dreams, visitation dreams, super dreams, and theophanic ("from the Source") dreams. Below is a sampling of dream types that have special relevance to our journey:

- *Recurrent dreams* might suggest that you're not a good listener. In my experience, when you get the message the dream contains, the dreams stop. Recurrent dreams are useful for extracting dreamsigns, and therefore triggering lucidity. Recurrent dreams can also be the product of things like post-traumatic stress disorder, where trauma is deeply lodged in the body-mind matrix (the unconscious mind) and keeps dislodging to manifest in dreams and nightmares until the trauma is healed. These difficult recurrent dreams can still be used to trigger lucidity, which then allows one to be free of their traumatic content.

- *Prophetic dreams,* and the subset of *warning dreams,* arise from the substrate or below. Karmic "seeds" are stored in the substrate mind, and when they first start to ripen, that ripening can be seen in dreams before it's experienced in life. This suggests that if you have a refined relationship to your dreams, they can literally save your life. Countless stories tell of people having premonitions in dreams, only to have the premonition come true.[12] The night that my father phoned to tell me that my mom had just been diagnosed with Alzheimer's, I had a dream where she came to me and said, "I have three years left." Three years later, within a week of the date I had the dream, she died.

- *Witnessing dreams* are a type of lucid dream where you prefer not to engage in the dream. You're lucid, but you prefer to just watch what unfolds without changing anything.

- *Luminous dreams* are a particular type of prophetic dream, mentioned by Traleg Rinpoche, that portend self-development. The dreams I alluded to in the introduction, which seemed to foretell my two-week breakthrough, were of this variety.

- *Incubated dreams* are dreams that we seed during the day and that germinate at night. Many ancient cultures practiced dream incubation, including the Greeks, who worked with it for healing. Asclepius is the Greek god of medicine and healing, and his patients would enter a dream incubation chamber for several nights in an attempt to receive a healing dream from the "Divine Physician." Lucky supplicants would be healed directly in the dream state; others would be told what to do to cure the illness. Some patients would receive dreams that were more symbolic and required interpretation (dream interpreters are called *oneirokritai*) for healing to occur.

Carl Jung believed that the unconscious mind delivers information in three successive ways: psychically, as in dreams; through "fate," or coincidence; and through physical disorder. "Dreams sometimes announce certain situations long before they actually happen . . . What we fail to see consciously is frequently perceived by our unconscious, which can pass the information on through dreams."[13] To ignore our deeper dreams is therefore to court more drastic physical events. If we don't get it at the level of the dream, we will eventually get it in physical reality.

I have had incubated dreams for decades. During the second year of my three-year meditation retreat, which was done with a small group, we lost our retreat master. When you're working so intensely with your mind for so long, it's important to have a guide. Because I needed guidance, I began to supplicate for it in my dreams. And because my motivation was pure and my supplications so fervent, I had many powerful dreams that guided me for the remainder of the retreat. I even had some dreams that were meant for the group, and cautiously shared them to benefit our retreat.[14]

The Tibetan tradition, as well as other cultures, recognizes "surrogate dreamers": lamas who can incubate and interpret a dream for you.[15] A personal item from the one requesting the dream is often placed under the pillow of the lama. Within a few nights a dream is delivered. I have received Tibetan empowerments that include placing an object from the empowerment under my pillow, with the instruction to pay close attention to my dreams that night. Sure enough, I usually have a dream connected with the event.

Dream incubation is easy. Just cry out from the bottom of your heart for help, and for that help to come in your dreams. For me it doesn't matter if it comes from the deepest aspects of my own mind or from some external source infiltrating my dreams. The message is what's important, not the messenger.

You can ask for specific guidance, as I often did in my retreat, but many people report that a more general request—"Tell me what I need to know!"—leads to the most fruitful response. As Patricia Garfield says, "Every night, the station is broadcasting." We only need to tune in.

Purifying Dreams and the Measure of the Path

Purifying dreams are a more general class of dreams. The idea is that karma can be created or purified while you dream. Karma is perhaps the most complex topic in Buddhism. Only a fully enlightened Buddha can understand it. The point here is that whenever intention is involved, karma is created. So if you're lucid in a dream and intend to do something bad in your dream, there are karmic consequences, a topic we'll return to when we discuss the differences between lucid dreaming and dream yoga. As we've seen, if we use our dreams properly, we can create good karma and positively influence our lives, or we can purify karma altogether.

KARMIC WEIGHT

Karma is created at the level of mind, speech, or body, and carries progressive impact as it becomes more physical or fully manifest. For example, I can have a vague thought about killing someone. This thought has karmic impact because it can predispose me to have a similar thought again. It leaves an imprint or trace. Karma is habit, and any action of body, speech, or mind is habit-forming. Think, say, or do something once and it's easier to think, say, or do it again.[16]

Because it's left at the level of mind (it's just a thought after all), it doesn't carry that much karmic weight, unless we have that thought over and over. Perhaps we start to say to ourselves, or to others, that we want to kill someone. The action is now more fully manifest. It has impact and consequences, and it carries more weight. We can get arrested by saying we want to kill the president, but we won't get arrested for merely having that thought. If we were to actually kill someone, then the karma is fully loaded because the action is fully manifest. Compared to a featherweight thought, physical action is really heavy.

Because dreams are mental, the karmic weight of our intentions and subsequent actions in a lucid dream are not that heavy, unless we continue to add weight to the karma by intentionally repeating the same dream activity. Mental karma is the lightest karma. But it's not inconsequential. Our external life, what we end up saying or doing, usually starts with what we think. That is, it starts with the internal contents of our mind: our thoughts, emotions—and dreams. A central maxim in Buddhism is that "the mind leads all things."

One of the wonders of dream yoga, then, is that through your pure intention in a lucid dream, and by stabilizing and training your mind in the dream state, you can clean up your karmic act. Tusum Khyenpa, the first Karmapa, is said to have achieved the purification of much negative karma through dream yoga and thereby achieved his enlightenment through this nighttime practice.

You can also evaluate your progress on the spiritual path by noticing what kinds of dreams you have. Through spiritual practice you purify your substrate consciousness—also known as the "storehouse" consciousness, because it stores all your karmic seeds. Using this image, progress occurs as all the bad seeds in the storehouse are replaced with good seeds, and then even the good seeds are emptied out.

As you purify your substrate consciousness, bad dreams and nightmares diminish and then disappear altogether (bad seeds are purified). Good samsaric dreams increase (more dreams of dharma, teachers, teachings—good seeds are being placed in the substrate). Dreams of clarity begin and then increase. And ultimately clear-light dreams may begin and gradually increase. At the final stages of purification, as the storehouse consciousness is completely emptied out, dreaming stops altogether (even the good seeds have been purified into emptiness).[17] There's nothing left to seed a dream.

This final stage is Buddhahood, or complete awakening. Tulku Urgyen Rinpoche, speaking of a highly realized master, said, "She had reached the level known as *collapse of delusion,* at which point there are no more dreams during sleep; the dream state is totally purified . . . throughout day and night the continuity of luminous wakefulness is no longer interrupted."[18] The "collapse of delusion" is the collapse of the storehouse, which occurs when the psyche and substrate collapse into the clear-light mind. At this level, awakening is continuous because no gaps (bardos) exist in the awakened mind.[19]

When the psyche is out of the way, the substrate level of the mind is revealed and this substrate is what gives birth to samsara. It's the relative level of truth, and we can access it with dream yoga, "the measure of the path." But samsara itself is one big deception, fundamentally misleading from the perspective of absolute truth. With duality comes duplicity. It's only when we go beyond the dualistic levels of the psyche and the substrate—when we get these duplicitous levels out of the way and arrive at the nondual clear-light mind—that absolute truth is expressed. We can go further on the path, and access this absolute truth, with sleep yoga, an advanced practice that we will return to later. For now, however, let's look at a practice that is more accessible and straightforward: the daytime practice of dream yoga known as illusory form.

If we can see that things are not truly real—that they are mere appearances whose true nature is beyond all concepts of what it might be—then our experience of both good and bad events in life will be open, spacious, and relaxed.

KHENPO TSÜLTRIM GYAMTSO RINPOCHE, *The Sun of Wisdom: Teachings on the Noble Nagarjuna's Fundamental Wisdom of the Middle Way*, translated by Ari Goldfield

12

Breaking the Frame
An Introduction to Illusory Form

THE NIGHTTIME PRACTICES of dream yoga are relatively advanced, and we will address them in subsequent chapters. Some people have more natural talent for dream yoga than others.[1] But dream yoga has a rigorous daytime practice called illusory form that is something anyone can do, and it's an authentic way to practice the essence of dream yoga. If nighttime dream yoga doesn't work for you—even if you never have a lucid dream—you can still derive great benefits from dream yoga by applying the principles of illusory form to your life.

Lucid Dreaming and Dream Yoga: What's the Difference?

In addition to the meditations associated with dream yoga that we discussed earlier, a number of other things separate lucid dreaming from dream yoga. The differences are often fuzzy, and one could argue that engaging lucid dreaming for any level of self-improvement transforms it into a type of dream yoga. But dream yoga is ultimately about self-transcendence rather than self-improvement. It's more spiritual than psychological.

One big difference is that there is no overt spiritual practice in lucid dreaming. If you indulge your desires in a lucid dream, you may wake up to your dreams, but you'll remain asleep to your life. You will not wake up in the spiritual sense. In fact, a feeling of mastery over your dreams may lead to ego inflation, which is the opposite of the egoic deflation we seek through dream yoga.

Furthermore, lucid dreaming can be so entertaining that it's easy to stray and become fixated. And fixation on *anything* is a problem on the spiritual path. This is why it's so important to situate lucid dreaming in a fuller spectrum of nighttime practices. If you have no idea of anything deeper than lucid dreaming, it's easy to get swept away at this superficial level. But infatuation with lucid dreaming loses its luster if you know there's more. Lucid dreaming can be a step in the right direction, but it's just a first step.

Also, if intention is involved, karma is created. You're cutting deeper grooves and strengthening habitual patterns every time you repeat a mental act. As we've seen, indulged lucid dreams can create negative karma, whereas dream yoga is designed to accumulate positive karma, or purify it altogether.

While lucid dreaming can be engaged for psychological purposes, and therefore insights from a dream can be transferred to waking life, the whole purpose of dream yoga is to take insights from the night and bring them into the day. In other words, dream yoga applies to all experiences, dreams of the day as well as dreams of the night. It embraces a wider range of experience than lucid dreaming, and even includes the experience of death.

Furthermore, from the viewpoint of lucid dreaming, daily consciousness is as awake as you can get. Not so for dream yoga, where in daily life you're considered to still be "asleep," or unaware. You've left the double-delusion, the nighttime dream, but you're back in the primary-delusion, the so-called waking state. You've woken up from one level of dream merely to find yourself in another.

In the world of dream yoga, nighttime dreams are considered the "example dream," which implies that waking reality is the real dream. So a major difference between lucid dreaming and dream yoga is that dream yoga not only wakes you up from the dream of the night, but also from the dream of the day. Ponlop Rinpoche writes, "When dreams are recognized as dreams, they are antidotes. When they are not recognized, they are simply confusion on top of confusion."[2] Waking up from the dream of the day is the nature of the practice of illusory form.

False Awakenings

Waking up from one level of dream only to find yourself in another is called a false awakening. In the world of nighttime dreams, you may wake up from one dream into what you think is waking reality, only to discover that what you thought was waking reality is just another dream. This dream-within-a-dream effect can be compared to nested Chinese boxes or Russian dolls. I refer to this series of "false awakenings" as "recursive dreaming." Recursion is the process of repeating something in a self-similar way, like looking into two mirrors facing each other. When recursion is applied to dreams, you're dropping into a tunnel of illusion, or a fractal of deception, like Alice in Wonderland. The question of "what is real?" is at the heart of recursive dreams. As Edgar Allan Poe said, "All that we see, or seem to see, is but a dream within a dream."

I've had a number of recursive dreams, and experienced as many as three layers of false awakenings.[3] Some of my dream yoga friends report as many as seven. It's unnerving to have the rug of reality continually pulled out from under your feet: "Wait a minute, I thought I *was* awake!" The scholar Wendy Doniger O'Flaherty alludes to this as the "myth of the receding frame,"[4] which is when the frame of reality keeps shifting or receding as you awaken from one dream into the next, and the dreamer is never sure that they've finally landed in an irreducible reality, or truly awakened. Our charter in dream yoga is not to switch from one dream into the next, but rather to switch from dreaming into true awakening—which is realizing the dream-like or empty nature of whatever arises.

So in the practice of dream yoga, true awakening (in contrast to the experience of false awakening) is characterized by the way it brings a quality of equivalence and equanimity (what Buddhism refers to as "one taste") to any state of consciousness—waking, dreaming, or dreamless sleep. Rather than seeking to "bottom out" in any one state and stake your claim that this is reality, you wake up to the reality—or the unreality, the emptiness—of whatever arises.[5] In other words, you break the frame.

If there's no framework that reifies one state as being absolute and all the others as being relative—that is, no framework that regards these states as solidly real—then *every* state is seen as being relative (dependent on every other state), and *that*, ironically, defines the absolute. Discovering emptiness, or the dreamlike nature of everything, is what shatters the frame. This is what Trungpa Rinpoche was pointing to when he said, "The bad news is you're falling through the air, nothing to hang on to, no parachute. The good news is that there's no ground."[6]

The realization that there is no bottom may be disappointing to the grasping and reifying ego. Ego wants a frame; it wants something solid to stand on and proclaim as really real. It craves a ground, a bottom line. But this ultimate non-solidity of any state *is* reality. Dreams, and dream yoga in particular, can lead us to this awakening. As Doniger O'Flaherty says, "The dream is what helps us to crash through the frame of apparent reality—the last visible frame—even though the dream, too, is a frame, and not the last frame either."[7]

You may think this physical world is the last and therefore truly real frame, until this world dissolves at death and your experience doesn't. Your experience just switches frames—from being locked in the world of materialism, and "asleep" in the spiritual sense—into what Buddhism calls "the dream at the end of time." There are three kinds of dream realities in Buddhism: the "example dream," which is our nighttime dream; the "actual dream," which is our daytime experience; and the "dream at the end of time," which is our experience after death. In the "dream at the end of time," you'll find yourself falling through space without a parachute, and craving for ground—a body—so desperately that that very craving will hurl you into one, and into your next life, as we will see later in the chapter on bardo yoga.

For now, though, let's look more at the nature of lucid dreams and false awakenings. In a lucid dream you dream with the awareness that you're dreaming, but in a false awakening you dream with the mistaken belief that you're awake. The teaching of dream yoga is to take the experience of false awakening and apply it to waking life. In other words, when you wake up in the morning, how can you be sure it's not another dream? How do you know that you're not dreaming right now? False awakenings demonstrate that you can't verify that you're awake just by thinking that you are.

We could say that lucid dreaming emphasizes the *differences* between waking and dreaming, as exercised in conducting state checks, whereas dream yoga emphasizes the *similarities* between waking and dreaming—which brings us to the daytime practice of illusory form (and the fourth main difference between lucid dreaming and dream yoga).

Mindfulness and Illusory Form

As we've seen, dream yoga and illusory form support each other. Your practice of illusory form will strengthen your dream yoga, and your dream yoga will strengthen your illusory form. In many ways they are the same kind of practice applied to two different states of consciousness.[8]

Illusory form is closely allied to mindfulness meditation. Mindfulness is about being fully present with things as they are. Illusory form practice expands this mindful awareness so that not only do you continually come back to awareness of the present moment, but you continually come back to an awareness that what's happening in the present moment is illusory.

Seeing a solid, lasting, and independent world—the way things are *not*—is partly a product of mindlessness. Mindlessness is a lack of awareness that sees stability where there is none. It's associated with a discursive and speedy mind, a mind that glosses over the discontinuous nature of reality, stitching things together into a *seemingly* continuous whole—the world of mere appearance. In cognitive science, this stitching together of discrete information—which generates the illusion of solidity and continuity—is called "flicker fusion." Things appear to be stable, but they're actually fleeting and flickering.[9]

In other words, our brains make things seem solid or whole based on limited information; we fuse together pixels of experience to create the appearances we think of as reality. We fill in the blanks that are inherent in reality with the putty of ego, which fuses together our seemingly solid, lasting, and independent world.[10]

Discontinuity and fragmentation are central characteristics of dreams. In one instant something is happening, and in the next instant it's something else. The mind hops from one disjointed scene to the next. Continuity, on the other hand, is a characteristic of waking reality. We flow seamlessly from one moment to the next. One of the insights from dream yoga and the practice of illusory form is that the more we wake up to the dreamlike nature of waking reality, the more discontinuous it becomes.[11]

A central maxim of the dream yoga journey is also shared by physics: *the deeper you look into things the less you find.* Conversely, the less you investigate, the "more" you find—the more things appear to be solid. Those who don't bother to look closely at things continue to see the world as more solid, lasting, and independent. They remain asleep. Those who do bother to look are the ones who see through this trinity of false appearances and wake up. Seeing reality, which is synonymous with seeing emptiness, is in one sense about seeing *less.* Things are less solid, less lasting, and less independent. If you see no-thingness (emptiness), that's the very best seeing. So from the perspective of dream yoga, and Buddhism altogether, seeing things as solid, lasting, and independent is a dreamsign that you're asleep in the world of duality.

These dreamsigns therefore help us understand what it is that buddhas wake up *from,* and what they awaken *to.* They wake up from seeing the world as solid, lasting, and independent, to seeing it as open, impermanent, and dependently originated. They wake up from the delusion of materialism and into a dreamlike reality. It's the irony of spiritual awakening: we awaken to the opposite of what we consider normal awakening each morning. Every morning we wake up from the fluidity of our dreams and into the solidity of our daily lives; buddhas wake up spiritually from solidity and into fluidity.

In terms of mindfulness, the faster the mind moves, the more solid and continuous things appear. Slow the mind down, through the practice of mindfulness, and the gaps in reality that have always been there start to be revealed. The pixilated nature of reality is discerned. It's like taking a movie reel, where discrete images pass before the projector at twenty-four frames per second (creating the illusion of continuity), and slowing it down. What seemed so continuous is now full of holes. Flicker fusion disappears and appearance falls apart.

This is another reason why mindfulness meditation is so helpful for dream yoga. The more mindful you are the more you see the fleeting, ever changing, dreamlike nature of reality. The more you see the discrete flickers. Seeing change is all about seeing differences. If nothing is different, nothing is changing. And noticing differences—noticing altogether—is the essence of mindfulness.

Not noticing these flickers gives rise to a type of mindlessness called "change blindness," which is a close cousin to the inattentional blindness discussed earlier. Remember that with inattentional blindness you fail to notice (are mindless of) an object that is fully visible because your attention has been directed elsewhere. You've been distracted. With change blindness, you fail to notice (are mindless of) a change in a scene. Both of these forms of blindness are synonyms for being asleep to our world.[12] The world is constantly changing, impermanent, and therefore discontinuous—like a dream. Through our mindlessness we're oblivious to the fact that we're the ones that freeze it solid.

The Stable Mind

The practice of illusory form reveals our lust for stability and shows us the difference between apparent outer stability and authentic inner stability—what we think we want and what we truly want. Steven LaBerge offers the insight that "waking consciousness is dreaming consciousness with sensory constraints; dreaming consciousness is waking consciousness without sensory constraints." Or like flopping back and forth in bed from waking to sleeping, Inayat Kahn said, "In reality, sleep and the wakeful state are nothing but the turning of the consciousness from one side to the other." Sensory input is what constrains consciousness and creates the apparent stability that we ascribe to our conventional reality. If there is one single ingredient in any appearance that causes us to think of it as reality rather than illusion, delusion, or dream, it's stability. Stability is virtually synonymous with our sense of reality. As the philosopher Evan Thompson says, "*Real* is the name we give to certain stable ways that things appear and continue to appear when we test them."[13]

Stability is also a central ingredient in what we refer to as sanity. When we say someone is really stable, the implication is that they're really sane. Conversely, instability is associated with insanity. So "stable" not only suggests "real," it also implies "sane." From a spiritual perspective, ultimate sanity is a synonym for enlightenment, which can be described as the full experience of reality. This is why my favorite definition of Buddhism, which is designed to lead one to enlightenment, is that Buddhism is a description of reality. Ken Wilber writes, "Psychopathology has always been considered—in one sense or another—as resulting from a distorted view of reality. *But what one considers to be psychopathology therefore must depend upon what one considers to be reality.*"[14]

To bring this back into the world of dreams: when an unstable mind is released unconstrained during sleep, we call that unstable state a "dream." It's only a dream, and therefore deemed unreal, because it is set in contrast to our more constrained and therefore stable waking experience. But when the mind gets very stable through meditation, and that steady mind is then released unconstrained into the dream state, dreams begin to feel more and more real.[15]

This stable mind also works on waking experience to see it as more dreamlike. So it is through the practice of mindfulness (which stabilizes the mind) that we wake up from the illusion of stability in the outer forms of daily life, seeing it more like a dream, and we simultaneously stabilize our dreams, seeing them more like waking reality. Dreaming consciousness and waking consciousness become increasingly alike—irrespective of sensory constraint. It's the same mind, after all, expressing itself in different venues. Lopon Kalsang Dorje says, "People who are awakened, Buddhas and Bodhisattvas, experience no difference between dream and the waking state. They realize the sameness which is infallible."[16] Marcel Proust famously echoes this in *In Search of Lost Time:* "I was alarmed nevertheless by the thought that this dream had had the clarity of consciousness. By the same token, might consciousness have the unreality of a dream?"

As you progress along the path, you lose the stability of external appearances (they're no longer seen as so solid, lasting, and independent), which may be initially unsettling to your stability-craving ego, but you gain the stability of a strong and unwavering mind, which is ultimately very settling to your spirit, or true nature. This is a great tradeoff. Because when the instability of external appearances inevitably rears its ugly head as the natural display of impermanence and death (which are both the natural display of emptiness), your stable mind can ride that impermanence without being thrown by it. *The stability of your mind becomes your unwavering reality.*

You then take refuge in that internal stability, and not in fleeting external appearances. You're no longer dependent on external circumstances for your stability, your sense of reality, or your sanity.[17] You take your stable mind with you into any possible experience. Wherever you go, there you are. And that "you" has got it totally together—even when everything else is falling apart. Nothing, absolutely nothing, can shake you. This is the unflappable and indestructible mind of an awakened one (in Buddhism known as the *vajra mind*).

The central criterion for reality is still met (stability), but it is now met within. At the highest levels of mindfulness, the mind itself becomes what you've been looking for—something changeless and therefore deathless, two central qualities of the clear-light mind. If the terms are defined properly, you could even say that the mind becomes "solid" (something you can rely on), "lasting" (changeless or unwavering), and "independent" (of any external influence). It's everything you've been looking for outside.

So through the practice of illusory form, what you lose out there you gain in here. You're therefore liberated from the vicissitudes "out there." You come to prefer your own stable mind over all unstable appearances. And unlike anything else, this stability is something that you can take with you, even after you die—because it's the real you, the indestructible quality of your deepest mind and heart. In the next chapter we'll learn how to engage this practice.

The whole purpose of the Doctrine of Dreams is to stimulate the yogin to arise from the Sleep of Delusion, from the Nightmare of Existence, to break the shackles in which *maya* thus has held him prisoner throughout the eons, and so attain spiritual peace and joy of Freedom, even as did the Fully Awakened One, Gautama the Buddha.

W. Y. EVANS-WENTZ, *Tibetan Yoga and Secret Doctrines*

13

The Practice of Illusory Form

THE DAYTIME DREAM yoga practice of illusory form has three aspects: illusory body, illusory speech, and illusory mind. We relate to the world through body, speech, and mind, and we solidify our experience of the world with our thoughts, words, and deeds. Illusory form works directly with these three gates to loosen and then dissolve our solid world. It helps us develop a penetrating vision, a vision that allows us to see through mere appearance and into reality, cutting through the forms, sounds, and thoughts that otherwise trap us in the anguish and discontent of worldly life—the suffering of samsara.

It's not necessary to use a telescope or bend over a microscope to contemplate the spectacle of the universe. It is sufficient to refuse to perceive as true all the illusions that blind us . . . In everything in the world, nothing exists besides illusions. Everything, without exception, is illusion.[1]

ZEN MASTER KODO SAWAKI ROSHI

The Practice of Illusory Body
(Cutting Through Forms)

The practice of illusory body is easy to summarize: you continually remind yourself that the forms of this world are like a dream. The basic practice is to say, almost like a mantra, "I'm dreaming," or "This is a dream," as often as you can, and to really *feel* that what you're perceiving right now is a dream. It's that simple. But here are some things you can do to support this practice, and ways to elaborate on it:

- Say "This is a dream" aloud, not just mentally. Saying it verbally strengthens it. Set your watch to beep every hour and use that signal as a reminder to say, "This is a dream." Any other signal also works: for instance, every time you hear a siren or see a plane. This doubles with the practice of prospective memory.

- Look at the experience of yesterday from the perspective of today. When you were living it, yesterday felt so solid and real. But from the perspective of today, it seems like a dream, doesn't it? Now look at today from the perspective of tomorrow. Doesn't today appear more dreamlike from tomorrow's perspective?

- Look at things as if you were looking at them from the back of your eye. This is a deeper and more penetrating gaze, one that doesn't get caught up in mere appearance. It's almost as if the gaze of the psyche, our non-lucid gaze, comes from the outermost surface of our eyes, while the look of the clear-light mind comes from the very back of our eyes. Retreat to that deeper look.

- Mirror practice. Stand in front of a mirror and say to yourself that all appearances are just like this reflection. There's no substance to anything that appears in a mirror. Then praise your reflection (which conjoins the practice of illusory body with the practice of illusory speech).

Point at yourself and say, "You're the most amazing person!" "No one can do what you do!" Indulge yourself with lavish admiration and notice how this feels. Then look at those feelings and see them as illusory as well, which conjoins this with the practice of illusory mind.

- Next, blame yourself. Give yourself "the finger." Point at yourself and say, "You're a worthless piece of crap! A total loser." See how that feels, and then look into the nature of those negative feelings. When I did this meditation in the last year of my three-year retreat, I initially found it patronizing and contrived. It seemed stupid. But since I had to do it for days on end, I decided to put my heart into it. The practice came to life and slowly started to change me. Now when people praise or blame me, it doesn't lift me up or take me down as much. I still feel the impact of the words briefly, but I don't give them a place to land, and I see through them more quickly.

- Reflect on the analogies of illusion. Many of these analogies come from the *Diamond Sutra,* which is a "cutting through" sutra. Diamonds can cut through anything. This sutra says: "So you should view the fleeting world: a star at dawn, a bubble in the stream, a flash of lightening in a summer cloud, a flickering lamp, a phantom, and a dream." Or my favorite: like a rainbow. Rainbows arise as the play of light and space, form and emptiness. I continually remind myself that I'm sitting on a rainbow, I'm typing on a rainbow keypad, I'm living in a rainbow house in a rainbow world.

- Put up sticky notes around your house that remind you, "This is a dream" or "You're dreaming." Place them inside cabinets, drawers, or other places to help you flash on the illusory nature of things.

• Take the characteristics of your dreams and transpose them into waking reality. For example, most of my dreams are highly visual. While there may be sounds and tactile sensations, it's mostly about sight. By wearing earplugs during the day it's remarkable how quickly my waking reality becomes dreamlike. If I'm in a dream yoga retreat, I may do this for hours. But initially, just try it for a few minutes. To simulate the discontinuous nature of dreams, move your head in rapid jerky motions, or keep your eyes closed a bit longer as you blink. When I do all this at the same time I'm wearing earplugs, my world quickly becomes dreamlike. If I do it for too long, however, it gets unsettling, almost nauseating. But that itself is revealing. It exposes my craving for stability. Play with what works for you.

• Experiment with inexpensive prismatic, or refractive, lenses, the kind they often hand out at Christmas light shows. These lenses, especially when worn at night, create halos and rainbow-like images around objects that are very dreamlike.

• Go to magic shows. Great magicians are great illusionists.[2] Look at surrealistic art: Salvador Dalí, Joan Miró, Yves Tanguy, René Magritte, and Dada artists like André Breton. Pablo Picasso was a master of seeing reality in discontinuous ways, as were the impressionists and pointillists. M. C. Escher is one of my illusory heroes. Almost any nonrepresentational artist can help you look at reality in new and illusory ways. I also find that optical illusion books are great at tricking the mind into surreal states.[3]

• Watch dreamlike movies—for instance, *The Science of Sleep, Waking Life, Vanilla Sky, Inception, Mulholland Drive, The Truman Show, Jacob's Ladder,* or *The Last Wave.* A good movie will suck you into it just like a good non-lucid dream. Khenpo Rinpoche says that movies and video games are wonderful modern analogies of illusion. A movie, just like a dream, can seem so real. We cry, laugh, and even scream when all that's really happening is empty images are being projected onto a screen. But we buy into it, literally and figuratively. Watch yourself get pulled into a movie, then step back and become lucid to what's happening. Wake up. It's just a movie.

- Psychotropic substances like LSD, DMT (the "spirit molecule," an essential ingredient in the Amazonian brew called *ayahuasca*), psilocybin mushrooms, and the like can induce illusory experiences that could act as a glimpse into the nature of reality, and shamans have used them for millennia. However, psychotropic drugs can do more harm than good, and I cannot recommend them. Artificial is rarely beneficial. The organic approach of traditional illusory form practice is healthier and more sustainable.[4]

ILLUSORY FORM SONGS

You can sing the following verses from traditional Buddhist texts throughout the day as a way of joining the practices of illusory body, illusory speech, and illusory mind.[5] Put them to your own melody.

- From the *Knowledge Fundamental to the Middle Way:* "Like a dream, like an illusion / Like a city of gandharvas / That's how birth and that's how living / That's how dying are taught to be."

- From the *Entrance to the Middle Way:* "There are two ways of seeing every thing / The perfect way and the false way / So each and every thing that can ever be found / Holds two natures within / And what does perfect seeing see? / It sees the suchness of all things / And false seeing sees the relative truth / This is what the perfect Buddha said."

- From the *Guide to the Bodhisattva's Way of Life:* "Then, wanderers, these dream-like beings, what are they? / If analyzed, they're like a banana tree / One cannot make definite distinctions / Between transcending misery and not."

- Two verses on the *Samadhi of Illusion,* from the *Jewel Ornament of Liberation.* First verse: "Knowing the five *skandhas* are like an illusion / Don't separate the illusion from the skandhas / Free of thinking that anything is real / This is perfect wisdom's conduct at its best!"[6] Second verse: "All the images conjured up by a magician / The horses, elephants, and chariots in his illusions / Whatever may appear there, know that none of it is real / And it's just like that with everything there is!"

The Practice of Illusory Speech (Cutting Through Sound)

Words, like physical forms, can hurt us when they're solidified. They're not as solid as bullets and bats, but a properly delivered word packs a punch. Words can make our hearts flutter, like when someone says "I love you" for the first time. And they can smack us, like when someone shouts "Fuck you!" into your face. They may not literally kill (even though the shock of words delivering bad news could give us a heart attack), but they can incite us to kill. A "war of words" can spark a literal war.

We put value into the words of others. "What would people say?" carries weight. Reputations are created and destroyed with words. A vow can contain or restrict experience almost as much as a physical container. The Ten Commandments, for example, are powerful restraints.

Buddhism describes ten virtuous and nonvirtuous deeds, distributed between the actions of body, speech, and mind. Of those ten, four are allotted to speech: lying, slander, harsh speech, and idle talk.[7] Note that the category of "wrong speech" has more wrongful actions than either wrong physical or wrong mental actions. One of the most nonvirtuous paths of speech is gossip: a mixture of lying, slander, harsh speech, and idle talk. Gossip often involves trying to get others to agree with our views, to help us make our views more solid and real. When we're not sure about things, we solicit gossip to help us reinforce our unstable impressions.

Illusory speech practice is about seeing through the solidity of words, *cutting through* the auditory bullets or buttering-up that take us down or lift us up. The fruition of illusory speech practice is to hear everything with equanimity and therefore not to be so affected by what others say. We can still be moved by what we hear, words still touch us, but only if we let them.

From a modern perspective, the traditional techniques of illusory speech practice can seem archaic. I'll share them out of homage to the tradition, then show you more contemporary ways to work with this practice. The first practice the texts recommend is "echo practice." The idea here is to go to a canyon and shout into it. Curse at yourself; then listen to the words as they come back and relate to them as the empty echoes they truly are. Then do the same with praise. Few of us can get to canyons and actually do this, but you get the idea. These days you could record yourself, or someone else, praising or blaming you.

Some texts suggest getting your teacher to praise you and then blame you. Other manuals talk about "the marketplace test." Go to a public place, do something outrageous (but not dangerous), and see how you respond when others verbally assault you. If you remain unfazed you've passed the test.

Sociologist Bernard McGrane devised a similar exercise (that might feel more safe). Go to a public place and stand perfectly still in the midst of other people. If someone approaches you, don't engage them. Stand like a statue and remain silent. Observe the reactions of the people who walk by. More importantly, observe your own response as people give you strange looks or talk about you.[8] I've done this practice and it was difficult. I stood perfectly still in the center of a shopping mall and within seconds people were looking at me and kids came to check me out. I discovered that I *did* care what people thought and said about me. I failed the test.

If you're scientifically oriented, you can deconstruct the power of words by remembering the physics of sound. Words are just longitudinal (compression and rarefaction) waves that strike your ear, that cause your eardrum to vibrate, that transmit electro-chemical impulses to the auditory parts of your brain, that are mixed with signals from other parts of your brain, that you impute meaning upon. They're just vibrations. "Good" or "bad" are not intrinsic to longitudinal waves but are qualities we impose upon them.

Another exercise is to listen to your native language and try to hear the words as if they were a foreign language, or as mere sounds. "Defamiliarize" the word back to pure sound. This practice reveals how instantly we bring meaning to sound. The moment we hear a word, we already hear it infused with its meaning and our history of associating with that word. We "translate" mere sound into a word, and therefore into meaning, on the spot.

To help you strip words back to pure sound, take a neutral word, like "car," and repeat it out loud. Notice how after a minute or so of hearing the word, the meaning strips away and you hear "car" very differently. Now try a more loaded or solid word, like "rape," "nigger," "Jesus," or "God." See how much longer it takes to strip the infused meaning away from those charged words.

In a workshop led by LaBerge, participants listened to a recorded word over and over for several minutes, without being informed what the word was. Our task was to see how many words we could hear within the repeated sound. The word he used for the exercise was "words" itself. Try it for a few minutes and see what you hear. Our group came up with around two dozen different words that we all heard, none of which were actually there. People heard "sword," "wear it," "wore it," "swore it," "score it," "square it"—or "its," "squirts," "heads," "quartz," "forehead," and "Lawrence," to name a few. But "Lawrence" isn't there, nor is "quartz," nor "swore," nor anything else but "words." This is a kind of auditory Rorschach test, designed to expose how we project ourselves onto things. We hear things that aren't there, see things that aren't there, like spooked inhabitants in the haunted house of our own mind.

When I did this exercise, after about a minute the reiterated "words" melted back into pure meaningless sound. But soon after that I started hearing some of these other words. I stripped "words" down, then quickly dressed it back up.

As mentioned above, you can also join illusory speech practice to illusory body practice by doing it in front of a mirror. Praise and blame yourself until you can enter the marketplace and have the words of others affect you as much as they do a mirror. When you can relate to words directed toward you with equanimity, you have accomplished illusory speech.

The Practice of Illusory Mind (Cutting Through Thoughts)

In the progression from illusory body to illusory speech to illusory mind, we're going from gross to subtle to very subtle form and learning how to see the dreamlike nature of each. The contents of our mind are pretty formless, but they still have enough form to dictate our lives. While being the most subtle, they're ironically the most powerful. Everything we say (speech) or do (body) starts with what we think or feel. "Illusify" the contents of your mind, regard your thoughts and feelings as dreamlike, and watch your entire world soften. Your speech becomes gentler and your acts become kinder.

With illusory mind practice we focus on the projector, not the projection. We relate directly to the mind, which is what happens when we go to sleep. When we lie down to sleep, we retract from our bodily actions and our speech, and return to our mind. The mind stands up when body and speech lie down. Just look at your experience. When you lie down, the contents of your mind rise up. If you suffer from insomnia, they keep you up.

We suffer in direct proportion to how solidly we take the contents of our mind.[9] At extreme levels, total reification of our thoughts and emotions is one way to look at madness. We may not be completely mad, but we do go crazy whenever we take our thoughts and emotions to be real.

At the other extreme are the awakened ones. The same thoughts and emotions that arise in a madman can also arise in a buddha, but the *relationship* to those thoughts and emotions is very different. A deluded person, one who is asleep, buys into the thought (the same way they buy into a non-lucid dream), whereas a buddha sees right through it. This penetrating awakeness is what we cultivate with the practice of illusory mind.

Illusory mind practice is an intimate and immediate application of the cutting through meditations discussed earlier. With illusory mind, cutting through the psyche and the substrate takes place on the spot. It's what Dzogchen Ponlop Rinpoche refers to as "wild awakening." We can cut through false appearances to glimpse the clear-light mind every time we see through a thought. Stabilizing that glimpse into a gaze takes time, but cutting through to the clear-light mind can happen in a flash. The path, as religious scholar Huston Smith put it, is to transform those flashes of illumination into abiding light.

Remember that thoughts are not the issue. Thoughts are the innocent play of the mind. If left alone, they naturally dissolve, or self-liberate, back into the clear-light mind from which they arose. But, of course, we rarely leave them alone. *That's* the problem. We pour the gasoline of attention onto these tiny sparks of mind, and they ignite into the worries, dramas, ruminations, anxieties, expectations, hopes, and fears that comprise the entirety of our lives—all born from taking our thoughts to be solid and real—just like we take our non-lucid dreams to be solid and real.

With illusory mind practice, the things we took so seriously—our ambitions, trepidations, anticipations, and doubts—are seen to be fleeting, ephemeral, and transparent, like harmless sparks dissolving into the nighttime sky. In a talk at Naropa University, Dzogchen Ponlop Rinpoche reminded his audience, "Try to see how you solidify your experiences—how you solidify your pain, your happiness, your joy—and how these experiences become so important to you that you can't even sleep at night. Our experience is so real, so important, and so bothersome to us that we cannot even have a good night's sleep."

If we solidify *any* experience, the result is samsara, sleep, and suffering. If we soften the contents of our mind, the result is nirvana, awakening, and the end of suffering. Many standard meditations work to help us see through our thoughts and emotions, and here we will use some of those meditations in the context of the mind aspect of illusory form.

Illusory mind practice starts with mindfulness *(shamatha)* and awareness *(vipashyana)*. Shamatha slows the mind down; vipashyana allows us to see through it. When thoughts are streaming through the mind, we tend to get swept away with the torrent. It's hard to see through the current. When the mind slows down, it gets "thinner" and more transparent. Vipashyana means "insight," and with illusory mind practice it refers to taking the mind's eye and turning it back in. This is the gaze of the "insider" mentioned earlier, and it allows us to see the outer layers of the mind for what they truly are—mere clouds floating through the vast open space of the mind.

While it does help to slow the mind down, we don't have to stop it. We don't have to get rid of a single thought or emotion. Thoughts are never the problem. Believing everything we think or feel (reification) is the problem.

On one level, illusory mind practice is easy. Just don't buy into everything you think. Try it and you'll see how easy it is. Watch a thought come up, look right at it, then watch it melt before your eyes. But because of a lifetime of taking thoughts to be real, it's hard to sustain this penetrating gaze. There's so much history of reification, so much karma and habit that keeps on solidifying everything that pops up. Constancy is therefore the difficulty.

With illusory mind practice we're adapting the sitting meditation discussed earlier by replacing the label "thinking" with "see through it." It's the same, remember, as saying "wake up." When a thought arises and distracts you, mentally say "see through it." Don't try to stop the thought, just cut through it with your X-ray vision. As Sogyal Rinpoche says, "Recognize them [thoughts] instead for what they truly are, merely experiences, illusory and dreamlike." In this way, the mind gradually becomes transparent to itself, like a fog melting away from the rays of the morning sun.

When you see the illusory nature of the contents of your mind, thoughts and emotions no longer have power over you. That's what spiritual liberation means. You're finally free from relating inappropriately to the contents of your mind. Thoughts and emotions now become adornments of the mind instead of obscurations.

If you continue to solidify your thoughts, and therefore buy into them, you will continue to buy into everything else. The seduction of outer forms starts from within, with the lure of our thoughts and emotions. This consumerism may sustain samsara, but it bankrupts nirvana. All the traditional practices come to the same point: everything in your mind is fleeting and empty, like a dream.

> When we look back, at the time of death, the experience of this life will seem like a dream. And—just as with our nighttime dreams—it will seem useless to have put so much effort into it. The fear we experience in a dream is gone when we wake up; feeling afraid was just an unnecessary exertion of effort causing us to lose sleep! When we look back on our lives at death, the amount of time we spent in hesitation, aggression, ignorance, selfishness, jealousy, hatred, self-preservation, and arrogance will seem like an equally useless exertion of energy. *So be able to regard all of these illusory thoughts and concepts as dreams* [emphasis added]. Within this illusory existence, what, if anything, is the logic behind any stubbornness, distraction, hesitation, or habitual emotions of aggression, desire, selfishness, and jealousy?[10]
>
> KHANDRO RINPOCHE

How you relate to your mind naturally extends into how you relate to your speech, your body, and its actions. How you relate to your speech and your body also extends into how you relate to your mind. These three aspects of illusory form therefore bootstrap each other. They lift each other up. The better you get at one, the better you'll get at the others. The result of these practices is to discover that there is a dreamlike eye consciousness that sees dreamlike forms, a dreamlike ear consciousness that hears dreamlike sounds, and a dreamlike mind that perceives dreamlike thoughts.

Trungpa Rinpoche summarizes all three aspects of illusory form:

> Whatever is seen with the eyes is vividly unreal in emptiness,
> yet there is still form.

Whatever is heard with the ears is the echo of emptiness, yet real.
Good and bad, happy and sad, all thoughts vanish into emptiness like the imprint of a bird in the sky.[11]

What Do You Really Want?

A central theme of dream yoga is that people, things, or events do not have the inherent power to affect you, unless you solidify them and therefore give them that power. Illusory form practice reinforces this idea by showing you that people, things, or events aren't even what you really want. External forms (people, things, events) aren't the point. It's the relatively formless states of mind they evoke that's really the point. Illusory form points out the difference between what you think you want (some external form) and what you really want (an internal formless state of mind). It's therefore another way of separating appearance from reality, and waking up to the truth.

Take a close look. When you want to get away from someone (or something), what you really want to get away from is the state of mind you allow them to evoke. When you want to move toward someone (or something), it's a pleasurable state of mind you allow that person to evoke that is really what you want to move toward. Otherwise that disagreeable person would always be repulsive, and the pleasurable person would always be attractive. If you think someone has that kind of power, give them some time and watch that power fade, like in a long-term relationship. The ability of an object to instill happiness or suffering also comes into question when you realize that what one person finds attractive another might find repulsive, or vice versa.

When you say something like "That person is really *hot*!" what you're really saying is that you're allowing that person to ignite a feeling of heat or passion within you. When you say, "I want that car!" what you're really saying is that you want the state of mind you're allowing the car to provoke. This discovery moves your focus from outside to inside. It's a tectonic shift that deposits responsibility for your suffering and happiness squarely where it needs to be: within yourself and with how you relate to the contents of your mind.

My friend Peter was going through a rough time in his marriage. In an effort to lessen his pain, Peter bought a big boat and took emotional refuge in his new vessel. Every free minute was spent polishing and maintaining his new toy. The boat gave him the solace he so desperately needed. He often slept in it, or took it out to the open waters to escape his problems. Peter came to associate his expensive toy with peace of mind. His wife was equated with misery; his boat was equated with happiness. He conflated, and therefore confused, an external object with an internal state of mind.

Peter didn't realize it, but he didn't really want to spend time on the boat. That's just how things appeared. The reality was that he wanted to spend more time in a happy state of mind. Peter learned this lesson the hard way, as most of us eventually do, when his boat started to have as many problems as his marriage. The propeller broke. Then the engine blew a gasket. Finally the hull cracked. It went from a happy place to another place of misery. Suddenly his wife didn't look so bad. If Peter had bothered to take a close look, he would have realized that his boat, let alone his wife, doesn't have the power to make him happy or sad—unless he gives those entities that power.

To reach any level of unconditional happiness, or *formless* happiness, Peter needs to tease apart appearance from reality and wake up to the heart of what he's really after. Until he does so, just like the rest of us, Peter will spend the rest of his life striving to reproduce the conditions (forms) that seem to make him happy, unaware (asleep to the fact) that unconditional, or formless, happiness is what he really wants. This is why true renunciates and ascetics (not the false ones who just want to run away from things) are on to something. They've woken up to the fact that external objects are not what anybody really wants.

This is also why people can be happy with completely different things. A native in the jungles of the Amazon might find happiness by hunting for wild boar, while a fashion model in Paris finds happiness when she's featured on the cover of a magazine. It's not the boar, or the magazine cover, that does it. The mind does it. The common denominator is the state of mind, not the state of any object. The teachings on dream yoga drive home the point: "Wake up! Can't you see it's all about working with your mind?"

This is why engaging in the practice of illusory form, and especially the practice of illusory mind, is so valuable. This is why meditation is not some mystical thing. It's the most realistic and practical thing possible. Instead of working indirectly with people, objects, and events outside, you're working directly with the true source of your pleasure or pain. Nothing has the power to make you happy or sad, unless you give it that power. And that power is unwittingly conferred when you take it to be real.

The Fruition of Illusory Form

As "outsiders," in the Buddhist sense, we're always projecting onto the external world, creating and sustaining our sense of self based on the echoes that come back. It's a kind of psychological "echolocation," or finding our way in the world based on the feedback we get from projecting ourselves onto it.[12] These echoes are all contingent on having something solid "out there" to bounce off of. If there's something solid out there, the immediate implication is that there must be something solid "in here." Where there is other, there is self. And the more solid the other, we surmise, the more solid the self.

This echolocation happens psychologically (How am *I* doing?), and even deeper, spiritually (or ontologically—the confirmation of my very sense of "I," or existence itself). In other words, the psychological feedback we crave is already a secondary reflection, which comes from what the psyche projects onto the world. The primary reflection arises from the illusion that there is even something out there to begin with, and this comes from what the substrate projects (the illusion of an outside world altogether). We first have to have an "out there" to bounce our psychological projections off of. The practice of illusory form works with both layers of solidity (the seemingly solid outside world, and then the seemingly solid feedback we get from it), but focuses more on the spiritual level by softening and then dissolving any notion of "out there" (and therefore duality).

When I did my first thirty-day group meditation retreat over twenty-five years ago, I was humbled to discover how much I craved these forms of feedback. It was a silent retreat, with instructions to even avoid eye contact, and there was absolutely no interaction with the outside word. I related to these restrictions as a kind of diet, or fast, which led me to discover how much I feast on outside feedback. Within a week of meditating twelve hours a day, my solid sense of self came into question. As my ego slowly dissolved, I found myself starving for feedback, for something to reestablish my existence. I kept the discipline of silence, but tried to cheat by catching the eye of somebody—anybody!—as they walked by during breaks from our formal sessions. When someone happened to look up (perhaps they were feeling the same existential anxiety) and we exchanged a glance, I breathed a sigh of relief. Someone acknowledged me! But most of the time my furtive glances fell on lowered heads, and this lack of feedback was deflating.

We all know what it feels like to be ignored, like when you send an email or text message and never get a response, but this level of dismissal was primal. It wasn't just my sense of performance in the world that was ignored, but my very sense of being in the world. As unsettling as this was, it revealed just how much I longed to be affirmed—not just psychologically, but ontologically. Trungpa Rinpoche once said, "The universe will not blink when you die," which was an exhortation to get over our inflated sense of self and the feedback it feeds on.

The less solid the universe, the less solid is the feedback that generates our sense of self. When we see through the apparent solidity of the outside world, we become aware of a larger context—that context of awareness (lucidity) that we discussed earlier. We're no longer boxed in by a box we didn't even know we made. Our attention still goes out, but it doesn't bounce back to us in the same way. It doesn't rebound to create and then sustain the very sense of "us." In psychological terms, we're no longer starved for egoic feedback, like a child constantly exclaiming "Mommy, Mommy, look what I can do!" What people say or think doesn't matter anymore. The fruition of illusory body (there's no-thing "out there") therefore gives rise to the fruition of illusory speech. We've seen through it all. It's fantastically liberating, because we're no longer confining ourselves by (or *to*) the outside world.

We continue to attend to things, but that outward attention, which is usually tainted with projection, transforms into radiance.

It's the difference between attending to something in the hope of getting something back (and fearing that we might not) and attending to it out of pure love, expecting nothing back. We put it out there, and then let it go. This is when we finally start to shine.

How often do people really start to shine when they give up worrying about what others say or think? How often do we blossom when we finally trust our inner light, and become fearless in expressing it, often outshining those still boxed in by hope and fear? Trusting your shine gives birth to authentic presence and confidence, as you live your life free from external constraints. When fully turned on, this liberated light radiates as majesty. You've come into your own. It's then, as widely attributed to the poet Maya Angelou, that "nothing can dim the light that shines from within."

When you're free of these external constraints, it's as if the clear-light mind can finally shine clearly without hesitation or doubt. If you're around someone whose light is fully transparent, you can feel the glow, the warmth, the egoless confidence. And you want to be around it. This solar energy is magnetizing, like the splendor of the sun, and can draw others into its sphere of influence to help them. This is real charisma, the blazing light of our heart-mind free of the projecting substrate and psyche.

I have felt this illumination and warmth, this wisdom and compassion, with the great masters of our time, from His Holiness the Dalai Lama, the Karmapa, Sai Baba, Father Thomas Keating, and other luminaries from other traditions. These masters do not market their solar energy (which is the clearest indicator of a charlatan), but live humbly to wake us up to our own internal light, what Shambhala Buddhism calls the Great Eastern Sun within. And they do so by freeing us from the solidity of the "eight worldly concerns," which is the way Buddhism articulates the external constraints that box us in.

These eight worldly concerns are actually eight mental prisons that confine our lives: praise and blame, fame and shame, loss and gain, pleasure and pain. With the practice of illusory form we see right through these prison walls and the folly of spending our lives scrambling to acquire praise, fame, pleasure, and gain, while struggling to avoid blame, shame, loss, and pain. The origin of these eight concerns is hope and fear; we hope for the former and fear the latter.

Understanding illusory form is what keeps us from going *out* and getting lost in our projections. It interrupts the "outsider" trajectory that hurls us into endless dissatisfaction, and allows us to see through the futility of this way of life. As Socrates said, "The secret to happiness, you see, is not found in seeking more, but in developing the capacity to enjoy less."

If thoughts and things are fundamentally illusory, there's no need to grasp after them. If there's no grasping, no relentless psychic effort of attachment and fixation, there's no fatigue. If there's no fatigue, there's no need for sleep. This is one reason why the buddhas don't sleep, in the conventional sense.[13] Khenpo Rinpoche summarizes the heart of illusory form:

> The appearances of this life—all the various appearances of forms, sounds, smells, tastes, and bodily sensations we perceive—seem to truly exist. But life's appearances do not say to us, "I am real." They only seem to be real from our confused thoughts' perspective when we think, "Those things really exist out there." *That is like what we do in a dream when we do not know we are dreaming* [emphasis added]. Similarly, we mistakenly believe that aging, sickness, and death are truly existent . . . but this is just confused consciousness at work. The buddhas' perfect wisdom does not view this life, or the aging, sickness, and death that occur within it, as truly existent. The noble buddhas and bodhisattvas with wisdom that sees genuine reality do not see these events as real.[14]

Finally, if the world is a dream, what is it that dreams this world? It is dreamt by the clear-light mind. The practice of illusory form is to keep dropping into the perspective of the clear-light mind, from which it is absolutely true to proclaim: this is a dream.

> At this time when the transitional process of dreaming is appearing to me, I shall abandon negligence and the cemetery of delusion. With unwavering mindfulness, I shall enter the experience of the nature of being. Apprehending the dream-state, I shall train in emanation, transformation, and the clear light. I will not sleep like an animal, but practice integrating sleep and direction perception!

GURU RINPOCHE, *Natural Liberation: Padmasambhava's Teachings on the Six Bardos,* translated by B. Alan Wallace

14

Advancing to Dream Yoga
First Stages and Practices

THE RELEASE OF a brilliant bolt of lightning requires the right atmosphere: the right temperature, the right altitude, the right humidity, the right electrical potential, and then suddenly, BANG, there's a flash of lightning. Our approach to dream yoga in this book has been a similar process: we've gathered the right view, the right meditations, the right attitude, the right motivation, and the right preliminary practices so that one day the thunderbolt of lucidity will flash within your dreams. This approach is called "the gradual path to sudden awakening."[1]

As we've seen, in Buddhism the preliminaries are more important than the main practice. For our purposes here, this means that if you do the preliminaries properly, dream yoga is more apt to "just happen." It's like when you go to sleep under normal conditions. You can't will yourself to sleep. The effort keeps you awake, and the harder you try the more you stay awake. "Try to relax" is an oxymoron. What you do to go to sleep under normal conditions is create the proper environment. You turn off the lights, lie down, close your eyes, make yourself snuggly, and then wait. If the proper environment is there, assisted by fatigue of course, sleep "just happens."

With our dream yoga journey so far we've been creating the proper environment. And like the transition from effortful to effortless mindfulness, most of the effort comes up front.

Getting to a level where dream yoga "just happens" requires deep inner work and may be inconvenient. Spiritual practice is often unreasonable and inconvenient. It doesn't always make sense from ego's perspective, and it doesn't always play into the hands of conventional reason. This is especially true for nighttime practice. Ego just doesn't want to go there. As we've seen, darkness (ignorance) is where ego takes ultimate refuge and finds its deepest shelter. Piercing light can be irritating for that which lives in the dark. It requires advanced spiritual techniques to penetrate this darkness, the underground shelter of ego, and reveal that light. Dream and sleep yoga are therefore advanced bunker busters that the stronghold of ego may not welcome.

Because these practices are subtle, it's easy to get discouraged. You'll need to maintain an attitude of determination. (Advanced practitioners never give up. That's how they advance.) You also have to become your own meditation instructor. Of course you can talk to other practitioners and dream yoga instructors, but this journey is a very private one. You have to be honest with yourself and be willing to go deep into the darkness of this truth-telling practice.

Some people are afraid of the truth even more than they're afraid of the dark. Many of us are afraid to look into the truth-telling mirrors of our life because we're afraid of what we might find. A psychologist once told me that alcoholics often can't look themselves in the eye when they gaze into a mirror, because they can't bear what they see. For many of us, we're not just afraid of physical mirrors but also emotional ones—like what our intimate partners reflect—or spiritual ones—like being with a guru or spiritual community. All of these mirrors have the potential to reflect our neurosis and therefore help us grow. Dream yoga is another such mirror—"the measure of the path," reflecting the measure of our spiritual practice. It's a mirror that we may not want to see.

Dzogchen Ponlop Rinpoche said with frankness that if you are satisfied with being stupid, then don't bother getting on the spiritual path. Just continue with your sleepwalking and pray that you don't stroll off a cliff. But if you're not satisfied with pain and suffering, and you prefer to wake up, sooner or later you have to face the deepest facets of your being. You have to bring up every hidden aspect of yourself, make friends with it, and then let it all self-liberate in the light of awareness.

The stages of dream yoga go right to the heart of this deep and dark place, working directly with ignorance (spiritual sleep), the root of all suffering. Ignorance is powerful because it's so insidious. It's hard to see. But it's also the most active force in samsara. If you see things as solid, lasting, and independent, you're under the attack of ignorance. It's like a background roar that's been going on from time immemorial, so you've adapted to it. Imagine being in a room for a long time with a huge ventilation system that is suddenly turned off. Until the background noise is extinguished, you have no idea it's even there.

Because ignorance is so constant, we never see it. We don't have the contrast (generated by a temporary cessation) to see that we're suffering from active ignorance. We don't have any other state of consciousness that allows us to detect that we're asleep. The master Orgyenpa said,

> The waking experience has been going on since a period
> of time that never began and is never really interrupted
> except by the additional overlay of dreamtime confusion.
> We know that dreams are not real because we wake up
> from them periodically, and therefore have contrast.
> However, *we have no such contrast by which to recognize the
> unreality of conventional appearances* [emphasis added].[2]

In the Four Noble Truths of Buddhism, the cessation of ignorance is the equivalent of the third truth, "the cessation of suffering," or *nirodha* (which means "cessation, extinction"; *nirvana* is a form of *nirodha*). With dream yoga, we develop the awareness that allows us to turn off the ignorance that we never knew was on.

If dream yoga is so subtle, you might ask, why bother? Well, most people don't. They prefer to sleep. The reason dream yoga is worth bothering with is that everything you do on the surface of your life is dictated by these subtle deeper levels. As we've seen, we're dealing with the tectonic plates of our lives here, and the tiniest movement "down there" can have enormous repercussions "up here." When literal tectonic plates move just a few meters, the earthquakes on the surface can be monumental. The same small shifts at unconscious levels can have similarly potent effects on our conscious lives.

By bringing the unconscious processes that control our lives into the light of conscious awareness, we can become free of them. This freedom is what much of psychology is about; Buddhism just goes deeper. Both traditions show us how we sleepwalk through life, guided in our slumber by the force of the unconscious mind, and give us the choice of waking up.

In particular, the path of dream yoga can create that flash of spiritual awakening to illuminate the fact that we're sound asleep.[3] When we're asleep, we don't look *at* (and therefore see) our ignorance; we look *through* it (and are therefore obscured by it), like seeing through dark sunglasses we don't even know we have on. In other words, we don't see that we don't see. We usually don't see things because they're too far away. But with our ignorance—or in the terms of dream yoga, our lack of lucidity—we don't see things because they're too close. It's like trying to see the inside of our eyelids. What we're doing with dream yoga is pulling our eyelids back so we can see exactly what it is that keeps us in the dark.

In our approach to the practice of dream yoga, we have moved from basic Western practices of lucid dreaming and on to forms of meditation and lucid dream induction, and beyond that to more advanced and subtle concepts of Tibetan Buddhism, such as the practice of illusory form. With the stage set, we are finally ready to explore the nighttime practice of dream yoga.

Phases and Stages of Dream Yoga

Traditionally, the practice of dream yoga is viewed as having three phases, and the practitioner usually moves through these phases in stages. The first phase is *recognition*. Recognize the dream to be a dream. The second phase is *transformation,* which roughly corresponds to stages 1 through 7 presented here and in the next chapter. The third phase is *liberation,* which relates to stages 8 and 9 in the next chapter. This numbering implies a developmental approach, but the practice is not necessarily linear. You can move back and forth between stages. Stages 1 through 7 can be viewed as somewhat dualistic; they involve working with the objects in your dreams. Stages 8 and 9 are more nondualistic, transcending any sense of subject and object altogether. From gross to subtle, from duality to nonduality, just like the spiritual path itself.

The stages outlined below are in general alignment with the classical stages, but the presentation is my own and the stages are more gradual and user-friendly than the traditional stages. Explore them and see what works best for you. You may have a strong connection or ability in one stage and no connection with another. You might skip stages entirely, or discover your own. How long you stay at a stage may also vary. Someone might stay at the first stage forever and make that their entire dream yoga practice. Others may systematically progress through these stages, spending weeks, months, or years on each one. Still others may bounce all over, one night finding themselves able to do some of the more advanced stages, and the next night coming back to stage 1. Some people might shift the order of the following stages, and start with a higher one.

At times I'll work on the higher stages, and other times I'll relax my efforts and drop back to early stages. At other times I'll indulge my fantasies at the start of a lucid dream and then shift into practice mode. Some nights I don't want to work at all and prefer to just sleep. Dream yoga has no hard and fast rules except this: go slow and easy. Your dreams are your own, informed by your personal background and expectations. Trust your experience and have fun. Everyone's journey is unique.

From a psychological (lucid dreaming) perspective, the point of the stages that follow is reconciliation and integration with dream elements, and therefore with the elements of your unconscious mind.[4] From a spiritual (dream yoga) perspective, the point of the practice is to gain mastery over the dream elements: once you recognize that you're in a lucid dream, you add more advanced ways of working with the dream, with the ultimate potential of enlightenment. The final stages of dream yoga are aimed at cutting through your unconscious mind to the clear-light mind below.

In lucid dreaming we *befriend;* in dream yoga we *transcend.* One could argue that befriending is transcending, and is a more peaceful approach, while purely transcending is a more wrathful (cutting through) approach. From an integrated point of view, in which we can honor and incorporate all aspects of nighttime practice, they both have a place.[5]

Stages 1 through 5, discussed in this chapter, are the beginning and intermediate levels of dream yoga. These practices could easily constitute an entire dream yoga curriculum, and can lead to profound changes not only in your nightly experience, but in your daily life. For those who want to go even further, stages 6 through 9 in the chapter that follows will show you just how far dream yoga can take you.

Stage 1

Fly in your dreams. Once you become lucid, take off and fly. Go for a joy ride. Because I often trigger lucidity by doing the state check of jumping up, it's natural to just keep going. This is a good first stage because it's fun. It's a bridge between standard lucid dreaming and dream yoga. Some traditional texts don't recommend flying as a first stage because people might be afraid of flying or of heights. If that's the case, then either don't do this or else try taking one step into the air and just hover above the ground. If you are afraid, it's a good way to work with fear, which would blend this stage with stage 4, as described below.[6]

Stage 2

Put your hands through things, walk through walls, or drop below the earth like a mole. This is a literal exercise in "cutting through," or seeing through appearances. I've been doing dream yoga and studying the teachings on emptiness for many years. I'll still approach a dream wall fully lucid, with the intent of putting my dream hand through the wall, and just not be able to do it. Even though I know I'm dreaming, I'll still bump up against the dream wall and perceive it as solid. My habitual pattern of taking things to be real is still operative, and this habit is revealed at this stage of practice.

If I up the ante and try to walk through a wall, I'll often bump my big dream nose against the dream wall and bounce back. Here's a trick: if you want to walk through a dream wall, turn around and walk through it backward. Because you don't know when you're going to hit the wall, you might find yourself suddenly going through it! In my dreams the wall turns out to be made of strange Jell-O, a gooey substance that I eventually slog through. I continue to chuckle in my dreams when this happens, both at the pathetic power of my habit in reifying things, and the funny nature of this trick.

My friend Patricia Keelin, a seasoned oneironaut, shared this tip with me: "If you're attempting to go through a wall or ceiling, try going hand-first. There's something in our evolutionary makeup that warns us not to bump our heads too hard. In my experience, going hand-first usually buys my mind just enough time to fully accept the shock of comprehending the illusory nature of that wall or ceiling I've come up against."

This stage starts to expose the strength of our habitual patterns. It's a potent truth-teller. After doing this stage for years, I can put my hand through a dream wall more quickly than before. My habit of reification is softening, and therefore so is my wall. This carries a double meaning: I'm no longer as "walled in" by events in my life, and I can see through barriers more readily. I'm becoming softer—and so is my world. Truth-telling is not always bad. Dreams also reveal good habits that are developing and that can inspire us to persevere.

This points to how failures in dream yoga can lead to success, the success of insight. My inability to control aspects of my dream, at any stage of practice, shows me where I'm stuck. These failures help me become aware of deep habitual patterns that still rule my conscious and unconscious life. Failures can also point out the disagreement between my conscious and unconscious intents. My conscious mind may intend something but my unconscious mind may not want to go along. Exploring this internal conflict of interest is always fruitful. Is it out of fear, loss of control, or laziness? Is it due to opposing beliefs, desires, or the raw power of habit-karma? Maybe I still want to feel walled in. Maybe my ego feels safe when it's surrounded by solid things.

This leads to an even deeper question: if the conscious dreamer isn't controlling the entire dream, who is? You can learn a lot about your deeper self by observing the dream environment and your failure to control it. It's your deeper self that creates the stage and truly runs the show. Until all the unconscious elements are brought into the light of consciousness, it's still the "night" (the unconscious) that rules the day. These unconscious habits run very deep. If you believe in rebirth, they run lifetimes deep. It takes time, and therefore patience, to bring them to light and to be free of them.

Success and failure at conscious control in a lucid dream has immediate implications for control in waking life. How successful are you in daily life when your conscious goals are opposed by unconscious forces with different goals? For example, your conscious self may want to become enlightened, but your unconscious self may not. Deep down inside, do you really want to wake up? Part of you may not. Maybe this is why the spiritual path is littered with obstacles, and why so many people give up. Let your failures teach you.

Stage 3

Change things. Turn a dream table into a dream flower; transform your boat into a car. Add and subtract things in your dreams, or shift their size. Expand your house into a mansion, then shrink it down to a doll house. Take that cactus and make five of them. What I often do is hold up my right hand and say to myself, "Let's make three of these." Just like with stage 2, it usually doesn't happen right away. I have to stare at my hand, focus the intent to multiply, and eventually several more hands do appear. Why do you want to do this? Tenzin Wangyal says,

> Just as dream images can be transformed in dreams, so emotional states and conceptual limitations can be transformed in waking life. With experience of the dreamy and malleable nature of experience, we can transform depression into happiness, fear into courage, anger into love, hopelessness into faith, distraction into presence.

What is unwholesome we can change to wholesome. What is dark we can change to light. *Challenge the boundaries that constrict you* [emphasis added]. The purpose of these practices is to integrate lucidity and flexibility with every moment of life, and to let go of the heavily conditioned way we have of ordering reality, of making meaning, of being trapped in delusion.[7]

While these practices are fun, they're also foundational. By transforming your mind (what else are these dream objects made of?) in the dream, you're learning how to transform it altogether. You're literally learning how to "change your mind." As Tenzin Wangyal suggests, the point is to take seemingly solid entities—which in the dream manifest as objects, but in life manifest as emotions, prejudices, attitudes, self-imposed limitations, biases, and so forth—and realize they're not as solid as they appear.

> Every time we change our dreams we increase our capacity to change our conscious experience while we are awake.
> TRALEG RINPOCHE, *Dream Yoga*, an audio course by Traleg Rinpoche

As the Tibetan master Padma Karpo said about this stage of dream yoga, we make big objects small and small objects big in order to realize "the nature of dimensions." And we make one object into many and many objects into one in order to comprehend "the nature of plurality and unity." In other words, through these practices we discover the *empty* nature of things—that dream phenomena have no inherent existence from their own side. If it were really real, I couldn't change it. So this is another way to work with emptiness, the central theme behind all these stages.

Stage 4

Create frightful situations, then work with your fear. The pioneering researcher Paul Tholey suggests that if you want to grow, you should seek out threatening situations in your lucid dreams and work with them. If you're already in a nightmare, work with the fear instead of running from it. This is an important and more advanced stage, for several reasons. First, because they're so charged, lucid nightmares initially tend to resist modification, and therefore control. Second, who wants to voluntarily generate a nightmare, or stay with one? Stephen LaBerge counters the first reason by stating that fear in a lucid dream is a reflection of marginal lucidity. This resonates with my experience. If I'm barely lucid, fear takes over. If I'm very lucid (which implies more control), I take over the fear.

> ❨ It is not the events in our nightmares that horrify us; it is our attitude of taking these events literally that scares the wits out of us. Once one realizes, "I am having a nightmare," one is no longer having a *nightmare.* Lucidity calms the mind and body and *makes* dreams safe. *Learning that dreams are safe, involves, in effect, learning not to fear one's own mental activity* [emphasis added]. This fearlessness should lead to a relaxation of defensiveness in encountering oneself. When students learn that the mind is a free, safe, and private "space," permitting many options, they may use dreams . . . to generate new ideas and solutions to problems.[8]   JUDITH MALAMUD

When you become familiar with your mind in meditation, and therefore discover the basic goodness of your mind, you make that crucial step into learning not to fear your own mental activity—as it's revealed in meditation, dream, or life. You learn that your dreams are safe and basically good because your mind is safe and basically good. You've made friends with your good mind. The master Tsongkhapa offers the essence of this stage:

> Whenever anything of a threatening or traumatic nature occurs in a dream [or you generate it] such as drowning in water or being burned by fire, recognize the dream as a dream and ask yourself, "How can dream water or dream

fire possibly harm me?" Make yourself jump or fall into
the water or fire in the dream. Examine the water, stones,
or fire, and remind yourself of how even though that
phenomenon appears to the mind, it does not exist in the
nature of its appearance. Similarly all dream phenomenon
appear to the mind but are empty of an inherently existent
self nature. Meditate on all dream objects in this way.[9]

In other words, realize that on an absolute level, you have nothing to
fear. This practice connects to bardo yoga, where a central teaching
of *The Tibetan Book of the Dead* is "Emptiness cannot harm emptiness." You don't have anything to fear with the "terrifying visions of
the intermediate state" once you wake up to the fact that they're all
projections of your own mind—just like in a dream.

Fear is the primordial emotion of samsara. It generates the
defensive self-contraction that gives birth to samsara, because fear
gives birth to the defensive ego, the false contracted sense of self.
When the Upanishads say, "Where there is other, there is fear," the
immediate implication is that "where there is *self,* there is fear." You
can't have one (self) without the "other." Self and other (duality)
co-emerge. While we may not be working directly with this primordial fear at this stage of dream yoga, we are engaging an expression
of it and beginning the path of transformation. We're getting close.

Fear is also the active emotive expression of ignorance, so we can
use fear as a way to transcend ignorance. As we saw earlier, it's very
difficult to detect ignorance directly. It's a blind spot. While ignorance may be hard to spot, fear is not, so we can use fear to lead us to
ignorance and help us transform it. Fear and ignorance are virtually
synonymous. We're always afraid of what we don't know. For example, we might be afraid of going to a dangerous country, or having
surgery, because we don't know what might happen. Fear also manifests as anxiety. We feel anxious about a job interview, a blind date,
a big trip, or a performance because we don't know how it will go.
With this stage of dream yoga practice not only are we able to transform our nightmares, we're able to work with the essence of any
nightmare (which is reification), and that includes the nightmare
of samsara.

Stage 5

When you become lucid, arise as a deity, or whatever sacred image has meaning to you. See yourself as a sacred form. Unlike the previous four stages, which emphasize outer dream objects, with this stage you're working directly with your dream body. For Buddhists who already do deity yoga, or generation stage meditations, this is a great way to extend that practice into the night. As a second step, if somebody else appears in your dream, transform *them* into a deity or sacred image.[10]

Guru Rinpoche said, "While apprehending the dream-state, consider 'Since this is now a dream-body, it can be transformed in any way.' Whatever arises in the dream, be they demonic apparitions, monkeys, people, dogs, and so on, meditatively transform them into your chosen deity. Practice multiplying them and changing them into anything you like."[11]

Why do this? To change the way you view yourself and others—to elevate your sense of identity, and to actualize the divinity within yourself and others. This is called practicing the "pride of the deity," and it's a more accurate way to view yourself and others.[12] We're always taking ourselves and others down, exercising a poverty mentality. We constantly berate ourselves with self-deprecating "mantras" like "I'm a loser. I can't do anything. No one will ever love me. I'm worthless." And we often feel the same toward others. We malign people, gossip, and engage in all manner of criticism. We use our profane outlook to degrade ourselves and others.

Visualizing yourself and others as a deity in your dreams counteracts this destructive view. Instead of dragging everybody down, you lift everybody up. In Vajrayana Buddhism this is also called the practice of "pure perception," or "sacred outlook," where your normal poverty mentality is transformed into a wealth mentality. You practice seeing people and things as perfectly pure, as they truly are, which is what the deity represents.

This stage of dream yoga is a "fake it till you make it" practice. It's hard to immediately see ourselves and others as deities, as expressions of perfect goodness (the clear-light mind), so we fake it. But we're using an imaginary template that matches reality. This dream appearance is in harmony with reality. In other words, you really are a deity, and so am I. The world really is sacred. If you could see things in the light of the clear-light mind, not only would you see yourself and others as illusory, you would also see yourself and others as perfectly pure, like a deity. This practice helps us recover our true identity. It doesn't mean people literally appear as sacred cartoon images or any version of what you think a deity might look like. It means that you see through their gross material forms and into their innate divinity. W. C. Fields once said, "It ain't what they call you. It's what you answer to." This stage helps you answer properly.

With this stage of practice, we're replacing our normal view of inherent existence, which stains reality and renders it impure, with the elevated view of inherent emptiness, which cleanses reality and reveals its intrinsic purity. In other words, spiritual purity (egolessness, or emptiness) means things are purified of inherent existence (ego, or thingness). That's what it means to "wake up." Buddhas wake up *from* the impurity of seemingly inherent existence and *to* the purity of inherent emptiness. The Buddhist scholar Christopher Hatchell says this about the generation stage yogas, or what is essentially "transformation yoga," which is what we're working with at this level of dream yoga:

> Generation stage yogas are typically methods through which one begins to "generate" or "give birth" to oneself [and others] as a buddha. One method of accomplishing this is to transform one's self-image: cutting off the idea that one is an ordinary, deluded, neurotic being. This ordinary self-perception is then deliberately replaced with the "divine pride" of being a buddha who is capable of performing enlightened deeds.[13]

At a book signing years ago I asked Ken Wilber, the most widely translated philosopher in America, this question: If you suddenly realized you only had a minute left to live, what would be the irreducible expression of your teaching? Ken is famous for his vast intellect and complex theoretical mind. What he said surprised me. "Hug the person next to you and realize you're hugging a deity."

The power of this stage of dream yoga became apparent to me about twenty years ago when I was studying Carlos Castaneda. I was reading about "inorganic beings," those otherworldly creatures in the world of Don Juan (Castaneda's teacher) that feed off of fear. One night I had a dream where I was standing on the shore of Lake Michigan, on the beach where I grew up. As I was looking at the lake, a chilling and unusual offshore breeze whipped up. The wind was blowing off the land and out onto the water. I became lucid because this was a dreamsign. Winds don't normally blow this way. The gale churned up whitecaps, and an eerie feeling came over me. I knew something bad was about to happen. As I looked across the lake, I could make out the form of something about to emerge from the water. Suddenly this hideous monster appeared, like a creature from the black lagoon of my mind, and came directly toward me. I backed away from the shore terrified, and as I did so the creature came at me faster. It was then that I realized this was an inorganic being who was feeding on my fear.

Because my lucidity was fairly strong, I had the presence of mind to visualize myself as the wrathful Tibetan deity Vajrayogini, and I morphed my dream body into this wrathful form. Vajrayogini is a major deity in Kagyu Buddhism, and it was a deity yoga I had been practicing for months. As I arose in that wrathful form, a sense of immutable strength arose with it, and the inorganic being who was now just a few feet away dissolved before my dream eyes. At that moment I woke up. My heart was pounding from the mixture of fear and the thrill of my inner sense of power.[14] I woke up and realized that there's an indestructible aspect of my being, the Vajrayogini within, that nothing can harm.

I have no idea if that was an inorganic being (I doubt it, because I don't believe in them) or merely an aspect of my unconscious mind arising in that terrifying form. It doesn't matter. What matters was what I was able to do with my fear. Even though I backed away from it initially, I took my stand and faced it directly with a truer aspect of my being—the indomitable Vajrayogini within me.[15]

On a more earthly level, another aspect of stage 5 is to exercise flexibility in identity. So in addition to morphing your body into a deity, morph it into *any* other body. Then take that dream body and make it tall, short, fat, or skinny. Once again, becoming more flexible is the product of good yoga.

In daily life you can be many things to many people. Depending on the situation, you can "arise" as a father, husband, son, brother, uncle, nephew, boss, employee, friend, or enemy. This happens instantaneously. You can be manifesting as a husband to your wife when your child approaches. In an instant, you transform into a father in an effort to relate better to your child.

This capability to manifest in whatever form is needed is the essence of the Buddhist concept of *upaya,* or "skillful means." Upaya is the ability to see others eye-to-eye, to meet them where *they* are, instead of where we want them to be. George Bernard Shaw said, "The single biggest problem in communication is the illusion that it has taken place." If we want to reach somebody, let alone teach them, we have to connect. That won't happen if we talk over their heads and preach our ideologies, or talk below them in a patronizing or condescending way. If we have the flexibility to manifest in a way that speaks to someone, we can truly help them. This often means becoming more like them. For example, to communicate with a child, we temporarily become childlike; to relate to an executive, we become more professional; to connect to a blue-collar worker, we speak their language.

Dream yoga can show you that you're not just one fixed being, but a spectrum of beings. By imagining yourself as another being in your dreams—not even a deity, just another persona—you're exercising your ability to present yourself differently. Dreams can therefore open us to seeing things, and expressing ourselves, in ways that we might never conceive of in the rigid waking state.

In our context, "persona"—and its cognate, "personality"—refers to all the different masks, or forms, we put on the formless awareness of the clear-light mind. We don these different masks anyway as we walk through life—why not take control over the ones we put on?

Changing our body in a dream has another application on the path. One way to dissolve a singular sense of self (ego) is to don multiple selves, and to therefore witness how fluid, and therefore erroneous, our solid, lasting, and independent sense of self truly is. Like a good actor, we take on the roles necessary to live successfully on the stage of life. In a lucid dream, we can switch our entire body as quickly as we switch thoughts, and we can therefore see just how malleable and expansive our sense of identity is.

This malleability is an expression of emptiness, or egolessness, which has the potential to be anything. When you realize the no-thingness of your self, you can express that no-thingness *voluntarily* into any thing (form) you want, which is what's exercised at this stage of dream yoga. The delightful Lama Yeshe, upon hearing that one of his students was a filmmaker, said to him, "Oh, you make TV, movies? I good actor. I best actor!" he laughed. "I can be anything, you see, because I am empty. I am nothing."[16]

So when a moment of poverty mentality sweeps over you, remember that you're not a loser, a failure, or any other derogatory epithet you fixate upon (and therefore continue to reify) through habitual patterns of negativity. You're a buddha, a deity, or any other nickname for the divine. You are divinity, period. You just don't know it. This stage helps you to know it by removing the fixations you have about yourself.

Change the way you see yourself. Expand your sense of identity.[17]

> The main focus of dream yoga is to realize the union of relative truth and absolute truth, appearance and emptiness.

DZIGAR KONGTRUL RINPOCHE

15

Higher Attainment
More Stages of Dream Yoga

THE FOLLOWING STAGES represent graduate school dream yoga, so don't worry if these advanced stages never enter your practice. But if you have had success with the earlier stages, you might be surprised how accessible these final stages can become. With perseverance and practice, you might find yourself in graduate school.

Stage 6

Enter into the body of another dream character. See through their eyes, feel with their body. This takes expressions like "step into their shoes" or "I'm just not that into you" to a new level, because you're stepping into another person's entire being. Why do this? Because it develops empathy and compassion.

A girl who was struggling with why a boy wasn't interested in her reports the following dream that helped her understand. Before going to sleep she was wondering why the young man was so reserved toward her. Whether she knew it or not, she was practicing a form of dream incubation. When she became lucid, she floated out of her dream body and into his dream body.

> I saw how he perceived me, the effect I had on him,
> and the feelings he had for me. I saw the conflict he
> was in . . . When I had watched his thoughts and seen
> myself through his eyes, I understood why he had been
> so reserved with me, and I realized that he would never
> return my feelings.[1]

The dream helped her resolve her feelings and develop empathy for the boy. It also brought a more realistic relationship.

I find this stage very difficult. It poses challenging questions for me. Is there a "they're" there, or is the dream person totally a projection of my mind? Is this stage a truth-teller for me? Does it reveal my inability to feel empathy and compassion? Even though I can't do it, I still try. Just attempting to step into another person's shoes gets me out of myself and into others. I'm still practicing empathy, even though I can't accomplish this stage. I'm allowing my failure to teach me, and to reveal my blind spots.

This brings us back to an important point. For many people, enlightenment, or nonduality, is a vague concept and an even more vague potentiality. We don't really know what it is, or how realistic it might be. We think maybe it's just a myth, for those in the glorious past, or for the spiritually elite. If enlightenment exists, it surely doesn't exist right here and now. We think maybe we can glimpse it toward the end of our life or in some future life. Just like we don't take responsibility for how we actualize our confusion and its resulting view of duality, we don't take responsibility for actualizing wisdom and its view of nonduality.

Because of our foggy view, we unwittingly defer enlightenment. We forget that nonduality—just like duality—is something we *practice*. Enlightenment is the stabilization of enlightened qualities that you can cultivate now. Whenever you act with kindness and compassion, whenever you display generosity and peace, whenever you manifest virtue and goodness, you are becoming increasingly familiar with, and therefore stabilizing, the enlightened state. All the noble qualities that comprise enlightenment are within us at this instant, and pop up now and again. Our task is to have them pop up more frequently and to keep them up.

This view of the immediacy of enlightenment is both a blessing and a curse. The blessing is that enlightenment is available. It is not a myth. It's temporarily realized whenever we express it, or practice the enlightened qualities that comprise it. This means that the sooner we make enlightenment a conscious practice—the sooner we cultivate enlightened qualities of love, selflessness, patience, compassion, and the like—the sooner we'll realize enlightenment. So the blessing is that it's up to us. It's our responsibility. And we can do it.

The curse is that it's up to us. It's our responsibility. And most of us only half-heartedly want to do it. Enlightenment sounds good on paper, but not if we have to give up so many comfortable bad habits and work to replace them with good habits. No one is going to give us enlightenment. No one is going to stabilize our mind, open our heart, and inject us with wisdom. We have to earn it.[2]

Many times I realize I have a choice, but because of the power of habit, I default into my established practice of samsara. I often prefer to sleep and to practice duality with my mindlessness and self-ishness. But as I progress along the path, and replace unconscious habits of confusion with conscious habits of wisdom, those times become less and less. I'm gradually defaulting into the good habit of selflessness, because I'm actively practicing it.

When we venerate the buddhas, we're paying homage to the extraordinary discipline, perseverance, tenacity, courage, and raw effort that went into stabilizing their enlightened qualities—the exact same qualities that are within us right now and that await our development. Buddhas are people who woke up to the fact that in order to attain enlightenment they had to practice it. They worked hard to counteract their selfish tendencies until selfless tendencies took over. When they felt the urge to grasp, they replaced that with the practice of release. When they felt the tendency to succumb to mindlessness, they replaced that with the practice of mindfulness. Just like with mindfulness, illusory form, and any other spiritual practice, they realized that the effortful stage matures into the effortless stage and eventually into the spontaneous stage, when they "suddenly" realize they've become a buddha.

So even though I fail miserably at this stage of dream yoga, I continue to work at it because I realize that enlightenment is more about mechanics than it is about magic. It's about deliberate choices, and deciding to act in an enlightened way now.

Stage 7

Create a special dream body. The last three stages of dream yoga require stability, focus, and vivid lucidity. In the spirit of advanced yoga, they are a stretch. Even if we can't do these final stages, they show us what we can aspire toward.

At stage 7 you create a special dream body, which is made out of prana-mind, and project it to different places.[3] Remember that this is what the Buddha reputedly did as he slept, often traveling to Tushita heaven to teach his mother. The idea is that you can project your dream body to distant places on this earth, or into other dimensions. The Dalai Lama says, "There is such a thing as a 'special dream state.' In that state the 'special dream body' is created from the mind and from *vital energies* (known in Sanskrit as prana) within the body. This special dream body is able to disassociate from the gross physical body and travel elsewhere . . . This is not just imagination; the subtle self actually departs from the gross body."[4]

How does one practice this? The details are best left for those who do the Vajrayana meditations that describe it, such as the practice manuals for the Six Yogas of Naropa. The basic idea is that during the day, you work to become familiar with the place you want to go, almost stamping your mind with the landscape. Then, drawing on the power of intention or aspiration, you say, "I will recognize my dreams to be dreams. I will transfer my dream body to [fill in the blank] and receive teachings to benefit others." The intention to benefit others is helpful, because it conveys that you're not doing this for your own entertainment. Kongtrul Rinpoche says that devotion, faith, and intention are the keys to this celestial form of travel. These ingredients provide the postage. You then go to sleep, and when you become lucid, you Fed-Ex your consciousness, your special dream body, to virtually any place you can imagine. You quite literally "overnight" it.[5]

Understanding the empty, and therefore magical, nature of reality is central to success at this stage. It is often taught that with an understanding of emptiness, almost anything is possible. Without it, not much is possible.

The special dream body can observe physical beings, but most beings cannot observe the dream body. Some teachers whimsically state that this would make the special dream body the perfect spy.[6]

Stage 8

Meditate in your lucid dream and achieve self-liberation. This advanced stage is especially subtle. It reveals how stable your mind truly is. While you're awake, you can meditate using the anchor of your body or an external object. There's something steady to return to. But in dreams you have a fickle mental body that flickers about like a candle in the wind and "external" dream objects that change as rapidly as the mind that observes them—because they are the display of that very same mind. There's nothing externally steady to come back to. There is no hitching post. The only stability in a dream is the stability of your mind. But with increasing steadiness and lucidity, developed by your daily meditations and the previous stages of dream yoga, you can start to meditate in your dreams.

A general rule for sustaining lucidity in a dream is to keep engaging the dream and to keep moving; a general rule for meditation, by contrast, is stillness. Reducing dream content and activity therefore tends to dissolve the dream. So in this stage, you really have to walk the fine line of "not too tight, not too loose."

Start your meditation by practicing a witness awareness. Watch what appears in your dream, but without getting sucked into it. This is akin to witnessing the contents of your mind dispassionately in your daily practice. Let whatever happens happen. You're practicing a type of witnessing dream, but without any entertainment value. It's more objective. If you feel yourself being pulled in, gently back out and watch the dream images arise and dissolve impartially, without grasping onto anything.

Why do this? Because witnessing the contents of your mind with equanimity—with disinterestedness—is the secret to liberation. Disinterestedness is not apathy, but detachment. This stage therefore works with grasping and fixation, which are the basis of our suffering.

I've tried to hold my mind onto lucid dream images for as long as possible, like a nightly version of practicing mindfulness meditation with an object ("referential shamatha"). While the dream image does get more vivid and intense for a few seconds, it tends to make my dreams fall apart, and I end up either waking up or slipping into a non-lucid dream. You can see how difficult this is when you realize that one technique for waking yourself up from a lucid dream is to stare at a dream object, and therefore stop your dream eye movements. Keeping your dream eyes fixed also keeps your physical eyes fixed, which stops the REM that defines most dreaming and causes you to wake up.

Holding my dream eyes onto a dream object is akin to what happens if I try to hold a thought or image during the day. It fades away. Deity yoga during a dream is different because I'm moving my mind across the image of myself as a deity, and because there's often the sense of being the deity (pride of the deity) without focusing too intently on any aspect of it. But some texts do say that one should generate a dream object and concentrate on that. If you can do it, try to remain free of all mental content other than the image. It would be like visualizing an apple now and holding that visualization as clearly and persistently as you can.

Another initial practice is to work with walking meditation, or some other mindful movement, in your dream. Participation or movement helps sustain the dream, while mindfulness of that movement turns it into a meditation. Try slowing down the mindful movement and see what happens. Does the dream fall apart? Can you keep the lucidity as the movement diminishes? Once again, you become your own meditation instructor.

Why do you want to meditate in your dreams? Namkhai Norbu Rinpoche gives one reason:

> Many of the methods of practicing Dharma that are
> learned during waking can, upon development of
> dream awareness, be applied in the dream condition.
> In fact, one may develop these practices more easily
> and speedily within the dream if one has the capacity
> to be lucid. There are even some books that say that

> if a person applies a practice within a dream, the
> practice is nine times more effective than when it is
> applied during the waking hours.[7]

This brings us back to an important central theme and another reason why dream yoga is so valuable. Meditation in general is about working *directly* with the mind. Most of the time the mind "works us," or more accurately, it works us over. We're constantly battered around by the contents of our mind. If we work with our mind at all during life, it's mostly indirectly. In other words, we usually relate *from* our mind instead of *to* it. Relating from our mind is no relationship at all. A thought or emotion pops up and we just go with it. That's what defines non-meditation, non-lucidity, and most of life. This is the classic "outsider's" approach.

Meditation, the way of the "insider," shows us how to relate to our mind directly. Now we're working with the internal blueprints of experience instead of the external constructs. When we work with our mind in meditation during the day, we're mostly working at the level of the psyche, which is as direct as most of us can get. It's a start. But the psyche is already a projection of both the substrate and the clear-light mind, which are the foundation of both samsara and nirvana, respectively. It's a level of mind at least twice removed from the source mind. If you can work with the substrate *directly,* let alone the clear-light mind—and these are the opportunities provided by dream and sleep yoga, respectively—you're getting as direct as you can. Now you're a real insider, totally getting the inside scoop. You're facing your mind point-blank.[8]

These dream yoga practices are exceptionally transformative because you're not working with the leaves and branches of the tree of samsara (the domain of psychology or other self-help methods). You're not even working with the trunk (classic meditation). You're working with the very roots of your entire experience. Transform the roots and you transform everything above. Patricia Garfield says, "By deliberately changing elements in your dream life, you can learn to confront many of your problems at their origin—in your own mind, rather than years later in the therapist's office."[9] Evan Thompson writes, "From a scientific perspective, lucid dreaming offers a kind of distilled consciousness, a way to examine consciousness in a preparation unmixed with current sensory input."[10]

Pierre-Simon Laplace, the French mathematician and astronomer, famously said that "the weight of the evidence must be in proportion to the strangeness of the fact." Proclaiming that you can evolve faster with practices like dream yoga is indeed a strange and radical fact, so let's add some weight. Traleg Rinpoche says that dream yoga can unleash potentials that have not been previously accessed, tapping into untapped reservoirs of wisdom. He relates that there are many stories of dream yoga practitioners maturing dramatically *in one night.* They go to sleep confused and wake up transformed.[11] The literature is replete with stories of rapid and enduring transformation. In the 2014 anthology *Lucid Dreaming: New Perspectives on Consciousness in Sleep,* Mary Ziemer says, "[Transformation] which can take years in waking physical reality, can be greatly accelerated as the psyche understands this process inwardly within a single dream."[12] In the same volume, Ryan Hurd writes, "Powerful lucid dreams stay with us for the lifespan, and may even permanently transform the personality structure."[13] Ted Esser adds, "That night—the results were immediate and life changing . . . How could it be so easy to have such a powerful experience? . . . most people who lucidly dream have the potential in short order to have experiences of their innermost selves that are consistently meaningful, inspiring, pragmatically useful, and potentially life-altering."[14]

The inner yogas of dream and sleep work with aspects of the mind that are the shortest distance between you and awakening. They are so direct, so face-to-face with the roots of samsara and nirvana, that they can offer a virtual shortcut to enlightenment. As we've emphasized before, just understanding the view alone can transform you. However, although the practice of meditation within a lucid dream is quite direct, it's also quite difficult. Quick doesn't necessarily mean easy. But if you've come this far on the dream yoga path, the potential for rapid and enduring transformation might inspire you to undertake these meditation practices and stick with them.

It is easier to develop your practices in a dream than in the daytime. In the daytime we are limited by our material body, but in a dream our function of mind and our consciousness of the senses are unhindered. We can have more clarity. Thus there are more possibilities.[15]

NAMKHAI NORBU RINPOCHE

All the stages prior to stage 8 involve some level of transformation, which is a central theme of the Vajrayana school of Buddhism. Stages 1 through 7 involve transforming the content of your dream, and therefore the contents of your mind. As profound as transformation is (it's really about changing the way you relate to your mind), it's still not the highest level. The highest levels of dream yoga (stages 8 and 9) involve self-liberation, which is associated with Dzogchen or Mahamudra, and is sometimes referred to as the "fourth vehicle (yana)," the Sahajayana, or the "vehicle of self-liberation."[16]

You can practice self-liberation in a lucid dream by either seeing right through whatever dream images arise (the apex of stage 8), liberating them on the spot, or dropping below the lucid dream altogether (stage 9). You're not interested in transforming anything. You're interested in seeing the perfect purity (the emptiness) of those contents, which instantly liberates whatever arises. With dream self-liberation, you penetrate the content with your X-ray vision and watch it vaporize before your mind's eye, like snowflakes hitting a hot rock. But vaporize does not mean euthanize. You're not trying to get rid of anything. Dream contents still appear, but they're now recognized as the empty forms of the clear-light mind that they truly are.

Khenpo Tsültrim Gyamtso Rinpoche comments,

When you are able to meditate on the inseparability of appearance and emptiness in a dream exactly as you would in the waking state, you have mastered meditation. If you can only meditate on the inseparability of appearance and emptiness during daytime experience, then your meditation does not give you [total] independence. You do not have power over your own mind . . . *Meditation is perfected only when you're able to meditate during dreams just as you meditate during the day* [emphasis added].[17]

One permutation of the self-liberating meditations is not to vaporize the content, but to follow it back to its source. This is the nighttime application of the daytime meditation we discussed earlier, where you follow your thoughts back to their source like following the rays of the sun back to the sun. Here you do the same thing, but now it's a dream image that you follow in. This is another way to dip into the clear-light mind, the never-setting sun at the core of your being, and transform dream yoga into sleep yoga, which will be the next stop on our journey. Dream images are the rays of this inner sun, and can direct you to it. Don't follow these rays out (which usually results in non-lucidity); allow them to lead you back in (which results in spiritual awakening). The central theme of "insider" versus "outsider" still applies at this most subtle level. Follow the dream image in and watch it dissolve into imageless (formless) awareness, which leaves you with nothing—the precise content of the clear-light mind.

The "sun and its rays" is a classic image in Buddhism, and suggests how infinite rays radiate from a single source but remain in constant contact with it, even in their apparent separation from it. Once again, appearance is not in harmony with reality. Thoughts and dream images are not separate from the clear-light mind. They are forever the shine of that mind, but they lose their luster and connection as we lose ourselves in them and head out and away from that luminous source.

> One benefit of meditating in your dreams is that you can literally start to practice 24/7. You no longer have an excuse that you don't have time to meditate, though this subtle practice may well reveal that you *want* an excuse!

Stage 9

Rest in the clear-light mind. The last stage of dream yoga is to drop below the psyche (which means any level of dream), and then below the substrate (the relative source of the dream), to finally rest in the pristine awareness of the clear-light mind. You let go of all dream images and rest in the awareness of awareness. Dzigar Kongtrül Rinpoche says that the apex of dream yoga is to dissolve all dream appearances and rest in the nature of mind. (For those who do form-less meditations like Mahamudra or Dzogchen, this is where you can practice these advanced "completion stage" meditations during dreams.) This final stage of dream yoga bridges into the domain of sleep yoga, which we'll discuss in detail in chapters 17 and 18. It also reaches into bardo yoga, where this dissolution of all form into formlessness (formless awareness) occurs spontaneously when we die, which we'll discuss in chapter 20.

What do you do once you reach the clear-light mind? Just relax, or "die," into the absolute nature of your mind. Rest in absolute peace, a state of effortless non-distracted non-meditation. You can then pop back up (take "rebirth") into a dream and do whatever you want as you form that formless awareness into countless dream forms. When you take the clear-light mind with you, dreams are instantly lucid. Then you can drop back down and rest again in the sumptuous bed of the clear-light mind.[18]

If these ultimate esoteric stages feel like more than you bargained for when you picked up a book about dream yoga, don't worry about them. Don't worry about any stage that doesn't resonate with you. If you can engage any stage and make it your practice, celebrate that. But this is a glimpse of what's possible. Now you can see why His Holiness the First Karmapa realized enlightenment via dream yoga. It is a complete path.

We don't say that what you experience in your
waking state has greater reality than what happens
in your dreams. Both experiences are equally real.

LAMA YESHE, *Life, Death, and After Death*

16

Near Enemies and Other Obstacles

EVERY DREAM PRACTITIONER faces common challenges.
One pervasive and insidious challenge is that our culture doesn't
support dream practice. "It's just a dream" is usually a dismissive
comment. As psychologist Rubin Naiman says, we have a "wake-
centric cultural bias." What would happen if we shifted to embrace a
"sleep-centric" attitude as being equally valid, and fully incorporated
this large aspect of our lives onto the path?

Many of the dream scientists I know were strongly discouraged
by their mentors and peers from making dreams the focus of their
work, because the academic community tends to similarly dismiss
the importance of dreams. Because dreams are unreal, they're considered unimportant. Our journey has been to reverse this stance.
In an effort to do this, we're challenging the status of waking reality,
cutting it down to size, while simultaneously elevating the importance of our dreams. If we're careful, we can almost say we're trying
to reify our dreams as a way to de-reify waking reality.

In the West, dreams for the most part are seen as entertaining,
disruptive, or mildly informative—but fundamentally inconsequential. We're never taught how to dream or how to nurture this
rich inner world. We're never told that dreams can be engaged for

self-fulfillment, let alone self-transcendence. Most Westerners have no idea that they can use the night to radically transform the day.

This unfortunate relationship to dreams is slowly changing as science continues to substantiate the power of lucid dreaming. It will continue to improve as dream yoga gains a stronger foothold and as therapists continue to help people with dream interpretation. But as a culture, the West has been asleep for a very long time and is slow to wake up to the transformative power of dreams.

In the indigenous Senoi culture of Malaysia, dreams play a central role. Children are taught to honor their dreams, and every morning the discussion at breakfast is, "What did you dream last night?" A Senoi boy is not considered to be a man until his dream characters cooperate with him, and eventually serve him. Because the dialogue is so open to the dream world, this deeper aspect of mind has a respected podium to inform waking life. At the same time, violence is almost unheard of within the Senoi people. They are unusually peaceful, cooperative, and highly creative. It's difficult to determine how much of this can be attributed to their sophisticated interrelationship between dreaming consciousness and waking consciousness, but the correlation is striking. In most cultures, dream life is lifeless. As Senoi children mature, it grows more positive and influential every year.[1]

Near Enemies

The path of dream yoga, and spirituality altogether, is littered with booby-traps called "near enemies." They are insidious snares, because they're so near to the virtuous qualities they shadow. Every noble quality has an ignoble side. Wherever you find light, you will find shadows. For example, the near enemy of compassion is pity, the near enemy of confidence is arrogance, with intelligence it's hyper-criticality, with equanimity can come apathy, with spaciousness you often find spaciness. Once you're sensitized to them, you'll start to find near enemies everywhere.

Nihilism

One of the principal near enemies of dream yoga and illusory form is nihilism.[2] When we say that "Everything is a dream" or "It's all an illusion," we might easily append that with "So who cares?" or "It doesn't matter what I do." This is called "losing the conduct in the view." We need to integrate view and conduct. Guru Rinpoche said, "Your view should be as vast as the sky, and your conduct as fine as barley powder."

Nihilism is an obstacle to spiritual practice because it doesn't acknowledge the immutable laws of karma, or relative truth. Things do appear, and those relative appearances follow strict physical and karmic laws. Although everything is illusory from an absolute perspective, this view has to be balanced with relative truth and a life that's lived within the realm of appearances. Mistaking the difference between nihilism and the understanding that everything is illusory, a naïve oneironaut could end up shirking their worldly responsibilities, doing whatever they want, and accruing vast negative karma as they go merrily down the stream and eventually down the karmic toilet.

Dream yoga may wake you up to a world where nothing is real, but once again that no-thingness is not nothingness. The dreamlike nature of reality is fluid, but it's not sloppy. When you finally wake up spiritually, the razor-sharp mind that cut through appearances and led you to awakening is called "discriminating awareness wisdom." It's a quality of mind that is extremely precise and discerning.

On a practical level, without discriminating awareness wisdom, someone with a spiritually nihilistic tinge might tell a person who is suffering that their pain is an illusion. That's an expression of ignorance, not compassion. Use the illusory worldview gained through dream yoga to inform you of the absolute nature of things, but then conjoin that vision with the granularity of relative life. True wisdom (the absolute) is always in union with compassion and skillful means (the relative). You want to transcend but include the relative, not transcend and exclude.

Spiritual Bypassing

"Spiritual bypassing," a term coined by the psychologist John Welwood, is another near enemy, and an obstacle in the practices of dream yoga and illusory form. Spiritual bypassing is when you use spiritual ideas or practices to avoid, or prematurely transcend, relative human needs, feelings, personal issues, or developmental tasks. Nonduality needs to honor duality, or it becomes sterile and disconnected. It becomes, as Welwood puts it, "A one-sided transcendentalism that uses nondual terms and ideas to bypass the challenging work of personal transformation. It uses absolute truth to disparage relative truth, emptiness to devalue form, and oneness to belittle individuality."[3] It abuses the dreamlike nature of reality to dismiss difficult relative concerns. The spiritual is used to degrade the material. Spiritual bypassing engenders spiritual elitism, and an even more hazardous escapism.

The spiritual psychologist A. H. Almaas says, "When we embark on a spiritual path, we unconsciously believe that we are setting out for heaven."[4] In other words, most of us want out of the bitter experiences of life, and a dreamlike reality sounds delicious. We enter the spiritual path to get out of our suffering, but in our desire to get out, we often cop out. We lose touch with the relative world as we ascend toward our version of heaven. Because spiritual practitioners often associate suffering with materialism, anything anti-matter sounds good. Dream yoga and illusory form do transcend matter, and therefore suffering, so they're easy prey for this disorder.

Differentiation Versus Dissociation

Dissociation is the near enemy of differentiation. Spiritual practices, such as dream yoga and illusory form, allow us to differentiate, rather than dissociate, from the world of form and the suffering associated with it. We also differentiate from the superficial psyche, and then the substrate, as we descend into our absolute identity as the clear-light mind. This is the inner meaning of "retreat," which means to "draw back." We're drawing back, or differentiating, from these false levels of identification. But we don't want to slip into dissociation and the rejection that is virtually synonymous with it. We don't want to dissociate, and therefore reject, project, or repress the psyche and the substrate. Cutting through the psyche and substrate does not mean cutting and throwing away.

Turning Near Enemies into Near Friends

At the highest levels of spiritual accomplishment, when we realize our absolute identity as the clear-light mind and become a buddha, we then use that light (and its penetrating insight) to illuminate the psyche. We transform an obstacle to the clear-light mind into an opportunity that can lead others to it. In other words, we continue to engage the psyche as a way to communicate with others still exclusively identified with it.

If you try to communicate with others who are still asleep (stuck at the level of the psyche), and you're operating from the perspective of the awakened clear-light mind, they may not hear you.[5] So you engage the psyche of others, meeting them where they're at, with your own awakened psyche. Just because you've seen through it doesn't mean you should reject it, or that you can't use it. Indeed, you use the psyche to its fullest capacity as a vehicle for reaching others. You use it, but you no longer let it use you. That's skillful means.[6]

The idea here is that every near enemy has a near friend. This is another beautiful two-way (bi-directional) street. Once you're sensitized to the idea of near enemies, you'll also start to discover near friends. With every shadow element there's always light. And with the vision of the clear-light mind, you can find it. Look for the light within the dark. It's there.[7]

For example, when someone is angry, look for the sharp mind behind the critical statements. That sharp and incisive quality is healthy. When someone seems arrogant, look for the confidence. Within apathy lurks the potential for equanimity; behind pity is the promise of compassion. This doesn't mean you're blind to the confusion, but it does suggest you don't buy into it.

How do you manage nihilism, spiritual bypassing, and other near enemies? First, be aware of them. When you identify them in your life, shake hands with them. This alone can turn enemies into friends. For example, when you notice you're starting to dismiss the world with your illusory form practice, smile at that tendency and realize it's a common trap. Then work to dismiss the *solidity* of the world, not the world itself.

Second, realize that the final stage of the path is not some distant heaven, but finding heaven on earth. In other words, return to this material earth—to your thoughts, your relationships, your job, and your daily life—infused with your spiritual realization. Know that in order to complete the path, you have to pull a U-turn and head back into that which you initially fled. You may have started the path unwittingly setting out for a distant heaven, but with genuine awakening you wittingly realize heaven is within yourself, and right here on earth. This is how to unite heaven and earth, the absolute with the relative. Bring your nirvana back to samsara and realize their ultimate inseparability.

REALITY IS NOT A DREAM

Even the most perfect analogy is still not the real thing. So proclaiming that "reality is a dream" holds a subtle danger. It's almost unavoidable to take our reifying tendencies, the very ones we're trying to transcend with these practices, and transfer those tendencies to solidify the notion that reality is a dream. Reality is not a dream. It is completely ineffable. Whatever we can say about it, it isn't.

Emptiness is the antidote to seeing things as truly existent, but emptiness itself is also empty. This is called the "emptiness of emptiness." You can't hang your hat on anything, not even emptiness. Don't shrink reality into any concept, analogy, metaphor, doctrine, or philosophy. Khenpo Rinpoche writes,

> Not to know the equality of appearance-emptiness
> And get attached to appearances alone is delusion
> But to get attached to emptiness alone is delusion too
> If you know the equality of appearance-emptiness
> There's no need to get caught up in or give up phenomena
> Those appearances and emptiness
> What you must do is rest in the spaciousness
> Of the equality of appearance-emptiness.[8]

Experience, especially of absolute reality, is inexpressible. Even on a relative level, experience is fundamentally indescribable. You can try to describe the taste of a Snickers bar, for example, till you're blue in the face. But until someone actually takes a bite, they'll never know what you're talking about. Writers do their best, as do poets, musicians, dancers, or artists. But reality can never be captured in something as tiny as the written word, or a poem, a symphony, a dance, or a painting. Try describing an orgasm or snow to someone who has never felt the bliss or experienced the cold. How much more difficult it is to describe the nature of mind and reality to someone who has never experienced it.

Reality is dream*like*. It is not a dream. Reality is not an illusion. It is illusory. As the masters warn, "Self-liberate even the antidote." Saying that reality is like a dream is the antidote to saying that it's solid, lasting, and independent. Now release that antidote. The Dzogchen master Khenpo Tenpa Yungdrung says, "Always remember that illusion itself is an illusion."

We're trying to melt our solid view of reality, a view that causes so much unnecessary suffering. Replacing that view with one that is dreamlike is not the definitive view. There is no definitive view, because any view will always be conceptual and therefore provisional.[9] Seeing reality as dreamlike is a big step on the progressive stages of meditation on reality, but if we reify anything, we're still missing the mark. The mark can only be hit with direct experience, not with any doctrine. Doctrine points us in the right direction, like a finger pointing to the moon. But don't mistake the finger for the moon.

The best thing that any teaching can do is inspire you to meditate. It's only when you transcend concept altogether that the experience of reality unfolds. That's another definition of emptiness: things are empty of our ideas about them, reality is empty or free of our conceptual imputations. Then you truly see. And when you try to convey what you see, you might say to others, "Well . . . it's like a dream."

Overcoming Some Practical Obstacles

From these general obstacles let's turn to some practical ones. In dream yoga, we're dealing with subtle states of mind, and we're trying to turn around a lot of momentum behind seeing the world as solid, lasting, and independent. It's hard to wake up from the force of these bad habits. You can't stop a freight train on a dime. Dream yoga takes patience, perseverance, and the willingness to be exposed.

View, Meditations, Attitude, and Motivation

If you're feeling impatience and discouragement in your practice, an immediate remedy is to strengthen your view. Even if that view is initially a conceptual one, it's a start in the right direction. The map is not the territory—but it can lead to the territory. Read books about lucid dreaming and dream yoga. Look closely at how your old view has amounted to nothing. Develop renunciation. Take seminars and meet like-minded friends. While dream yoga is a solitary practice, you're not alone in practicing it. Others can guide you, and there are Internet forums and other "nightclubs" on lucid dreaming you can join. If your view becomes strong enough, it will cut through any obstacle.

To stay inspired, delight in small successes. If you're remembering more dreams, celebrate that. If your dreams are clearer and lasting longer, that's fantastic. If you've had your first lucid dream, rejoice in that. Reflect on the Dalai Lama's advice for anything worthwhile: "Never give up!" Merely attempting these practices reaps benefits. The nighttime meditations are about increasing awareness, which will improve even if you never have a lucid dream.

Guru Rinpoche says that the remedy for many obstacles is to train more in illusory form:

> Dreaming is induced by latent predispositions, so regard all daytime appearances as being like a dream and like an illusion . . . In particular, it is crucial to practice the instructions on daytime appearances and the illusory body. At this time, powerfully imagine that your environment, city, house, companions, conversations, and all activities are a dream . . . train in Illusory Form during the day, and accustom yourself to envisioning the dream state. As you are about to sleep, do so with the yearning "May I know the dream state as the

dream state, and not become confused." Also cultivate mindfulness, thinking, "When I am apprehending the dream state, may I not become confused."[10]

The Nyingma master Namkhai Norbu agrees, saying, "If you have not mastered the lucidity—awareness that one is dreaming while doing so—then during the day you should continually remind yourself that all that you see and all that is done is not other than a dream. By seeing everything throughout the day as if it were a dream, dream and awareness are thoroughly mixed."[11]

Lucidity practice is cumulative, which means that every night of practice, whether it ignites a lucid dream or not, adds more momentum. Just the intention to wake up in your dreams adds more weight. You're using the immutable laws of karma to your advantage. Give your mind a push toward lucidity every night, and that will eventually push open the door to the world of lucid dreams. But like any endeavor, if you stop accumulating momentum, it will fade, and the door can close.

If I don't practice formal induction techniques, my lucid dreams decrease. As a long-time meditator, however, I've seen a gradual increase of lucidity over the years as a result of my meditation and illusory form practice. I may not practice dream yoga every night, but I do meditate every day and flash onto things as being illusory as often as I can. These practices bear natural fruit at night, so this cumulative aspect continues.

So another remedy is more mindfulness meditation. Once again, if you become lucid to the contents of your mind during the day, you will become more lucid at night. Along with this, consider expanding your motivation. Persevere at dream yoga with the idea that this is not just for you; you're fundamentally doing this practice for the benefit of others. This bigger picture helps you situate any dream yoga problem, which suddenly gets smaller and more workable.

Other Tricks and Tips

A common problem with dream practices, especially at first, is getting so excited about being lucid that you wake yourself up. To prevent this, temper your emotions, look down at the ground or floor of your dream when you first become lucid, then engage the dream. Sensory engagement with the dream discourages the brain from changing states to waking consciousness. Look, listen, and feel the dream. A classic tip is to rub your dream hands together. Just as engaging your waking world in the morning pulls you out of your dream and into the world, engaging in your dream world pulls you into your dream and out of waking reality. The beginning of lucidity is also a good time to remember your goals for the dream—for instance, what stage of dream yoga you want to practice.

Another skill is that of learning to prolong the dream when it starts to fade. After some practice you'll be able to tell when the dream is starting to come apart. Often the visual aspects change by fading, losing color, or becoming more cartoon-like. The crux of sustaining lucidity, according to Scott Sparrow, is this:

> The duration of a lucid dream . . . becomes dependent upon the ability of the dreamer to maintain a balance between waking and dream consciousness. If this balance is to be achieved with any regularity the dreamer must learn to recognize and hold in abeyance the forces impinging upon him from both the waking and dream state which tend to upset the delicate balance of lucidity.[12]

It's the "middle way" theme again, which is like walking a tightrope. If you slip off the rope one way, you'll drop back into a non-lucid dream. If you slip off the other way, you'll wake up. Just like when a fantasy sucks you in during the day, if the dream draws you into its content, you'll become non-lucid. You've become too involved with the contents of your mind, which are now arising in the form of dream images. And just like in life, it's usually *movement* that sucks you in.[13] To prolong a lucid dream that is sucking you into non-lucidity, the first thing you can do is direct your attention toward unchanging aspects of the dream, like the dream ground as suggested above. Ground yourself into the dream, then look up and engage the dream.

This one-pointedness is simultaneously the product, and practice, of mindfulness. After you've grounded and "pointed" your awareness, you can look up into the dream environment without losing yourself in it. Your pointedness (mindfulness) will weaken the distracting influence of movement. With this stability, you're better equipped to engage the dream and start to work with it. If you begin to lose it, narrow your vision to one spot in the dream, or otherwise ground your awareness, and start over.[14]

This is standard meditation instruction: when you get distracted on the cushion, "lower your gaze." Instead of looking *out* and getting distracted, turn your attention *in* and re-collect. In general, balanced attention developed through mindfulness and insight meditations will contribute to your success with dream yoga. "In prototypical lucid dreaming we find the development of a simultaneous capacity for detached observation or self-reflection along with a continued 'dreamt' participation," explain the dream researchers Harry Hunt and Robert Ogilvie. "This development of a capacity for sustained self-reflection for its own sake, and the difficulty of its integration with complex ongoing involvements, also describes the goal and difficulties of the 'mindfulness' or 'insight' meditative traditions."[15]

As an alternative to grounding your awareness and practicing one-pointedness, LaBerge offers another trick to sustain lucidity when dreams start to fall apart: spin your dream body (like a whirling dervish) or move your arms around like pinwheels. You will be loading the perceptual system so it doesn't switch states from dreaming to waking. Adding a reminder that the next scene will be a lucid dream scene is also helpful in sustaining lucidity.

These techniques emphasize different approaches to sustaining lucidity. The first one emphasizes grounding your awareness with one-pointedness; the second one emphasizes bodily movement. Experiment. See what works for you.

If the dream dissolves and you find yourself awake, don't toss and turn in bed, or otherwise move your body. Movement will engage the waking state and draw you into it. Instead, vividly imagine spinning or rubbing the hands together of the dream body you just left. It's also important to add the resolute reminder that you'll soon be dreaming and that the dream will be lucid. Otherwise you may end up reestablishing the dream, but not recognize it as such.

With these tips it's possible for lucid dreaming to begin anew—that is, as a waking-induced lucid dream.

Spinning in a dream can also be used for changing scenes. While your dream vision blurs from the spinning, you can envision a scene that you'd like to be in once you stop spinning. For example, if you intend to have a healing dream, but find yourself in a scene that's too chaotic, you can conjure up an environment that feels more appropriate.

Getting involved with the dream in an effort to sustain lucidity has to be balanced with a sense of perspective, or objectivity, or you'll slip back into a non-lucid dream. Get involved, but not too involved. The more emotionally intense the dream, the worse people do at maintaining lucidity because they tend to get sucked in. So remind yourself, "This is a dream. I'm lucid in this dream. I know I'm dreaming." In the world of lucid dreaming, rationality and objectivity trumps emotionality.

Continue to convince yourself that you're dreaming by doing things you couldn't do in waking life. This is where the practices of dream yoga come in. Not only do these practices transform lucid dreaming into dream yoga, but they also help you stay lucid in the dream because you're actively working with it, and doing things that are impossible in waking reality, things that remind you it's just a dream.

The Dalai Lama offers this general tip: "If your sleep is too deep, your dreams will not be very clear. In order to bring about clearer dreams and lighter sleep, you should eat somewhat less. On the other hand, if your sleep is too light . . . you should take heavier, oilier food." I've found that to keep my dreams clearer, and my sleep lighter, there's nothing better than to sleep sitting up. Namkhai Norbu shares these tips about how to avoid sleep that seems dreamless because it is too deep:

> In this case, place the pillows higher using lighter or
> fewer covers, let more air and/or light into the sleeping
> place or move to a more open spot. If dreams do not
> come regularly, you may experiment by sleeping in
> whichever way you find comfortable, on either the
> right or the left side. If dreams still do not come,

concentrate on the throat chakra, and visualize a red "A"; if this is difficult, a red ball will suffice. If you still do not remember dreams, visualize the red letter or bead as increasingly more luminous each successive night. If difficulty persists, think of a white bead on your forehead, at the location of the third eye. If there is still nothing, visualize the white bead with increasing radiance each successive night.[16]

Once you start to believe in your dreams and initiate the dialogue, you can expect to find a ready conversationalist in your deeper self. Experiment with the tips and techniques in this chapter to see what works for you. Respect your dreams and you'll bring them to life. If you strengthen your view, practice meditations such as mindfulness and illusory form, and fortify your motivation, you will succeed. No obstacle can withstand these antidotes.

There is that most divine knowledge of God which takes place through ignorance, in the union which is above intelligence, when the intellect quitting all things that are, and then leaving itself also, is united to the superlucent rays, being illuminated thence and therein by the unsearchable depth of wisdom.

DIONYSIUS THE AREOPAGITE quoted in *The Principal Upanisads*

17

An Introduction to Sleep Yoga

JUST AS DREAM yoga is a step beyond lucid dreaming, sleep yoga is a step beyond dream yoga. It's called "sleep yoga" because it brings lucidity or awareness into deep *dreamless* sleep. And while lucid dreaming constitutes partial lucidity, lucid sleep constitutes full lucidity. Dreaming is sometimes called the "gateway" to infinity; the subtle practice of sleep yoga fully deposits you into infinity. In the education of the night, accomplishing sleep yoga is like getting your doctorate. The Dalai Lama said, "Going through this transition without blacking out is one of the highest accomplishments for a yogi."[1]

MIND WITHOUT DISTRACTION

Practitioners who are not distracted (lost in "sleep") during the day are also not distracted (lost in mindless sleep) at night. We have this account from the seventeenth-century master Samten Gyatso:

I really have no great qualities, nothing marvelous to boast of, except that my distraction has vanished . . . I still have one problem, though: maintaining awareness in the brief period between falling asleep and actually sleeping. There are a few moments in which I still lose presence of mind and the awakened state is briefly lost. But once sleep begins, the awakened state is recognized and remains stable through the whole night. The only challenge left now is that one small gap just as I fall asleep.[2]

And another from the master Karsey Kongtrul some four centuries later:

I have reached a level where the entire valley of Tsurphu appears as the mandala of Chakrasamvara and with each passing day conceptual thoughts are fewer and farther between. Now there is only one problem left: I still lose presence of mind in the moment of falling asleep. It lasts no more than a couple of seconds, but I am sorry to admit I do become unaware. Apart from that, this mind no longer gets distracted at any time, day or night.[3]

Mind of Clear Light, Mind of Awareness

The Dzogchen teachings say that dream yoga is a secondary practice to sleep yoga. The primary practice is "the practice of natural light"—another way of saying "the practice of the clear-light mind." Dream yoga is considered secondary because if you accomplish sleep yoga, dream yoga naturally occurs. You're automatically lucid in your dreams. There may come a point where sleep yoga develops spontaneously for you, but don't worry if it never enters your meditative curriculum. It's not for everybody.

While lucid dreaming and dream yoga work mostly with levels of the unconscious just below the psyche, sleep yoga works mostly with the deeper levels of the substrate and the clear-light mind.[4] This is why in the Tibetan tradition, sleep yoga is referred to as "luminosity yoga": it's dealing with the luminous nature of the awakened mind. Almost everywhere you look in Buddhism, you'll find terms—such as "clear-light mind," "luminosity," and "enlightenment"—that suggest the intimate relationship between awakening, light, and mind.[5] In Buddhism, "light" is virtually synonymous with "awareness."[6]

It bears repeating that when we talk about the clear-light mind, we are *not* talking about physical light. What we are talking about is the light of the mind, which is difficult to describe. It's not a light that is seen in the usual sense (which would be dualistic), but it's a light that sees itself, illumination that illuminates itself, awareness that is aware of itself (which is nondualistic). In this case the light is nondual awareness, or reflexively aware wisdom, as described in the *Kena Upanishad:*

> What no speech can express, but what expresses speech . . . What none can comprehend with the mind, but by which, the sages say, the mind is comprehended . . . what none can see with the eyes, but by which one sees . . . what none can hear with the ears, but by which hearing is perceived . . .[7]

During the day we see the things of the world illuminated by the sun. In the darkness of sleep, what illuminates the objects in our dreams? For that matter, what allows us to "see" our thoughts and emotions? The objects of mind are illuminated by the luminosity of the mind itself. Unlike the outer sun, which dualistically shines upon its objects, the inner sun doesn't shine from somewhere within, casting its light upon mental objects. The inner sun, the clear-light mind, nondualistically takes on the form of mental objects, which means that the contents of mind illuminate themselves.

While the ego (psyche) can experience states of consciousness associated with dream yoga, ego cannot experience the clear-light mind. Deception cannot experience truth; delusion cannot see reality. For the ego, the "experience" of the clear-light mind is no experience. It's utter blackness, complete unconsciousness. It's essentially the experience of the death of ego, and as Trungpa Rinpoche said, "You can't attend your own funeral."

The clear-light mind, and therefore sleep yoga, is about realizing nonduality, or wisdom. Ego, or the psyche, is virtually synonymous with duality, or consciousness. Duality cannot experience nonduality;

consciousness cannot experience wisdom. We cannot see the clear-light mind as an object. Remember that "consciousness" is a pejorative term in Buddhism because it's always dualistic. We are always conscious of some thing, which means that consciousness is always based on subject and object. When consciousness dissolves into wisdom as we descend into dreamless sleep, we (ego) descend into darkness and go unconscious. Dzogchen Ponlop Rinpoche says, "The essence of deep sleep is, in fact, great luminosity, the true nature of mind. It is utterly bright and utterly vivid. It is a dense clarity, and because its clarity is so dense, it has a blinding effect on the confused mind."[8]

We (ego) always identify with forms that arise in awareness, with the thoughts and things of this world. That's what ego *is:* exclusive identification with form. We don't identify with formless awareness itself, which is another term for the clear-light mind. Formless awareness is no-thingness, which from ego's perspective is experienced as nothingness. How can some thing (ego), indeed the mother of all things, relate to nothing? It can't. So when no-thingness (formless awareness, egolessness) arises, we black out and fail to recognize dreamless sleep.

This is a bitter irony, because formless awareness is who we really are. It's only because the identity theft of the psyche has been going on for so long, and the crime is so perfect, that when our true identity is finally pointed out, we don't recognize ourselves. "That's not me!" is what we unconsciously cry out when we drop into dreamless sleep. "I'm not nobody! I'm somebody!" Just as thoughts and emotions (mental forms) steal our awareness during the day, and we therefore falsely identify with them, so it is with the images that arise in our dreams at night. What is found then is found now. Or more accurately, what is *not* found then is not found now. The theft simply continues.

Because there are no thoughts (forms) in dreamless sleep, there's no sense of "me."[9] When awareness is dislocated onto form and that form is lost as we descend into sleep, our awareness is lost. From a materialistic perspective, we lose it (consciousness, our false identity) when we fall asleep. But from a spiritual perspective, sleep offers an opportunity to find it (wisdom, our true identity). The spiritual path, and the nighttime practices, help us relocate ourselves. We lose consciousness but have the opportunity to gain wisdom. It's a grand game of lost and found played out in the darkness of the night.

We also relocate our identity in terms of moving (relocating) our center of gravity, or locus of identity, from the psyche to the clear-light mind. With this seismic shift, we then live our life not from the dislocated psyche, but from the relocated clear-light mind. People often feel the need to discover who they are, or to "find themselves." Countless books and movies address finding your true self, which is an authentic itch that longs to be scratched. But every temporary relocation of identity in the conventional world is but a substitute for this fundamental move back to the irreducible Self. You'll never find your real Self in any level of form, no matter how subtle, because your real Self is selfless/formless.

If we return to our astronaut-oneironaut analogy, we can learn something about deep inner space by looking at deep outer space. Imagine floating in outer space, where the light of the sun is constantly streaming. If there's no object placed in that light and space, then nothing is actually seen. The only thing you see is the blackness of outer space. You don't see the light. But the instant you put an object into that streaming light, both the light and the object suddenly appear.

Shine a flashlight up into the night sky. Without dust particles, smoke, or haze to reflect the light, the light isn't seen. The physicist Arthur Zajonc says, "How does light look when left *entirely* to itself? . . . Absolute darkness! . . . without an object on which the light can fall, one sees only darkness. Light itself is always invisible. We see only things, only objects, not light."[10]

It's exactly the same with the darkness of the deep inner space of your own mind. The light of awareness, the clear-light mind, is constantly streaming. But if an object—in this case a thought form, dream image, or emotion—doesn't arise in that light and space of the mind, nothing is seen. It's perceived as a total blackout, complete unconsciousness, which is exactly what we perceive in dreamless sleep. Let's replace a few words in Zajonc's statement to illuminate this assertion: How does awareness look when left entirely to itself? It is absolute darkness! Without a mental object upon which awareness can fall, we see only darkness. Awareness itself is always invisible. We see only thought forms, not awareness itself.

The Seduction of Thought

We grasp desperately to the forms of our mind because, for the ego, there's nothing else. It holds onto thought for dear life. Ego's gaze is so solidly fixed outside—which at this inner level means fixation on the contents of our mind—that it never bothers to look deeper inside. It forever chases the rays of light sent out by the clear-light mind, rays which are frozen into form by the substrate mind. If we looked deeply within, we would find what we're really looking for, what we truly want. Nothing.

Sleep yoga, as part of the family of formless meditations (including Mahamudra and Dzogchen), can help us understand the irreducible mechanics of happiness, and therefore what it is that we irreducibly want, a topic we've been circumambulating throughout this book. Once again, these impractical nighttime meditations lead to very practical discoveries. The esoteric informs the exoteric.

We can get to the bottom line of irreducible happiness by looking at what it is that the buddhas want. Those who are spiritually awake don't want anything. They're utterly content with resting in pure awareness.[11] As we've discussed, for the enlightened ones, external things are finally seen for what they really are, mere shadows of the clear-light mind. And who wants shadows when you can bask in the sun?

The discovery of no-thingness is the definitive discovery. It's the ultimate satisfaction. From this perspective, all external pursuits are mere substitutes. It's such an irony. You think you want something, which always means something external (at the level of sleep yoga, even thought and emotion are external). But if you take a close look, what you really want is no-thing. What you really seek is to dissolve into the formless (thingless/emptiness) clear-light mind. Our genuine longing is therefore a kind of spiritual "death wish," for it's the longing to transcend (die to) the fully formed ego. As we've seen, until you find this original mind, the painful game of hide-and-seek that is samsara—the sport of throwing yourself out into form and then hiding from yourself, the diversion of losing the essence in the display—continues forever.

Formless Mind, Deathless Mind

Because it's formless, the clear-light mind is also deathless.[12] This is the deepest part of you that doesn't age and die. It doesn't enter the world of space and time, and it doesn't get cancer, AIDS, Alzheimer's, or Parkinson's. It is unborn, and therefore undying. It is the true immortal You.

Everything "above" this formless awareness that is born into the world of form (the substrate and psyche) and that therefore lives in the world of space and time, will die. If you identify with these formed aspects of your *relative* self, you will suffer in direct proportion to that level of identification when those aspects inevitably decay and disappear. But if you realize the formless nature of your being, you will transcend death. The *Kena Upanishad* says, "It is the ear of the ear, the mind of the mind, the speech of the speech . . . the eye of the eye. Knowing thus, the wise have relinquished all false identification [with the psyche and substrate] . . . [and] become immortal when departed from this world."[13] This is the opportunity that sleep yoga presents each night. This is also where sleep yoga bridges into bardo yoga, the final yoga of the night. By working with sleep yoga, you are directly preparing for death.

Formlessness is virtually synonymous with death, and for the fully formed ego, there's nothing more frightening than that. Sleep yoga (and bardo yoga) is the practice where "fearless in the dark" reaches its apex. This is where you can discover that there's absolutely nothing to fear. There's everything to look forward to. You "die" into formlessness every night only to be "reborn" into conscious form the next day. You're already experiencing a mini-death every night; you just don't know it. By coming to know your formless nature, and becoming increasingly familiar with it (the definition of meditation), you can begin to transform the darkness of dreamless sleep into the deathless luminosity it truly is. The Taoist master Lao-tzu wrote,

> Seeing into darkness is clarity.
> Knowing how to yield is strength.
> Use your own light and return to the source of light.
> This is called practicing eternity.[14]

That's why even the view of sleep yoga is so profound. This view sheds light onto your deathless nature and your true identity. The light of this view can illuminate every other aspect of the nighttime practices and shine upon every step you take during the day.

The Experience of Lucid Sleep

What's the experience of lucid sleep like? Being nondual, and therefore non-representational, it is difficult to describe. Here are some accounts that hint at the experience. Tenzin Wangyal Rinpoche says, "When we refer to the 'experience of clear light,' what do we mean? It is not really an experience at all, but rather [a recognition of] the space in which subjectivity, sleep, dream, and waking experience occur."[15]

In an essay titled "Hyperspace Lucidity and Creative Consciousness," Fariba Bogzaran says of transpersonal dreams and other ineffable nighttime experiences: "The dreamer does not have visual, kinesthetic, or auditory references from waking life." Instead, these dreams "are a construct of unknown and never-before-exposed experiences . . . of the phenomena of light, void and emptiness, unity consciousness, and other nonrepresentational transpersonal experiences."[16] How much more ineffable, then, are dreamless experiences without any content?

In *Lucid Dreaming: Gateway to the Inner Self,* Robert Waggoner describes his experience: "As if a floating point of light in an expanse of aware, living light, the self-less awareness exists. Here, all awareness connects. All awareness intersects. All knowledge exists within the brilliant, clear, creamy light of awareness. Awareness is all; one point contains the awareness of all points; nothing exists apart. Pure awareness, knowing, light."[17] It might be surprising to learn that Waggoner is not a Buddhist, and writes with no reference to sleep yoga, as he continues:

> Within the aware light, there was no idea of self, or me,
> or mine. There were no thoughts, memories, or analysis;
> no Robert—only a light-filled knowing. Though I
> had no broader context from which to consider it, it
> seemed like my awareness had finally arrived at its

source: pure awareness, the reality behind the manifest appearances and symbols. The ultimate homecoming. In that aware light, All Is—the essence of everything seemed contained in an ever-present Now. All awareness connected in that pure awareness. In that great nothing, Everything Is.[18]

And in her essay "Lucid Surrender and Jung's Alchemical Coniunctio," Mary Ziemer shares this experience:

When the dreambody seemingly dissolves on the cooling, black light and winds, it feels like what the alchemists describe: the soul becomes free of the body—the spiritualization of matter. Depending on my state of mind, I have found that this dissolving process can feel like either an ecstatic death dominated by Eros or an annihilative sensation dominated by a feeling of mortification.[19]

It's hard to say exactly what Ziemer is experiencing, but the sensation of annihilation can only arise if the psyche is still involved, and therefore fearful of its own transcendence (death). When the descent into the clear-light mind occurs without any reference, it's a blissful dissolution. But if the psyche tries to grasp, there could be the sensation of falling in a dark abyss, and the corresponding fear of annihilation.

Remember the relative defense that the psyche puts up as you head toward the truth. For a slimy creature that lives and thrives in the dark, the ego responds to light and its revelations (that the ego doesn't truly exist) as a terrifying venture. With the proper view of where you're going, however, anxiety turns into anticipation, darkness transforms into light, and fear transforms into fearlessness.

The soul, having entered the vast solitude of the Godhead, happily loses itself; and enlightened by the brightness of most lucid darkness, becomes through knowledge as if without knowledge, and dwells in a sort of wise ignorance.

LOUIS OF BLOIS, quoted in *The Principal Upanisads*

Silent night, holy night. All is calm, all is bright.

JOSEPH MOHR

18

The Practice of Sleep Yoga

SLEEP YOGA, SIMPLY put, is the practice of sustaining awareness as we go from waking consciousness to dreamless sleep. I recommend sliding into the practice of sleep yoga with a three-stage progression of daytime mindfulness meditation. These stages will help you develop stability, and sustain awareness, as you drop into sleep.

Daytime Meditations for Achieving Lucid Sleep

The first stage is *mindfulness of form,* which involves placing your mind on any external form, like an object, your body, or your breath. It's an easy first step. The second stage is *mindfulness of mind,* which is when you begin to transition from gross outer things into more subtle inner thoughts. The practice here is to witness all mental events—thoughts, emotions, images—without getting involved in them. As we've seen, the contents of our mind tend to suck us in, just like the contents of the world, and so we become non-lucid to what's happening in our mind. Mindfulness of form and mindfulness of mind help us wake up to (and therefore *from*) outer and inner forms. As we progress from the former to the latter, we're sliding down from gross to subtle, from form to formless.

The third stage is *formless mindfulness*. This is the main preliminary daytime practice for sleep yoga and is also known as non-referential shamatha, objectless shamatha, shamatha without a sign, or awareness of awareness. With this practice, instead of placing your attention onto any form, inner or outer, attention is placed on awareness itself. Awareness simply rests within itself. Chökyi Nyima Rinpoche says that in objectless shamatha, attention should rest "free from focus, in a total openness free from reference point" and should remain "totally undisturbed by emotions, thoughts, and concepts."[1] One way to do this is to find and then rest in the gap between thoughts. Find the gap now, in daytime mindfulness meditation, and you will be better able to find it in dreamless/formless sleep.

Another way to rest free from reference point is to "slide down from the top," descending through the three stages. Start by paying attention to twenty-one breaths, or however long it takes to settle your mind. Then move your attention to the contents of your mind without getting drawn into them. Watch thoughts and images float by like clouds in the sky-like nature of your mind. After a few minutes, settle your awareness into the state of being aware. Drop the clouds and dissolve into the sky. At this point your awareness is directed nowhere, but simply rests within itself.

If a thought arises, or something external distracts you, let it go and return to awareness itself. Release anything that interrupts the clarity of your open awareness. It's called "non-referential shamatha" because you're not returning to any referent, any object, any thing. You're coming back to formless (thingless) awareness itself.

At this point, in one sense, there is no such thing as distraction because distraction *becomes* your meditation. In other words, when something captures your awareness, you briefly rest on that. It only becomes a distraction when you don't release it for the next "distraction" (anything that grabs your attention), and instead allow yourself to spin off on it. For example, you're sitting in non-referential shamatha when you hear a plane. Recognize the sound without commentary. Notice your tendency to comment about the plane, how loud it is, where it might be going, what kind of plane it might be, and so forth, and then release. Catch and release. Then a dog barks, so now rest your mind on that. In the next moment you smell breakfast cooking downstairs ("breakfast cooking downstairs" is already a commentary; the instruction is to just smell). So rest on that.

With this open approach to whatever arises, there's nothing to interrupt your practice. This brings one of my favorite definitions of meditation as "habituation to openness" to a fruitional level. The key is to let your mind naturally recognize whatever sensation arises, but without letting yourself drift into any mental story about that sensation. Let it come and then let it go. With this formless refuge, you're now indestructible; your mind becomes unflappable. Nothing can distract you, because there's nothing to be distracted from. You'll accept, without indulgence, whatever arises, and take fleeting refuge in that.

This open approach to experience has practical applications when it comes to things like unconditional happiness. At the end of his long life, the sage Jiddu Krishnamurti was asked about his immutable serenity. His answer is really the secret to happiness: "I don't mind what happens."

With practice, you will come to rest in the substrate consciousness, which is classically marked by the experience of bliss, clarity, or non-thought. Even though you're not at the clear-light mind yet, you're getting close. You're starting to smell it. This is a pivotal experience. Resting in this ground state of consciousness is so pleasant, complete, and satisfying that any level of distraction or entertainment pales in comparison. *Awareness comes to prefer itself rather than any external form.* This is the pivotal point that swings your life from being an "outsider" to an "insider." Everything outside is seen to be the mere shadow that it truly is, and lounging in the light of the mind, awareness itself, is the only place to be.

Because the practice of non-referential shamatha is so subtle, how do you know you're actually doing it? B. Alan Wallace offers this advice:

> It is helpful for any kind of practice to know what the extremes are so you can cleave a middle path between them. For this one, if you try too hard, this gives rise to agitation and if you don't try hard enough, you fall into dullness. Once you recognize the two extremes, you want to do

something in between, which means bouncing off of those extremes more and more lightly. If you are focusing on any object, a thought or an image, this is one extreme, on the agitation side. The other extreme, which is more elusive, is sitting there with a blank mind not aware of anything. You are not attending to any object—just vegetating. What is in between is a quality of freshness because you are located in the present moment and vividly aware. You are not attending to any object at all but are aware that awareness is happening. It is wonderfully simple but subtle. It is like slipping into an old pair of shoes. When you are in it, you really know you are there. You need to develop a confidence that you know when you are doing it correctly. This is how it is done.[2]

Resting in awareness of awareness is natural, relaxing, and settling. It's like coming home.

For more advanced students, the apex of daytime meditations for sleep yoga are the formless meditations of Mahamudra and Dzogchen. These are the practices that introduce you to the clear-light mind itself, and then show you how to stabilize that recognition. The main practice of Dzogchen is *trekchö,* or "cutting through," which refers to cutting through both the psyche and the substrate to arrive at the bed of the clear-light mind. These meditations need to be learned and practiced under the guidance of a genuine master. They're extremely subtle, and fall under the classification of "ear-whispered lineage," which means they are intended to be whispered into your ear directly from the master. I will maintain the integrity of that lineage and invite you to explore these most refined levels of formless awareness with a meditation master.[3]

Namkhai Norbu drives home the importance and challenge of working to attain daytime stability in the levels of shamatha presented above: "Being aware of continuing our awareness in dreamtime means maintaining the same awareness we have during the daytime. If we have no capacity to be in the state of Rigpa [the clear-light mind], the state of real knowledge, in the daytime . . . we cannot have it in the nighttime either."[4] We may not be able to recognize the clear-light mind initially, but access to the substrate consciousness, via non-referential shamatha, points us powerfully in the right direction.

Nighttime Meditations for Attaining Lucid Sleep

Perhaps the easiest way to enter dreamless sleep consciously is to close your dream eyes when you're in a lucid dream.[5] By doing so, the mind is no longer drawn out to dream images. When I close my dream eyes, sometimes I just see black, which is what happens when I close my daytime eyes. Other times (as I'll describe below) closing my dream eyes does send me toward the dreamless state. Dream images are images of the mind, and therefore part of mindfulness of mind, or mindfulness of mental objects. By closing your dream eyes, the mind (awareness) turns in on itself, which is akin to non-referential shamatha. Try it and see what you see.

A method recommended by the Dalai Lama for entering dreamless sleep is that when you find yourself in a lucid dream, "focus your attention on the heart center of your dream body and try to withdraw the vital energy into that center. That leads to an experience of the clear light of sleep, which arises when the dream state ceases."[6]

Using the inner yoga approach (see "Throat Visualization" in chapter 5), we can practice a technique similar to the throat visualization for dream yoga, one that expands on the Dalai Lama's method. Remember that when we fall asleep, the bindus (consciousness) descend from the head to the heart, which is also where they go in deep formless meditation and death. Practicing a heart visualization engages this process and helps us maintain awareness as we fall asleep. This also connects us to our very subtle body, the body associated with sleep yoga, which resides at the level of the heart.

We discussed the subtle body—the bridge between mind (the formless) and body (fully manifest form)—in chapter 5. The very subtle body, being formless, is harder to describe. It resides at the center of the heart, and is composed of a very subtle wind inseparable from the very subtle mind it "supports." Described as the "indestructible bindu," it is sometimes visualized as a sesame-sized bead of light. The very subtle body is eternal and unchanging. It continues from life to life without beginning or end. It's the light of mind that never turns off.

The heart chakra is blue, and its frequency, or "sound," is HUM, which is often referred to as the sound of the awakened mind. Close your eyes, slowly recite HUM for a few minutes, and feel what it does to your heart. For me, the HUMS are like subtle depth charges that go off at the level of the heart.[7] The blue heart chakra exists about twelve finger-widths below the red throat chakra (that distance also separates all the other chakras along the central channel from their neighboring chakras), or underneath your sternum on a line that connects your nipples. (Don't worry about being too precise with the location. It's more important to *feel* the heart center.)

I spontaneously located my heart chakra many years ago when I was going through a heart-breaking separation. One evening as I lay down to sleep, I felt an itch in the center of my chest. As I reached down to scratch it, I was startled at the sensation when I hit that spot. It was exquisitely tender, almost painful to touch. It was my first experience of "opening a chakra," which is common parlance in spiritual circles. In my case, it had been broken open.

Among a number of variations in the actual visualization, my favorite is to visualize a four-pealed blue lotus at the heart (see figure 7). On the top petal is a yellow bindu, or mind pearl, which represents earth; on the right one is a blue bindu, representing water; on the bottom one is a red bindu, which represents fire; and on the left one is a green bindu, representing wind. In the center is a whitish-blue bindu, representing space. Visualize these bindus as shimmering pearls of light. Just as with the throat visualization, sleep yoga uses the bindus to support consciousness as we lose contact with the world of form. The mind must have something to hold as it falls asleep. If it doesn't have the light pearls, it will grab something else, like a stray thought.

As you fall asleep, guide your mind around the lotus exactly the same way you did for the descent visualization (at the throat) in chapter 8. But in the heart visualization you will have the added sense of dissolving the elements from fully formed earth into formless space. If you circumambulate the petal successfully, by the time you get to the center you're no longer visualizing the bindus. You've *become* the whitish-blue bindu, the clear light itself.[8] You drop through these stages of sleep whether you know it or not. With this visualization you can bring this unconscious process into conscious awareness. Then as the body slides into sleep, you slide into the clear light.[9]

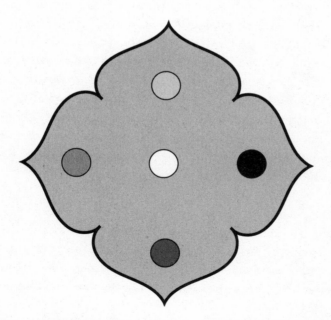

FIGURE 7   **Blue lotus with bindus.** Visualize this lotus with deep-blue petals, each holding a bindu, or pearl. Imagine that the bindu on the top petal is yellow (earth), the right bindu is blue (water), the bottom bindu is red (fire), and the left bindu is green (wind). In the center is a whitish-blue bindu (space).

CLARITY AND EMPTINESS

Guru Rinpoche says,

> At first when you fall asleep . . . earth is dissolving into
> water. At that time, train in the vivid sense of clarity and
> emptiness, and focus your interest at the heart. Then
> when consciousness sinks, water is dissolving into fire,
> and at that time do not lose the vivid sense of clarity
> and emptiness. When the mind becomes agitated, fire
> is dissolving into air, and at that time, too, train in the
> vivid sense of clarity and emptiness. Falling fast asleep
> corresponds to air dissolving into consciousness, and at
> that time, too, clearly and vividly focus on your heart,
> without losing the earlier sense of clarity and emptiness.
> Then the state of dreamless lucidity corresponds to the
> consciousness dissolving into the clear light, and at that
> time your sleep will lucidly remain in the clarity and
> emptiness that is unborn and devoid of recollection. If
> you recognize the clarity and emptiness of that occasion,
> which is free of the intellect, this is called "recognizing
> the clear light." That is similar to the dissolution of
> consciousness into the clear light at the time of death, so
> this is training for the intermediate state between death
> and birth. The present recognition of the dream-state is
> the real training for the intermediate state [bardo].[10]

Here, "clarity and emptiness" refer to the two aspects of the
clear (emptiness) light (clarity) mind. They are not two separate things, but two aspects of the same thing. Clarity is
emptiness, and emptiness is clarity. The experience of emptiness is like the experience of space. In the recognition of that
space, the recognition itself is the clarity, or luminosity.

Another technique that I have found valuable is to drop through
the floor, or ground, of your lucid dream with the explicit intent

of reaching your heart chakra and entering dreamless sleep, or formless awareness. It's as if the bindus (consciousness) that are gathered in the throat literally drop into the heart. I find it difficult to consciously descend around the lotus directly into dreamless sleep. I usually lose it (I'm unable to attend my own funeral). But descending from the "halfway" point of a lucid dream does work. For me, lucid dreams are a type of "halfway house" on the way to my true home at the heart. They're also "halfway" in the sense that lucid dreams are partial lucidity (one-half), while lucid sleep is full lucidity.

When I close my dream eyes in a lucid dream, things do indeed go dark. But I can tell when I'm not in a lucid sleep (formless) state because there's still a vague reference point. I still seem to have a point of view, even though there's nothing to view. *I* am seeing the black. There's nothing out there, but there's still a vague sense of something in here. It's similar to closing your eyes in a sensory deprivation tank (or dark retreat). You can still locate yourself, a vague sort of "spiritual proprioception."[11] Even though I can't see my body when I close my eyes in a lucid dream, I still feel that I have one. There's still a subtle sense of duality.

When I close my dream eyes and drop through the dream ground—which I sometimes do while holding my dream nose or dream breath (it often has the same feeling as diving feet first into deep water)—I find myself losing myself. It's still dark, but with a luminous energetic tinge. There's awareness, but no point of view. It's a non-referential awareness. There's "seeing," but nothing to see and no-body to see it. The black light just knows and sees itself.

"I" can't see, feel, or locate any sense of body. Yet "I'm" aware. I can't say it's like floating in outer space (which I have not done), but there is nothing to float. I *can* say it's not like falling through space (which I have done while skydiving), because there's nothing to fall. Dualistic consciousness has fallen away. It's just formless space. Amorphous awareness. No center, no fringe, no-thing. This nothingness, of course, is the no-thingness of emptiness.

Sometimes when I drop from a lucid dream into dreamless sleep, from a mental body into no-body, I feel my dream body dis-integrate as I go down. I might see my dream hands separate and drift away from me, or find a limb here and another one there. Usually my awareness is simultaneously dipping in and out of formlessness. I'll "lose myself"—any sense of location, proprioception, or body—only to pop back up to a vague sense of lucid dream body, which is when I might see a body part here or there. Depending on how I relate to this disintegration, I'll either witness the carnage dispassionately and chuckle at this bizarre experience, or briefly panic and wake myself up.

So for me, the technique that works the best is to close my lucid dream eyes, hold my dream breath, and take the plunge through my dream ground with the clear intent that I want to dive into the center of my heart with full awareness.[12]

Finally, remember the technique of seeing through—or in our terms, cutting through—the dream state once you're in a lucid dream. After becoming lucid to the dream, try to see through the dream by dissolving it. You can practice this by releasing the dream images and then resting in the pure (formless) awareness of simply being aware without an object.

Some Practical Tips

Keeping a small light on while you sleep can help to instill a sense of alertness during your sleep yoga practice. You're using an external light to connect you to internal light. In sleep yoga, awareness must be stable without relying on any form, but until that happens, light is a useful support. It acts as a type of transitional object between form and formlessness. Light is mostly formless, but it still has very subtle form. Tenzin Wangyal says that external light provides the conventional mind with "a direction, a support, as it moves toward dissolution in pure awareness. External light can be a bridge between the conceptual world of form and the non-conceptual direct experience of the formless."[13]

The sleeping lion posture (see chapter 5) also works with sleep yoga, but I have found sitting up while I sleep (which is rather like sleeping on a plane) to be even better. Sitting up helps align the winds and channels in a way that is conducive to a lighter sleep, and it also infuses a heightened sense of awareness. Eating light, refraining from alcohol, and keeping the room cool are also helpful for supporting a lighter sleep—in both senses.

Reaching a state of literal exhaustion—for instance by staying up for a night or two—also helps to exhaust the conventional mind (psyche) and is another common tactic used to point out the clear-light nature of the mind. (Sleep yoga is great to do after international flights when you finally drop dead into bed.) The exhausted mind tends to drop like a rock into sleep, which means it's less likely to be distracted as it goes down.

If you can arrange it, a teacher or a good dharma friend could be at your side as you fall asleep, and either whisper into your ear, "You're sleeping, recognize the clear light," or periodically wake you up and ask, "Were you aware? Did you recognize the clear light? Were you lucid?" And you could do the same for them. If you've watched someone doze off, it's easy to tell from their breathing and eye movements when they fall asleep or start to dream. To get a better sense of where your sleep yoga partner might be, refer back to the stages of sleep and the bodily changes that occur from stage to stage (in chapter 3).

You can start to see why sleep yoga is a more advanced practice! Most people will probably draw the line at dream yoga, with its relatively minor inconveniences. Sleep yoga can be a major inconvenience, but it also leads to major realization.

As with dream yoga, one of the most important triggers for lucid sleep is strong motivation. You have to really want to wake up in dreamless sleep. If you have a connection to deities or higher powers, you can make heartfelt supplications for help in maintaining awareness as you sleep. Sleep yoga is a Vajrayana practice, which emphasizes devotion as a key to success. Even if you're not a Vajrayana practitioner, you can still use the power of devotion to help you wake up in dreamless sleep. You might cry out with heartfelt longing for help in waking up to your clear-light mind. Unite that devotion with the aspiration that you will succeed in sleep yoga for the benefit of others. Pray that you will become familiar with your clear-light mind as a way to help others wake up to their own enlightened nature. A little magic goes a long way with sleep yoga.

What to Do in Lucid Sleep

While it may be more difficult to induce lucid sleep, the good news is that once you're lucid in dreamless sleep, the actual practice of sleep yoga is extremely simple. Unlike the progressive stages of dream yoga, the only thing you do in sleep yoga is relax. You've consciously "died." Now rest in peace. Rest in the nature of your clear-light mind. What constitutes progress is the ease and frequency with which you can descend into dreamless sleep lucidly, and the length of time that you can remain there. But the practice itself could not be easier. Paradoxically, that's what makes it so hard.

The bulk of the sleep yoga journey is really post-sleep yoga, or what you do after resting consciously in the formless awareness of deep sleep. You can't rest in peace forever. Sooner or later you have to emerge from dreamless sleep and "reincarnate" into form again. With sleep yoga you *consciously* form your formless awareness as you emerge from dreamless sleep.

The post-sleep yoga practice is twofold. The first part of the practice is to sustain the clear-light mind as you emerge into the dream state, which results in instant and sustained lucid dreams. (As mentioned before, sleep yoga is considered the primary nighttime practice in Dzogchen because if you accomplish sleep yoga, you automatically accomplish dream yoga.)

What usually happens as we emerge from dreamless sleep into the dream state is that we bring our ignorance (our non-recognition of the clear-light mind) with us, which naturally results in non-lucid dreams, the dreams of ignorance. The "light" is turned off, or more accurately was never turned on, which results in "dark" (non-lucid) dreams. In other words, we continue our sleep (non-recognition) into the dream state. The darkness extends "up."

So the first part of the post-sleep practice is to emerge from dreamless sleep into the dream state with the clear light still turned on. This light then penetrates, infuses, and illuminates whatever arises, and results in clear-light dreams, as described earlier. As the *Brhad-aranyaka Upanishad* puts it, "When one goes to sleep (he) dreams by his own brightness, his own light." Dreams still arise, but they instantly self-liberate in the shine of the clear-light mind. You're stretching, or extending, the clear-light mind into your dreams, which is what good yoga is designed to do.

The second part of the post-sleep practice—and the ultimate goal of sleep yoga—is to continue this stretch as you enter the next state of consciousness, which is waking up in the morning. What usually happens as we emerge from dreams into daily consciousness is that we bring our ignorance (non-recognition) of the clear-light mind with us yet again, which naturally results in a non-lucid "waking" reality, or the sleep of ignorance from which the Buddha awoke. The clear light is turned off once again, or more accurately was never turned on, which results in "dark" (non-lucid) daily experience. In other words, we spread this darkness across our world, mis-taking things to be solid, lasting, and independent (our classic dreamsigns), and succumb to what one liturgy refers to as "the darkness of fright-ful existence."[14] We continue our sleep (non-recognition) into the waking state, and live our lives in the dark, sleepwalking through life. The opposite of "clear light" is "obscure dark," which aptly defines the samsaric daytime mind. And, of course, we also bring our distraction from the clear-light mind with us, which results in our moment-to-moment distractedness throughout the day. What is found then is found now.

MEDITATION MAGIC AND JOY

The dream researcher Clare Johnson shares her experience of what sounds like the clear light, and the joy of keeping it on as she enters her day. Her account also suggests the enhance-ment of meditation that can occur in sleep and dreams:

> I close my [dream] eyes. All imagery vanishes and it goes
> black. Instantly I am deeply relaxed, it's so much faster
> than meditation in the waking state and I marvel at
> how deep I go within seconds . . . I can't feel my dream
> body at all; I seem to be floating . . . I am now in a deep,
> trancelike state, my thoughts slowing . . . The darkness
> is turning to light and as I watch, I become surrounded
> by and suspended in golden light. It feels so wonderful,

> like being transformed into radiance . . . It no longer
> seems separate from me; I am the light and it is me . . .
> I eventually wake up feeling as I am still bathed in it,
> refreshed and quiet and peaceful.[15]

So the second part of post-sleep yoga is to come up all the way
with the light still turned on. This light then penetrates, infuses,
and illuminates whatever arises, and results in illusory form, as
described earlier.[16] Thoughts and things still arise, but they instantly
self-liberate in the shine of the clear-light mind. More precisely, they
arise instantly recognized *as* the radiance of the clear-light mind.
There is no darkness, no shadows, no-thing to be found anywhere.
Nothing but light. The "darkness of frightful existence" has been
illuminated and therefore eliminated. Through sleep yoga, you've
stretched the clear-light mind into daily life. The result is described
in these words of the thirteenth-century Sufi master Najm Razi:

> If the light rises in the Sky of the heart . . . and, in the
> utterly pure inner man attains the brightness of the sun
> or of many suns . . . then his heart is nothing but light,
> his subtle body is light, his material covering is light,
> his hearing, his sight, his hand, his exterior, his interior,
> are nothing but light.[17]

The central practice of sleep yoga, as we said earlier about spiritual
practice, is to heal our primordial dismemberment—the fracturing away of our psyche from the clear-light mind—through
remembrance, mixing meditation and post-meditation together in
nonduality. Only the very highest practitioners can actually transition from one state of consciousness into another without losing
it (the clear-light mind), so don't despair. Most of us lose it, and
leave the clear light behind. But using the secret language of the
inner yogas, you'll gradually find your heart in your throat (lucid
dreaming), and eventually in your head (lucid living). As Dudjom
Rinpoche said, "Even though the meditator may leave the meditation, the meditation will not leave the meditator." (This is another

way to talk about the progression from effortful to spontaneous meditation described in chapter 6. At this point you don't have to return to the cushion, because you've never left it. It's forever in your back pocket.)

Sleep yoga, a journey into and then out of the clear-light mind, is a yoga of sustaining awareness as we go in and out of formless sleep. That's the practice. We take our dualistic consciousness as far as it can take us, which is right to the rim of dreamless/formless sleep. But dualistic consciousness cannot perceive nondualistic dreamless sleep, so we have to leave it at the door and "die" into the nonduality of lucid sleep.

If we're successful and can sustain awareness in dreamless sleep, the practice now becomes bringing this nondual awareness with us as we come back up. In other words, to be "reborn" in a nondual state as we come back to life (form) with (nondual) awareness instead of (dualistic) consciousness. So we practice taking (impure) consciousness with us as we go down, because that's all we have right now (it's all we're familiar with). We then replace it (transform it) with (pure) awareness once we are down, which is accomplished by becoming increasingly familiar with that awareness as we rest fully aware within it. Finally, we then work to sustain this (nondual pure) awareness as we come back up. It's consciousness going down, and wisdom coming up. Duality going down, nonduality coming up. This is why, if we're successful, we can be transformed so quickly with sleep yoga. We can go to sleep a confused sentient being and wake up a buddha.

The biggest obstacle to sleep yoga, of course, is discouragement. Tenzin Wangyal offers this encouragement: "Great masters have written that it has taken them many years of steady practice to accomplish sleep yoga, so do not be discouraged if you have no experience the first or the hundredth time you try it. There are benefits just from attempting the practice. Anything that brings more awareness into your life is beneficial. It takes long sustained intention and practice to realize the goal. Do not allow yourself to grow discouraged. Bring your entire being to the practice, with strong intention and joyful effort you will surely find your life changing in positive ways and will certainly accomplish the practice."[18]

Dropping into and recognizing the clear-light mind is like recharging our X-ray eyes. In post-sleep yoga, whatever arises is immediately seen through, and therefore instantly self-liberates. But these X-ray eyes are not a death beam. You don't have to vaporize every thought or thing to be free of it. You only have to see through it.

For most of us, the most important aspect of sleep yoga will be the view, the understanding of this potentiality or enlightenment. We can hold the aspiration to attain this level of awakening, we can reach toward awareness by continually seeking the luminosity of the clear-light mind, and we can try to stay plugged in to this source through the practice of illusory form. In this way, flashes of illumination can be transformed into abiding light.

Awareness nourishes the mind in a way that nurtures the whole living organism. Awareness illuminates previously unseen facets of the mind, and lights the way for us to explore ever-new dimensions of reality.

TARTHANG TULKU, *Openness Mind*

19

The Fruition of Dream and Sleep Yoga

THE PRACTICES OF dream yoga and sleep yoga, as we have seen, are not just for sleep. They prepare you for life, and especially for death, as we will see in our final chapter. The Buddhist path is to take these insights and spread them to "outsight." In other words, the practice and fruition of dream and sleep yoga is to see everything from the perspective of the clear-light mind. Once the clear-light mind is recognized, the meditation is to integrate the light with everything. When that's accomplished, it's called enlightenment.

Practical Benefits

Along the way toward this advanced aspiration, however, are many other worthwhile fruits of lucid dreaming and dream yoga, and you will surely discover your own. Paul Tholey offers this pragmatic list of the benefits experienced by lucid dreamers:

> "Normal" dreams were experienced as more pleasant and meaningful. Furthermore, 66% of the clients were able to resolve problems and conflicts of various kinds by means

of their lucid dreams. In waking life, they felt less anxious (62%), more emotionally balanced (45%), more open-minded (42%), and more creative (30%) . . . frequent lucid dreamers were less tense, anxious, and neurotic, and more likely to have more ego strength, emotional and physical balance, creativity, and risk taking ability.[1]

The dream pioneer Patricia Garfield has documented further benefits (most of which I have experienced in my own journey and which have been echoed by my lucid dreaming colleagues). She suggests that lucid dreams help:

- develop greater self-awareness

- banish nightmares

- test alternate behaviors in a safe environment and practice deliberate actions upon reflection, such as self-assertion

- accelerate activity of the immune system for physical healing

- enhance your ability to change waking life

- develop new elements of personality and facilitate a deeper understanding of yourself

- integrate conflictual aspects of the self and synthesize the personality

- explore the creative potential of the mind.[2]

I would add that lucid dreaming increases the power of choice, which is the basis of freedom. Prisoners have no choice, whether they're literal inmates or those held captive by the contents of their own mind. When you're stuck in a non-lucid dream, you're a hostage of your unconscious mind as it's played out in the medium of your dream. But once you wake up to the dream, you have the choice of indulging it, or going "back in" (and losing your lucidity), or standing back and witnessing the dream, or working to control it.

This same power of choice applies to life, and can keep you out of trouble as thoughts and emotions start to imprison you. For example, this morning I came close to being sucked into an argument with my wife. The energy was building, and I was just about to lose it in an angry outburst. But I stepped back, became lucid to what was happening, and made the choice not to indulge my anger. I could have gone "back in" and accelerated the argument, but my lucidity (new perspective) allowed me to make the better choice.[3]

Spiritual Benefits

The practices of dream and sleep yoga also have rich benefits in the transcendental realms, many of which we have hinted at throughout our journey.

Nocturnal yogas bring sleep and dreams fully onto the path.

Even if you just practice mindfulness while lying in bed, you're extending your practice. One-third of our lives is spent in near oblivion. We can change that and make better use of our precious life.

In twenty-five years as a meditation instructor, I have found that many people limit their meditation, and therefore their meditative mind, to formal sessions of sitting meditation. But by only practicing when you sit, it's easy to leave your meditation behind when you leave your meditation cushion. On one level, sitting meditation is just remedial work. Don't limit yourself to the cushion. Bring your meditation into bed and then into your daily life.

Dream yoga is part of Vajrayana Buddhism, which is called "the quick path." Another name for Vajrayana is "the path of skillful means." What defines this path is its vast display of different meditations. Vajrayana teaching has a meditation for every possible state of consciousness: waking, dreaming, dreamless sleep, sex, dying, and even meditations for after death. These meditations are skillful means that allow us to bring everything onto the path. So one reason the Vajrayana is the "quick path" is because everything becomes the path. When you're able to practice, or travel, all the time, you get to your destination faster.

Insights can be transposed from the night into the day.

Take what you've learned and bring it to life. Even if you don't do dream yoga per se, the practice of illusory form is immediately applicable to life. For example, says Tarthang Tulku Rinpoche,

> We can learn to change the frightening images we see in our dreams into peaceful forms. Using the same process, we can transmute negative emotions we feel during the daytime into increased awareness. Thus we can use our dream experiences to develop a more flexible life. With continuing practice, we see less and less difference between the waking and the dream state. Our experiences in waking life become more vivid and varied, the result of a light and more refined awareness . . . This kind of awareness, based on dream practice, can help create an inner balance.[4]

There's a gold mine down there in your deep unconscious mind. You can tap into the richness and bring it to the surface of your life.

By gaining mastery over dream and sleep, you gain mastery over your own mind.

The point of dream yoga isn't really about controlling your dreams. It's about controlling your mind. Until you transform the unconscious elements of your mind, they will continue to control your conscious life. By gaining mastery over your mind, you become fearless in the dark and eventually eliminate it. We're always afraid of what we don't know. By bringing the light of awareness into this darkness, we can conquer fear, the primordial emotion of samsara. And if we conquer fear, we vanquish samsara.[5]

By conquering fear, you can conquer the toxic hope of ego.

Hope and fear are the parents of the eight worldly concerns, so we can therefore transcend them. With no hope for pleasure, gain, fame, and praise, we no longer fear pain, loss, shame, and blame. As this equanimity matures, we eventually have no preference for samsara or nirvana, because both are seen to be illusory.

This means that appearances no longer have power over you, just like a non-lucid dream no longer has power over you. You still see the same appearances as everyone else, but because you see their illusory nature, you relate to them very differently. Thoughts and external appearances still arise, but they no longer have the power to move you. You see right through them.

By gaining mastery over your mind, you eventually gain mastery over the world.

Dream yoga is a classical way to develop the psychic powers called *siddhis* in Buddhism. Masters who have accomplished dream yoga, and who truly see the world as a dream, can manipulate the physical world as if it is no longer physical.[6] This power over the outside world is called "relative siddhi."

Miracles happen when you tune in to the miraculous and illusory nature of reality. Christ did it, the Buddha did it, and countless other masters from any tradition can do it. Khenpo Tsültrim Gyamtso Rinpoche says, "It is possible to trust such accounts if you understand that the nature of samsara is indivisible appearance and emptiness like a dream or a magical illusion. Without such understanding, it will be hard to believe them."[7]

Relative siddhi can be used to help others, but in the scheme of things it's not that important. If we're not careful, psychic mastery over the physical world can become a sorcerer's trap. Many people get stuck at the level of relative siddhi, thinking that's the point. The real point, however, is absolute siddhi—which is when the world no longer has power over you.

When we think of an experience as "just a dream," it's less real to us and loses power. The world only has the power we give to it. It's a power we unwittingly bestow when we project it to be real. If we freeze the world into concrete and steel, that reification can hurt us. If we melt the world into illusion, it can't hurt us. Emptiness cannot harm emptiness. We can still be physically dinged and egoically bruised, but if we no longer exclusively identify with these outer aspects of our being, we're not fundamentally hurt. Our deepest nature remains unscathed. We still feel things. Indeed, we feel them more because we're so awake. But they hurt us less.

Those awakened beings that contact reality have real power, because it's the power of truth. At a conventional level, this is why we respect scientists. Scientists work with the foundations of relative reality, which can literally have thermonuclear power. In modernity, scientists often displace religious authorities as the high priests of our age, because of the power invested in them from the truth of relative reality. In the same way, but even deeper, the masters that contact absolute reality have even more authority. The powers of the awakened mind, of a buddha, are inconceivable.

By becoming a child of illusion, you become more childlike (which is different from being childish).

Things no longer burden you once you've seen through them. You become lighter and more playful. Khenpo Tsültrim Gyamtso Rinpoche says, "Though shifting appearances ceaselessly rise, just be unattached as a child at play."

When your mind becomes more malleable and dreamlike, so does your experience. You may find that you're able to wrap your mind around things that were previously beyond your stretch. On an emotional level, things still touch you, but they don't get to you. Your mind becomes elastic, adaptable, and resilient. As the popular maxim asserts, "Blessed are the flexible, for they are never bent out of shape."

In this way, dream yoga brings you to life. Lifeless people, the spiritual sleepwalkers, are "stiffs." Stiff is the mind that cannot conform, contain, or adjust to its experience. Stiff is the mind that resists experience. And suffering is the consequence of this mental rigidity, because suffering comes from the mind's inability to accommodate its experience. With dream yoga, we stretch the conventional and contracted mind until it snaps out of itself. Small mind then expands into Big Mind. That open mind, like space itself, can hold anything without being affected by it.

What's the softest, most open, and flexible "thing" in the universe? Space. Nothing is softer than space. Yet nothing is more indestructible. You can't hit it, burn it, or cut it. That's the mind stretched open. That's the mind of a dream yoga practitioner.

You develop a quality of spontaneous humor.

Allied to the flexibility and adaptability that comes with dream yoga, is the discovery that everything is a big joke. Materialism is such a hoax. Jokes work by developing a narrative that sets you off in one direction then suddenly switches course with a timely punch line. The set-up allows the punch line to deliver its humorous crack-up.

The narrative in the cosmic joke that ego has constructed is that things are solid, lasting, and independent. We've been set up to believe this narrative by our parents, our society, and virtually the entire world. The punch line that the nighttime practices deliver is the sudden realization, or switch, that sets you in a totally different direction: the appearances that you've bought into are not fundamentally real.

"Humor" comes from a root that means "liquid," as in the humors (fluids) of the body. A liquid mind is fluid, flexible, and highly adaptable. Fluids never get bent out of shape. Like water, a melted mind can adapt to any container or environment. It's easy going because it goes with the flow of reality and not the dictates of mere appearance. This liquidity is the result of melting the unholy trinity of solid, lasting, and independent.

When we "break up" in laughter or "crack up" after a good joke, that light-hearted feeling comes from breaking or cracking our solid and serious approach to things. The more solid the setup, the bigger the crack-up. That's why the laughter of the buddhas shakes the universe. The great master Longchenpa said,

> Since everything is but an apparition,
> Perfect in being what it is,
> Having nothing to do with good or bad,
> Acceptance or rejection
> You might as well burst out laughing![8]

Over the past twenty years, I have spent countless hours around some of the most awakened people on this planet. A common characteristic is their ceaseless humor and playfulness. Quick with a pun, a prank, or a tall tale, these masters are constantly ribbing and razzing their students. They're able to poke fun at everything because they've poked through everything, and they delight in the levity of seeing things as they truly are.

You will gain compassion and the desire to awaken others.

Imagine being in a room full of hundreds of sleeping people. You're the only one awake, and you're wandering around the room. Some of the people are sleeping soundly, while others are writhing and moaning from an obvious nightmare. Your natural response, especially if it's a room full of loved ones, would be to rouse them from their slumber and say, "Wake up! It's just a bad dream. There's no need to suffer." This is how the buddhas spend their lives.

The awakened ones are full of empathy and kindness. They have tapped into the wealth within and want others to partake of these vast natural resources. It's like taking a journey to a place with breathtaking scenery and longing to share it with your family and friends. Writer Tiziano Terzani said, "It's not how far you've traveled, it's what you've brought back." Dream yoga travelers can voyage far into exotic inner terrain, but they always come back with wondrous insights to share.

Dream yoga and the practice of illusory form will simplify your life and save you lots of money.

What's the point in spending your life chasing apparitions? Why get hung up about finding that dream house, buying that dream car, or getting that dream mate? Chasing rainbows is futile and frustrating. This doesn't mean we shouldn't pursue our dreams and aspirations, in that noble sense, but that we should understand the fleeting nature of going after *things*. It means we shouldn't attach too much expectation in that pursuit.

When we're no longer caught up in appearances, we cease grasping after them. When grasping ceases, so does samsara. The end of materialism means the end of consumerism. Matter just doesn't matter as much. This has had a big practical impact on me. I'm no longer as interested in money, nor the illusory objects it allows me to buy. The X-ray eyes developed by dream yoga and the contemplation of illusory form have allowed me to see through all that. We're born owning nothing, and we can't take anything with us when we die. As George Strait sang, "I ain't never seen a hearse with a luggage rack."[9] Discovering that external appearances are a heap of nothin' is a magnificent consequence of the nighttime yogas. My life is freer, and certainly lighter.

Sleeping and dreaming are concordant experiences of death, so dream and sleep yoga prepare you to die.

Buddhas not only don't sleep, they also don't die, in the conventional sense. Their outer form dissolves, as does anything composed of form, but because they no longer identify with form, death no longer has any meaning. A number of years ago, just before I was about to teach a weekend program on death and dying, I met with Khenpo Rinpoche. I told Rinpoche about my program, and asked him if he had any suggestions on what I should convey to the participants. He said, "Tell them that death is an illusion."

Formless means deathless. In other words, by cutting through false levels of identity, the psyche and then the substrate, and fully identifying with the clear-light mind, there is no such thing as death. Remember that the clear-light mind does not enter the world of space and time. It is unborn and therefore undying. That means *you* are unborn and undying.

From Insight to Outsight

One of the most beautiful aspects of dream yoga is that it leads to the discovery of a sacred world. Here's how this magical discovery comes about. When you're in a dream, there seems to be a subject (you) perceiving an object (the dream). There's an unquestioned sense that the dream somehow appears on the screen of your mind, and you're sitting somewhere in this theater of the mind watching it. The screen and the dream images seem to be "out there" and you're somewhere deeper "in here." But take a closer look. Examine your dream experience from the perspective of waking consciousness. Look at the double-delusion from the perspective of the primary-delusion, and you'll discover that sense of duality to be illusory.

There's no overt dream yoga involved with this investigation. Anybody can do this. Look closely at last night's dream and you will discover that there is no subject, no object, and no act of perception. This is called "three-fold purity," which is another term for nonduality. In other words, nonduality occurs when we purify the illusion of subject, object, and the impure perception that seems to separate these two.

What's going on here? How is your nightly perception of the dream taking place? How do you know your dream? The answer is subtle, and the implications are profound. *The objects in your dream know themselves.* They are reflexively aware. They illuminate themselves. Everything that appears in the dream is the nondual radiant expression of the nondual clear-light mind. The dream has no dreamer.

We touched on this mind-bending conclusion in our brief discussion of "pure perception" and the reflexively aware wisdom of the clear-light mind. Now take this insight and extend it to your daily waking experience. Start by looking at your mind. For example, when you sit in meditation, who is it that sees your thoughts? Just like in a dream, it feels like there's someone (the real you) observing the contents of your mind. Thoughts seem to appear on the screen of your mind, and you're just witnessing them. But this too is an illusion. Thoughts have no thinker. The Zen master Thich Nhat Hanh lends a hand:

> When we look at an action we believe there needs to be
> a separate actor existing behind it. The wind blows, yet
> really there is no blower. There is only the wind, and if
> it doesn't blow, it's not the wind at all. When we have
> a thought, we may believe there's a thinker existing
> separately from the thought. As we cannot find a blower
> outside of the wind, nor a rainer outside of the rain,
> in the same way there is no thinker existing outside
> of a thought. When we think something, we are those
> thoughts. We and our thoughts are not separate. When
> we say something, those words are us; there is no speaker
> outside of the words. When we do something, our
> action is us. There's no actor outside of the action.[10]

This is why Suzuki Roshi said, "Strictly speaking, there are no enlightened people. There is only enlightened activity."[11]

Now take this insight yet again and transpose it to the final "out-sight," or the seemingly external world. Is your perception of the world fundamentally any different? When you see the world purely, from the perspective of the clear-light mind, you see right through duality, and appearances know themselves. Just like in a dream, there is no subject, no object, and no act of dualistic (impure) perception. Everything is reflexively aware, and therefore perfectly pure.[12]

Dream yoga seeds this vision and allows you to penetrate to the absolute nondual nature of mind and reality. Plant this pure perception in your dreams and watch it flower into daily experience. This is where you finally get rid of fear at its root, because where there is no *other,* there is no fear. By seeing through duality, you'll see right through fear.

This leads to the discovery of a sacred world, because when you see things from this perspective, they're no longer seen as independent things. You don't see the mountain. The mountain sees itself. It illuminates itself. When you wake up to things as they are, you don't see things. Things see or know themselves. They illuminate themselves. This is how you irreducibly illuminate your life through lucid dreaming and the Tibetan yogas of sleep. You illuminate your life by fundamentally transforming the way you see it, and the very way by which you know it. These nighttime yogas allow you to see everything in a new light—*as* that light—the light of your own mind.

Where are you in all this? Nowhere and everywhere. When you finally wake up, you become nothing. The psyche and substrate, what you know as "you," are gone. But by becoming nothing, you become everything. You dissolve into the clear-light mind that illuminates this entire universe. You *become* the mountain, the river, and every other possible thing. You become the entire universe, which is now held in a nondual embrace.

When things are discovered to be empty of self, they're simultaneously seen to be full of other. So this is the secret of emptiness, and the basis of compassion. This is also why we don't need to fear emptiness, for it's actually fullness. As your personal sense of self shrinks and eventually evaporates, your cosmic sense of identity pro-portionally expands. Kalu Rinpoche said: "You live in confusion and the illusion of things. There is a reality. You are that reality. When you know that, you will know that you are nothing and, in being nothing, are everything. That is all."[13]

Dream yoga eventually replaces the degraded and impure view of materialism with this elevated and pure view. It's a sacred view that allows you to see a sacred world. So the next time you wake up in the morning, look back upon the dream, the double delusion, from which you just arose. Then look out at the world and ask yourself: is *this* any different?

Someday, upon spiritual awakening, you will look back upon the dream of waking appearance, the primary-delusion, and come to exactly the same insight. Then you might say to yourself, "How could I have been so fooled, so asleep, for so long?"

> Death is not extinguishing the light; it is only putting out the lamp because dawn has come.
>
> RABINDRANATH TAGORE, quoted in *The Ultimate Journey: Consciousness and the Mystery of Death*

20
Bardo Yoga

WE'VE ARRIVED AT our final destination of the nighttime practices, and the end of our evolution of these nocturnal meditations. Bardo yoga is a contemplative practice that transcends but includes its predecessors, and shows you that the nighttime practices can take you all the way into, and through, the darkness of death. This final yoga involves more than dream and sleep yoga, but the nighttime meditations are an integral aspect of it. The bardo teachings are extensive, and dealt with thoroughly elsewhere.[1] We'll examine them briefly in the light of our nighttime practices.

With this material we're diving deep into the heart of Vajrayana Buddhism and the stretching aspects of these mental yogas. Bardo yoga extends awareness from waking to dreaming to sleeping and finally into dying. The Tibetan word *bardo*—which means a gap, an interval, a transitional in-between state—also refers to the gap between lives. Even doctrinally this material is a stretch. But the most realized beings on this planet have been teaching bardo yoga for centuries, and purely for our benefit. It may initially seem beyond our reach, but it's worth reaching for.

Lucid dreaming itself is a kind of bardo, or "in-between," awareness where the dreamer engages in aspects from both the dream state and the waking state. You maintain the awareness of the waking state while sustaining the environment of the dream state. You're not quite here (awake) nor there (asleep), but have one foot in both worlds. This "bardo" aspect is part of all three nighttime practices (dream yoga, sleep yoga, bardo yoga), which themselves are about bridging the gap between the conscious mind and every level of the unconscious. So even though bardo means "gap," and implies something that separates, bardo yoga is actually something that unites.

Bardo yoga bridges life and death, uniting both into a seamless whole. For an awakened one who has crossed this bridge, life and death no longer have meaning. One side is the same as the other.[2] Like everything else, these two disparate phenomena merge into nonduality. And just like the awakened ones don't sleep or dream, they also don't die, in the conventional sense.[3] This is why they have absolutely no fear of death, for as His Holiness the Sixteenth Karmapa said just before his physical body died, "Nothing happens." He had already crossed that bridge, and "died before he died."

While appearances (lies) die, reality (truth) does not. If you can identify with the truth of your clear-light mind before you die, "nothing happens" at death. Sogyal Rinpoche, the Tibetan master who has done more than anyone to bring the wisdom of the bardo teachings to the West, says,

> The fear that impermanence [death] awakens in us, that
> nothing is real and nothing lasts, is . . . our greatest
> friend because it drives us to ask: If everything dies and
> changes, then what is really true? Is there something
> *behind* the appearances? Is there something in fact we
> *can* depend on, that does survive what we call death?
> Allowing these questions to occupy us urgently . . .
> we slowly find ourselves making a profound shift in
> the way we view everything. We come to uncover in
> ourselves "something" that we begin to realize lies
> behind all the changes and deaths of the world . . .
> "something" that nothing destroys, that nothing alters,
> and that cannot die.[4]

When it comes to darkness, there's nothing darker than death. But just as with the other dark practices, we can transform that darkness into light and illuminate our way through an otherwise harrowing passage. With this light, the greatest obstacle transforms into the greatest opportunity. Many masters assert that there are *more* opportunities for awakening after death than in life—if you can shed some light and see where you're going.

On a general level, the Buddha taught, "Of all footprints, the footprint of the elephant is the deepest and most supreme. Of all contemplations, the contemplation of death and impermanence is the deepest and most supreme." Lucid dreaming has the ability to deliver us into this supreme contemplation, and place our lives in a larger context. "We are typically caught up in the events of our lives in such a way that we lose ourselves in them and literally forget or never notice that we *are* alive and that someday we will die," suggest the dream researchers Harry Hunt and Robert Ogilvie. They continue,

> This is the full human context to which, on rare occasions, we spontaneously "wake up" . . . In terms of common underlying processes indicated by the shared phenomenology of dream lucidity and such meditative realization, the formal parallel to the directly felt "this-is-a-dream" within REM is the fully sensed "this-is-a-life-and-some-day-it-will-end" within everyday living . . . The tenuous unstable quality of this "coming to" within daily living is formally identical to the instability of most dream lucidity.[5]

This chapter assumes, as does Buddhism, that something continues after death, just like something continues through the night. It's beyond the scope of this book to explore topics like reincarnation. We'll limit our discussion to a short survey of how sleep and dream relate to death and can prepare us for it.

The Universal Process

Euphemisms and idioms for death point to the intimate connection between the process of going to sleep, dreaming, and waking up and the process of dying, the after-death state, and being reborn. When a pet is euthanized, we say things like, "I had to put him to sleep." "Rest in peace" is commonly spoken as a wish for someone who has died. If it's a natural death, people usually die lying down, the same posture we assume when we sleep. The Spanish writer Cervantes said, "There is very little difference between a man in his first sleep, and a man in his last sleep." The Talmud says that sleep is one-sixtieth part of death. The connections are boundless.[6]

In Greek mythology, sleep and death are twins. Nyx, the goddess of the night, and Erebus, the god of darkness, gave birth to twin boys: Hypnos (the god of sleep) and Thanatos (the god of death). Hypnos then fathered Morpheus, the god of dreams.

The process of death and rebirth is also echoed in the arising, abiding, and cessation of each thought. According to some mystical views, the process is repeated yet again in the arising, abiding, and cessation of the cosmos. Sogyal Rinpoche refers to the recurring nature of this phenomenon as the "Universal Process."[7] It has an intuitive elegance and vast practical implications. Because these varied processes share similar characteristics, you can use one to help you understand another. For example, you can use your understanding of the arising, abiding, and cessation of a day to help you understand the arising, abiding, and cessation of a life, a thought, or a dream. Take your insights from one level of the Universal Process and use them to help you understand the others. In this way you can go back and forth between these different levels and strengthen your understanding of them all.

According to Khenpo Karthar Rinpoche and other masters, dream yoga came about principally as a way to prepare for death. The Universal Process illustrates the connection. The Dalai Lama says, "A well trained person can recognize a strict order in the four stages of falling asleep, and is well prepared to ascertain an analogous order in the dying process."[8] Bokar Rinpoche expands on this concept: "The energy governing each element ceases to be functional and is absorbed into the energy of the following element. This process of absorption of the four elements into each other does not occur only at death, it also happens in an extremely subtle manner when we fall asleep or when a thought is removed from our mind."[9]

The Three Bardos

The Tibetan conception of death involves a passage through three bardo states. The first is the "painful bardo of dying," which begins with a condition that will end in death.[10] It's called "painful" because it hurts to let go. This process is analogous to that of falling asleep, which generally isn't painful because it's easy to let go at the end of each day. For someone well versed in bardo yoga, that same ease is applied at the end of each life. They go easy into that good night because their view allows them to see that they'll wake up into the next good "day."[11]

At the end of the process of dying, the clear-light mind is laid bare. This is analogous to the moment of dropping into deep dreamless sleep, and it marks the end of the bardo of dying and the beginning of a state called the "luminous bardo of *dharmata.*" *Dharmata* means "suchness," "isness," and is virtually synonymous with the clear-light mind (as suggested by this bardo being "luminous").[12] Most people black out at the moment of death and do not recognize their clear-light mind (just as happens with dreamless sleep). This bardo therefore lasts for "the time it takes to snap your fingers."

The dead person's awareness then stirs, takes on a mental body, and moves from the clear-light mind (dharmata) into the "karmic bardo of becoming," which is analogous to dreams arising from dreamless sleep. This third bardo lasts about forty-nine days, where the mental body (like the body in a dream) is buffeted around by the winds of karma (habitual pattern), just like when we're tossed around by non-lucid dreams.[13] At the end of this bardo, the dead person's consciousness finally grasps on to a form and takes birth as that form. This marks the end of the bardo of becoming (you've finally become some*body*) and the beginning of the bardo of this life. It's analogous to waking up in the morning and entering your day.

The study and practices of these three bardos constitute the essence of bardo yoga. Bardo practices are those that help you recognize these bardo states of mind now—just as our nighttime yogas do.

The Measure of the Path

Dream yoga prepares you for the bardo of dying and the bardo of becoming. Sleep yoga prepares you for the bardo of dharmata. In the bardo teachings it is said that every night is a pop quiz that assesses your readiness, and also helps you prepare, for the final exam. Just like most of us do not recognize dreamless sleep or dreams (we're non-lucid to both), most of us will not recognize any of the death bardos. We will wake up after death into our next life, just like we wake up into our next day, non-lucid to what happened the "night" before. This is yet another instance of dream yoga as "the measure of the path."

When we come to recognize dreams as dreams, we'll recognize the bardo of becoming as the bardo of becoming. Then instead of being blown around involuntarily after death, we become lucid and take control over the post-death experience. Just like in a lucid dream, there may be limited control over the bardo content, but endless options for controlling how we relate to that content. In other words, we can have the power of choice, which can ultimately lead to choosing our next form, the next "scene" we wish to inhabit.

At an even more advanced level, someone who recognizes dreamless sleep will also recognize the bardo of dharmata. For that person, there is no bardo of becoming—no more "dreams" of any sort. If they (the issue of identity here is complex—"they" at this point refers to the clear-light mind or formless awareness) do dream, or take on form, they do so lucidly, and therefore voluntarily. They can "come back" in any form whatsoever, with complete freedom of choice, to help others wake up to the freedom they literally embody.[14] Without this lucidity and control, the rest of us reincarnate (re-form) involuntarily due to the force of habit, and will continue to do so ad infinitum until we become lucid to the process and take control. This control, of course, is nothing more than control over our own mind, just as the journey through the bardos is nothing more than a journey into our own mind. Once again, dream yoga isn't fundamentally about controlling your dreams. It's about controlling your mind.

There's a popular saying in Tibet: "Based on my experience last night, I can infer I'm going to have a hard time in the bardos tomorrow." This could be said by someone who has not prepared for the test. But for someone who has prepared, they can infer that they'll have a good time in the bardos tomorrow. Instead of dreading the final exam, they look forward to passing it with flying colors. Instead of stressing out about death, they can relax, which is the core instruction for life and death.[15]

How proficient does one need to be in lucid dreaming to experience lucid dying? Guru Rinpoche, the author of *The Tibetan Book of the Dead*, and therefore a primary resource in the bardo teachings, says, "If the dream-state is apprehended seven times, the transitional process (following death) will be recognized." To which Gyatrul Rinpoche adds, "The reference to recognizing the dream-state seven times implies that one can recognize the dream-state on a regular basis. If you maintain that ability throughout the rest of your life, then the chances are very good that you will be able to recognize the transitional process [bardo] following death."[16]

The threefold pattern we see in the bardo teachings, says Sogyal Rinpoche, "does not only unfold in the process of dying and death: It is unfolding now, *at this moment, at every moment,* within our mind." This, he says, "is a truly revolutionary insight, one which, when it is understood, changes our view of everything."[17]

And, of course, that pattern also unfolds each and every night. As we have seen throughout our journey, everything unfolds within our mind. Waking, dreaming, sleeping, and dying are all voyages of the mind.

I coincide with the world.

The French philosopher JEAN-LUC NANCY,
describing what happens while falling asleep

Epilogue

WE BEGAN THIS book talking about the commonality of sleep, how sleep is a unifying factor of humanity. It's not only human beings that share this experience, but all sentient beings. Now we can see that this biological camaraderie is just the outer level of a deeper spiritual union.

Here's the inner level, and a lovely way to come full circle. When we drop below the superficial psyche, where difference is virtually synonymous with division, where discrimination, strife, and warfare are sparked by the illusion of separateness, we start to descend to our common spiritual roots. We disconnect from the superficial layers of mind and connect to our shared awakened nature, our unified clear-light mind. As author Kat Duff says, "Our carefully constructed notions of ourselves, of where we end and the world begins, dissolve without our knowing."[1] Sleep requires that we forget our individual and superficial selves, and in doing so we can remember our unified and collective Self—who we truly are.

This commonality resembles Jung's "collective unconscious," but goes even deeper. When we wake up to the clear-light mind, this is our collective *super*consciousness, our shared buddha nature. So not only do we yoke with each other at this deepest level, we also commune with the divine, the Buddha within. As the dream researchers Jayne Gackenbach and Harry Hunt assert, "The further down the rabbit hole you go, the more collective the experience becomes."[2] And the more sublime.

We may not know it yet, this unified field of being may not be recognized yet, but this is where we go every night. This is what we fall into when we drop into the deepest sleep, and arise from when we enter each day. At this ground-zero level of being, ignorance is replaced with insight, consciousness is supplanted with wisdom, multiplicity is replaced by unity, and war is replaced with love. Duality melts back into nonduality. Every single night.

Remember that reality is what you attend to. Attend to the superficial psyche, which is always looking *out,* and you will skim the surface of life and forever remain asleep. You'll never know who you really are. You'll remain a victim of primordial identity theft, an attendant to the veneer of your being. Reverse your gaze and attend to your clear-light mind, which will always invite you *in,* and you will wake up to your true nature.

As we have seen, if we're aware of it, we're the most awake, the most enlightened, in deep dreamless sleep. Conversely, we're the most asleep, the most unenlightened, in so-called waking life. Even the French philosopher Montaigne said, "Sleeping we are awake, and waking asleep." Buddhas are those who wake up to this realization, sentient beings are those who do not. When we "wake up" in the morning and head *out* to the world, we've actually fallen asleep. We've stepped onto the path of the "outsider" and begin to sleepwalk. When we go to sleep consciously at night and head back *in,* we have a precious opportunity to wake up. We've stepped onto the path of the "insider" and begin the journey to awakening.

"Outsiders" arise every morning unaware of what they've just left behind. This is what creates the ineffable sense that something is missing, and therefore ignites the search to find it. The "it" takes many substitute forms—from the search for happiness to the pursuit of pleasure to the quest for meaning—until the authentic "it" is identified, and the misplaced clear-light mind is finally seen as what we truly crave. Something *is* missing. A theft has occurred. But in this crime nobody has taken the item, your precious true identity, from you. You just dropped it. It has fallen from the pocket of your memory.[3]

Here's the summarizing point. At our core, below any superficial language, beneath any gender, race, color, or creed, underneath even the slightest scent of duality and difference, we are absolutely all the same. The practices of the night lead us to this common ground and awaken us to the universality of the human condition. For you see, when you go to sleep, you're actually going to meet me—and every other sentient being on this planet—at this deepest possible level. We're going to sleep together, to rest in the same luxurious bed of the primal mind. Rumi put it this way:

> Out beyond ideas of wrong-doing and right-doing,
> there is a field.
> I'll meet you there.
>
> When the soul lies down in that grass,
> the world is too full to talk about.
> Ideas, language, even the phrase
> *each other*
> doesn't make any sense.[4]

Do you remember where the mind goes in deep dreamless sleep? It falls from the head and returns to the heart. Every night you and I meet at the level of our heart. Our practice is not to forget this nightly reunion when we come back to the surface of life, and to sustain our heart connection. As the philosopher Plotinus said, "They have seen God and they do not remember." We don't just see him—we become him. We're all God at heart. We just forgot.[5] "We may not remember that place of peace in the morning," says Kat Duff, "but I believe we can see it in the faces of those deeply asleep. There is an almost angelic look to those calm countenances . . . gazing upon the face of someone sleeping peacefully, it seems as though we are given the opportunity to see someone through the eyes of God."[6]

Yesterday a mouse was trapped inside my study, which faces out into a large yard. I opened the door and tried to coax him back outside, but he just kept racing back and forth along the back wall.

He finally settled into a corner, and I gazed at the terrified little guy cowering just a few feet away. I'm not afraid of mice, so after a few minutes of looking at my new friend, I slowly walked over and picked him up. As I held him I could feel his beating heart. In that instant I felt a heart connection, and realized he's just like me. He too wants to be happy. He too wants to avoid suffering. My warm beating heart is just like his, and so is yours.

I walked him to the edge of my yard and set him free. By feeling his heart I touched my own. I realized yet again that it's when I get stuck in only seeing outer forms that I lose inner connections. When I felt his tiny heart beating in my hands, my view immediately changed from outer to inner, from appearance to reality. I'm wearing a human costume, and he's clothed in mouse attire, but underneath the outfitting, we share the same naked heart. I may have set him free to run into the field, but he momentarily set me free from my exclusive identification with outer form.

So the next time you see me, my mouse, or anyone else, remember that we've met before. Just last night we were sharing the same primordial bed of mind and heart. Remember that at this most fundamental level of love, we're still together.

Acknowledgments

THE RESEARCH FOR this book was carried out over many years. While much of this research is listed and credited in the endnotes, a vast amount was provided in the oral teachings of meditation masters in India, Nepal, and throughout the United States. This oral transmission was profound because it came from masters who have accomplished the nighttime meditations. Khenpo Tsültrim Gyamtso Rinpoche, Kenchen Thrangu Rinpoche, Dzogchen Ponlop Rinpoche, Tenzin Wangyal Rinpoche, Dzigar Kongtrul Rinpoche, Khenpo Karthar Rinpoche, and Traleg Rinpoche are teachers who offered invaluable teachings that seeded this book.

An elite group of readers helped me shape this book into its final form. I'm grateful to David Berman, Jeremy Hayward, Karen Hayward, Jay Mutzafi, and Patricia Keelin for their insightful comments. Thank you to Haven Iverson and Tami Simon at Sounds True for believing in this book. Special thanks to my editor Gretchen Gordon, an absolute wizard in her craft. Her grand vision and attention to detail did much to improve this book.

Notes

Prologue

1. R. D. Laing, *The Politics of the Family* (New York: Pantheon, 1971), 82.
2. While Freud and Jung spent a great deal of time with dreams, they spent very little with lucid dreaming. The first edition of Freud's *The Interpretation of Dreams* (1899) has no overt reference to lucid dreaming, but the second edition does. Jung had little interest in the topic, at least as we are defining it. However, Jung did work with dreams in very creative ways. Jung said that he did not dream, but was dreamed. See Mary Ziemer, "Lucid Surrender and Jung's Alchemical Coniunctio," in *Lucid Dreaming: New Perspectives on Consciousness in Sleep,* vol. 1, eds. Ryan Hurd and Kelly Bulkeley (Santa Barbara: Praeger, 2014), for a good summary of Jung's relationship to lucidity in dreams.
3. See my article "Just When You Think You're Enlightened" for more on the dangers of sharing spiritual experiences (*Buddhadharma: The Practitioner's Quarterly* 12, no. 4 [summer 2014]: 31–35). Author Kenneth Kelzer shares this caveat: "It is difficult to talk about mystical experiences or even lucid dreams to people who have not had either . . . some people could easily become angry . . . insofar as they make no claims to having mystical experiences themselves and could easily feel alienated." (Kenneth Kelzer, "The Mystical Potential of Lucid Dreaming," in Hurd and Bulkeley, *Lucid Dreaming: New Perspectives on Consciousness in Sleep,* vol. 2, 301.) So while sharing can connect you to others, it can also alienate others.
4. A "performative contradiction" arises when the propositional content of a statement contradicts the presuppositions of asserting it. "I am dead" is one blunt example (you can't be dead and report it). On a philosophical note, the radical relativism of postmodernism is a raging example: everything is relative—except for my proclamation of this relativity. That's absolute. Performative contradictions are nasty blind spots, and blind spots are a topic we'll come back to again in this book.

INTRODUCTION Adventures in Consciousness

1. There are four main schools of Tibetan Buddhism. In order of emergence, they are the Nyingma, Kagyu, Sakya, and Gelugpa traditions.
2. Lama Thubten Yeshe, *The Bliss of Inner Fire: Heart Practice of the Six Yogas of Naropa* (Somerville, MA: Wisdom Publications, 1998), 27.
3. His Holiness the Dalai Lama, *Sleeping, Dreaming, and Dying: An Exploration of Consciousness with The Dalai Lama,* edited and narrated by Francisco J. Varela (Boston: Wisdom Publications, 1997), 45.
4. The dream researcher Ryan Hurd says, "If we grant that lucid dreaming may be powerful enough to heal, then we must also admit that it may also be powerful enough to do us harm." (G. Scott Sparrow, "The Argument

for Caution," in Hurd and Bulkeley, *Lucid Dreaming: New Perspectives on Consciousness in Sleep,* vol. 1, 328–329.)

5. Buddhist teachings are organized in a number of ways; the "Three *Yanas*" and "Three Turnings" are among the most famous. The Three Yanas, or "vehicles," are the Hinayana ("narrow or small" vehicle), Mahayana ("wide or great" vehicle), and Vajrayana ("diamond or indestructible" vehicle). The Three Yanas *(triyana)* and the Three Turnings *(dharmacakrapravartana)* are not the same. Hinayana is more or less the same as the First Turning, but both the Second and Third Turnings are part of the Mahayana. The Vajrayana is outside the Three Turnings; it is often considered a subset of the Mahayana. (The view is the same, but the methods to realize the view are different—sutra versus tantra.)

6. In Buddhism, *prajna* is translated as "wisdom," but is closer in meaning to insight or discriminating knowledge. It is the faculty of mind that apprehends the truth, how things really are, which is a central theme of this book. Although everyone possesses prajna, it's usually underdeveloped and needs to be cultivated through practices like insight meditation or other forms of mental training.

In Hinduism, prajna is the state of deep sleep in which the activity of the mind ceases and the *jiva* (one who lives in the outer body, or the self that identifies with outer body and mind, what we'll be calling the "psyche" in this book) momentarily and unconsciously unites with *brahman* (absolute consciousness, or pure transcendence, what we'll be calling the "clear-light mind"). The Upanishads (arguably the first written map of the mind) articulate four states of consciousness: *vaishvarana,* the waking state; *taijasa,* the dream state; *prajna,* deep dreamless sleep; and *turiya* ("the fourth"), the super conscious state of illumination. It's called "the fourth" because it transcends the other three. From a psychological point of view, it's called turiya; from a philosophical point of view it's called brahman. So turiya and brahman are Hindu correlates for the clear-light mind. In Buddhism, "the fourth" is connected to "the fourth moment," which is the timeless dimension that is beyond the other three moments of past, present, and future. In other words, the fourth moment refers to the experience of the clear-light mind.

7. Ken Wilber makes the important distinction between states of consciousness and structures (or stages) of growth. Traveling and evolving through states of consciousness will be our journey in this book. We will venture from gross states (waking consciousness) to subtle states (dreaming consciousness) to very subtle states (deep dreamless sleep consciousness) using the vehicle of meditation.

States of consciousness are the great contribution of the East. Structures of development are the great contribution of the West. Structures are developmental levels that we grow into as we age. Hundreds of Western developmentalists have mapped out these structures. One of the most famous articulations comes from the cultural historian and evolutionary philosopher Jean Gebser, who talked about five major structure stages through which we evolve: archaic, magic, mythic, mental, and integral.

CHAPTER 1   What Is a Lucid Dream?

1. A more technically accurate term for "lucid dream" would be "cognizant dream," used by Stephen LaBerge (see note 3 below). "Metacognitive dreams" is also used, where "metacognitive" means "thinking about thinking," or "reflecting on one's mental processes." Lucid dreams are also described as a "hybrid" state of consciousness, a hybrid of waking and dreaming. One problem with this term is that "hybrid" implies a disso-ciative combination of dreaming and waking, which supports the more Western scientific approach of the presence or absence of consciousness, versus a more Eastern approach of a spectrum of consciousness ranging from gross (waking) to subtle (dreaming) to very subtle (dreamless sleep), a view that is more resonant with this book.

   Still others use the term "integrative consciousness," again implying the integration of usually disparate states of consciousness, or "volitional dreaming," which implies conscious control. Some scholars look at the popular definition of lucid dreaming as a Western term, because it assumes a (monophasic) culture where waking and dreaming are distinctly different states, an assumption that is not held by many indigenous (polyphasic) cultures.

   The three principal states of waking, sleeping, and dreaming are not mutually exclusive. Like everything else in reality, they interpenetrate. When you're having a daydream, you're dreaming in the waking state; when you're awake in a dream, you're lucid dreaming; when you're awake in dreamless sleep, you're lucid sleeping; and of course from a spiritual perspective, when you're "sleeping" in waking life you're a normal confused sentient being. Buddhas are simply those who remain awake in all states.

2. The neuroscientist J. Allan Hobson theorizes that recognizing that we're dreaming stimulates the dorsolateral prefrontal cortex, which is responsible for self-awareness and working memory. This area is usually deactivated during normal non-lucid REM sleep. The dorsolateral prefrontal cortex is also associated with the experience of when and how to act.

3. One cannot talk about lucid dreaming without honoring Stephen LaBerge. With a doctorate in psychophysiology from Stanford University, he has dedicated his life to the scientific exploration of lucid dreaming. His contributions are seminal and influence many pages of this book. The rigor that he brings to this field is important. Many books on lucid dreaming are available, and because dreams deal with highly personal dimensions of experience, almost anybody can say anything about dreams. In my reading of the literature, many books take artistic license in their accounts. It's difficult to substantiate subjective inner experiences. This makes the science behind lucid dreaming, let alone dream yoga, difficult. Lucid dreaming is still on the fringe of science and academic study, often relegated to the mystic, the poet, or the New Ager. In the face of many obstacles, LaBerge has doggedly spent his life bringing needed discipline to a field that is dom-inated by speculation and metaphysics. He is a pioneering voice of clear and precise thinking in a fuzzy world.

4. Flying and having sex are indeed the two most frequently engaged-in activ-ities for lucid dreamers. See Bahar Gholipour, "What People Choose to Dream About: Sex and Flying," LiveScience.com, July 10, 2014, livescience.

com/46755-flying-sex-lucid-dream-content.html. Other common adventures are doing things that are impossible in waking life: breathing underwater, talking with animals, time travel, and being someone else.

5. One neurological reason for this truth-telling is that the prefrontal cortex is deactivated when we sleep. This part of the brain is involved with "executive function," which relates to the ability to determine good and bad, to differentiate between conflicting thoughts, to predict outcomes, to apply moral values, and to moderate social behavior. (One reason adolescents and young adults get into trouble is because the prefrontal cortex isn't fully developed until age twenty-five, which leads to bad decisions and poor social control. Executive function is "parental" function.) During sleep, the brain is largely uncensored, and therefore even secrets we didn't know we held can leak out.

6. Though the two words are often used interchangeably, there is a difference between the "unconscious" and the "subconscious." "Subconscious" can be defined as "partial consciousness," or "pertaining to what is in the margin of attention; pertaining to that of which one is only dimly aware." In psychoanalytic terms, "it is a transition zone through which any repressed material must pass on its way from the unconscious to the conscious." (J. P. Chaplin, *Dictionary of Psychology,* 2nd ed. [New York: Dell, 1985], 452.)

The unconscious, in psychoanalytic terms, is the region of the mind that is the seat of repressions; it is also "characterizing an activity for which the individual does not know the reason or motive for the act," and "pertaining to all psychic processes that cannot be brought to awareness by ordinary means." (*Dictionary of Psychology,* 481.)

The philosopher Evan Thompson offers this comment, which is central to our journey in this book: "One way to think about the Indian yogic idea of subtle consciousness is to see it as pointing to deeper levels of phenomenal consciousness to which we don't ordinarily have cognitive access, especially if our minds are restless and untrained in meditation. According to this way of thinking . . . much of what Western science and philosophy would describe as unconscious might qualify as conscious, in the sense of involving subtle levels of phenomenal awareness that could be made accessible through meditative mental training." (See his *Waking, Dreaming, Being: Self and Consciousness in Neuroscience, Meditation, and Philosophy* [New York: Columbia University Press, 2015], 8.)

7. Tadas Stumbrys et al., "The Phenomenology of Lucid Dreaming: An Online Survey," *American Journal of Psychology* 127, no. 2 (summer 2014): 191–204.

8. Kelly Bulkeley, "Lucid Dreaming by the Numbers," in Hurd and Bulkeley, *Lucid Dreaming: New Perspectives on Consciousness in Sleep,* vol. 1, 1–22.

9. Viktor I. Spoormaker and Jan van den Bout, "Lucid Dreaming Treatment for Nightmares: A Pilot Study," *Psychotherapy and Psychomatics* 75 (2006): 389–394. This study showed that lucidity was not necessary for reduction in nightmare frequency. LDT alone was effective in reducing them. See also Antonio Zadra and Robert O. Pihl, "Lucid Dreaming as a Treatment for Recurrent Nightmares," *Psychotherapy and Psychomatics* 66 (1997): 50–55.

10. Patrick Bourke and Hannah Shaw, "Spontaneous Lucid Dreaming Frequency and Waking Insight," *Dreaming* 24, no. 2 (June 2014): 152–159.

"Results show that frequent lucid dreamers solve significantly more insight problems overall than non-lucid dreamers. This suggests that the insight experienced during the dream state may relate to the same underlying cognition needed for insight in the waking state."

11. Studies have shown that events in the dream body often coincide with corresponding events in the physical body. Most importantly, the brain can't tell the difference between something that is "real" and something that is dreamt. See Morton Schatzman et al., "Correspondence During Lucid Dreams Between Dreamed and Actual Events," in *Conscious Mind, Sleeping Brain: Perspectives on Lucid Dreaming,* eds. Jayne Gackenbach and Stephen LaBerge (New York: Plenum, 1998).

12. "Lucid Dreamers Are Using Their Sleeping Time to Get Ahead," *Business Insider India,* August 18, 2014, businessinsider.in/Lucid-Dreamers-Are-Using-Their-Sleeping-Time-To-Get-Ahead/articleshow/40376872.cms.

13. Janine Chasseguet-Smirgel, "'Creative Writers and Day-Dreaming': A Commentary," in *On Freud's "Creative Writers and Day-Dreaming,"* eds. Ethel Spector Person, Peter Fonagy, and Servulo Figueira (New Haven, CT: Yale University Press, 1995), 113.

CHAPTER 2   A Map for Practices of the Night

1. The Eightfold Noble Path constitutes the last of the Four Noble Truths (the truth of suffering; origin of suffering; cessation of suffering; and path leading to the cessation of suffering). The Four Noble Truths are the very first teaching of the Buddha, one that describes the path from *samsara* (suffering) to *nirvana* (happiness). The eight factors are: right view, right resolve, right speech, right action, right livelihood, right effort, right mindfulness, and right meditation. "Right" is sometimes translated as "complete."

2. Fear in a dream doesn't always disappear at the onset of lucidity. It's more the realization that no physical harm can come to us in that realm that provides an opportunity to continue exploring the dream despite a fearful reaction to its contents.

3. Matthew Kelly, *The Rhythm of Life: Living Every Day with Passion and Purpose* (New York: Touchstone, 2004), 298.

4. This, of course, is why we fear death. It's the ultimate blackout. "Right view" is particularly applicable when it comes to seeing into and beyond the darkness of death. Dream and sleep yoga can penetrate this darkness and can therefore remove the fear of death, which is why they're connected to bardo yoga.

On a different note, when astronomers talk about "dark matter" and "dark energy," "dark" refers to the fact that they don't know anything about this matter or energy, which constitutes the vast majority of matter and energy in the universe. "Darkness" is their code word for ignorance as well.

5. We can view the process of awakening in two ways: the relative, or developmental approach, and the absolute, or sudden approach. The relative approach, which is in resonance with Western psychology, is to make the unconscious conscious. It's a more gradual path. The absolute, or fruitional, approach is more about relating directly to whatever arises on the spot, and results in the ability to self-liberate anything that arises in our mind the

instant it manifests. The fruitional approach is not interested in history, but in instantly waking up from it (and from anything else that obscures the clear-light mind). In nearly thirty years of studying Buddhism, which specializes in the fruitional approach, I have never heard a Buddhist master say, "Tell me about your past," which is almost the opening line in many forms of psychotherapy.

6. C. G. Jung, *Collected Works,* vol. 8 (Princeton, NJ: Princeton University Press, 1969), 310.

7. The level of dream control is a controversial issue. Tibetan dream yogis claim that complete control over dreaming is possible. If you have complete control over your mind, you can control whatever arises within it. But many Western lucid dreamers claim that having control in a lucid dream doesn't mean you have total control over every detail of the dream. Control is limited to what you focus on in the dream. The dreamscape itself is created by a larger aspect of your unconscious mind, and while you can turn your attention to different aspects of the dreamscape and alter that, you don't control the background of the dream. This leads to a question: if the dreamer doesn't control the dream, who does? For a Western discussion on dream control, see Robert Waggoner, *Lucid Dreaming: Gateway to the Inner Self,* chapter 2, "Does the Sailor Control the Sea?" (Needham, MA: Moment Point Press, 2009).

8. If we can relate to *whatever* arises with complete equanimity, then there's no such thing as unwanted experience. If there's no longer unwanted experience, then there's no need to reject experience into the unconscious mind. If we stop the rejection, we stop stocking the unconscious mind (i.e., the "storehouse consciousness," or eighth consciousness of the Yogachara) and it eventually empties out. At this point the unconscious (unaware) mind disappears altogether because everything has been brought to light in the conscious (awakened) mind. Only consciousness (awareness) remains. So by saying yes to whatever arises, which is the essence of spiritual practice, we can potentially and gradually bankrupt the unconscious mind, and therefore samsara. This is how we purify karma. Equanimity purifies karma. At this point, sleeping and dreaming cease, and one attains the awakening of a buddha. Confusion has been transformed into wisdom; the unconscious mind has become fully conscious; darkness has been transformed into light.

9. Enlightenment, or spiritual awakening, remains a contested topic. In Buddhism, entire volumes (like the *Dasabhumika Sutra*) are devoted to the stages of awakening, and each of the Three Turnings has its own description, as well as varying articulations of the stages. A common classification is the ten *bhumis* ("levels" or "grounds") of spiritual development. If someone can attain even the first bhumi, it's an inconceivable accomplishment. This is not to discourage people from the path to awakening, but to simply put it in realistic perspective, and to temper the exaggerated claims of many Westerners that they have attained enlightenment. I'm in no position to evaluate levels of attainment, but it's safe to say that complete awakening in this modern age is exceedingly rare. It's much more fruitful to discuss the practical aspects of awakening, which is one mission of this book.

To make things even more interesting, and accurate, there is a difference between "waking up" and "growing up," or horizontal and vertical enlightenment, respectively. This includes the important distinction between realizing all states and structures of consciousness, as referenced in endnote 7 from the introduction.

10. "Ego" is used in this book as the sense of self, or what the American philosopher Daniel Dennett refers to as "some concentrated internal lump of specialness"—a sense of self that we will discover to be illusory. On an absolute level, there is no such thing as ego. Ego is just a funny way of looking at things, a form of arrested development. The Scottish philosopher David Hume (1711–1776) looked deeply into his experiences to try to find the experiencing self, but all he could find was experience itself. He concluded that the self is not an object but merely a "bundle of sensations." From this the British philosopher Derek Parfit distinguished between ego theorists, who believe there really is a self, and bundle theorists, who assert the self is an illusion. Parfit then goes on to say that the Buddha was the first bundle theorist. The self is just a bundle of illusions, with only relative status. (See Susan Blackmore, *Consciousness: A Very Short Introduction* [Oxford: Oxford University Press, 2005], 68.)

11. Dark retreat is a specific practice associated with *thögal,* one of the most advanced practices of Dzogchen. This retreat is also associated with the bardo teachings, and is sometimes referred to as "the bardo retreat." Traditionally (and only under the strict supervision of a meditation master), a meditator goes into total darkness for forty-nine days. During this period the shine of the clear-light mind manifests in various "visions," akin to what happens during the second phase of the luminous bardo of *dharmata* after death. If you take these visions to be real, instead of attaining enlightenment, you attain insanity. It's a potentially dangerous retreat. To a lesser degree, we suffer from varying levels of insanity when we take our daily "visions," the appearances of waking life, to be real. Dark retreat shows the meditator the roots of all this madness. See Chögyam Trungpa's introduction to his translation of *The Tibetan Book of the Dead* (Boston: Shambhala, 1975); Tenzin Wangyal's *Wonders of the Natural Mind: The Essence of Dzogchen in the Native Bon Tradition of Tibet* (Barrytown, NY: Station Hill Press, 1993); and Christopher Hatchell's *Naked Seeing: The Great Perfection, the Wheel of Time, and Visionary Buddhism in Renaissance Tibet* (Oxford: Oxford University Press, 2014).

12. See Chögyam Trungpa, *Shambhala: The Sacred Path of the Warrior* (Boston: Shambhala, 1984), for just one example.

13. See "Stage 8" in chapter 15 for more inspiration on why you should bother with these subtle practices.

14. Bruce Tift, *Already Free: Buddhism Meets Psychotherapy on the Path of Liberation* (Boulder, CO: Sounds True, 2015), 62–63, 70.

CHAPTER 3   Understanding Sleep Cycles

1. American Sleep Apnea Association, sleepapnea.org/i-am-a-health-care-professional.html, accessed March 22, 2014.

2. American Heart Association, "Sleep Apnea and Heart Disease, Stroke," heart.org/HEARTORG/Conditions/More/MyHeartandStrokeNews/Sleep-Apnea-and-Heart-Disease-Stroke_UCM_441857_Article.jsp#, accessed August 3, 2014.

3. David K. Randall, *Dreamland: Adventures in the Strange Science of Sleep* (New York: W. W. Norton & Company, 2012), 26.

4. National Sleep Foundation, "Sleep Aids and Insomnia," sleepfoundation.org/article/sleep-related-problems/sleep-aids-and-insomnia, accessed May 12, 2014.

5. Randall, *Dreamland,* 233.

6. Statistic Brain Research Institute, "Sleeping Disorder Statistics" (April 12, 2015), statisticbrain.com/sleeping-disorder-statistics, accessed July 14, 2015.

7. Medical Daily, "Nearly a Third of Americans are Sleep Deprived," medical-daily.com/nearly-third-americans-are-sleep-deprived-240273, accessed July 14, 2015.

8. In a *New York Times* op-ed column titled "To Dream in Different Cultures" (May 13, 2014), the anthropologist Tanya Luhrmann remarks on how our obsession with eight hours of continuous sleep is a product of our electrified age, and artificial light. In premodern times, she says, people engaged in "punctuated sleep," which is more akin to how our kindred animals sleep. She quotes Roger Ekrich, author of *At Day's Close: Night in Times Past,* who writes that people went to bed for the "first sleep" as the sun set, but then woke up throughout the night: "There is every reason to believe that segmented sleep, such as many wild animals exhibit, had long been the natural pattern of our slumber before the modern age, with a provenance as old as humankind," says Ekrich. In many ancient societies, what happened during the night was important, and because people woke up frequently, they remembered more of their dreams. Luhrmann goes on to quote the anthropologist Eduardo Kohn, who writes, "Thanks to these continuous disruptions, dreams spill into wakefulness and wakefulness into dreams in a way that entangles them both." And ways that inform them both. See H. R. Colton and B. M. Altevogt, eds., *Sleep Disorders and Sleep Deprivation* (Washington, D.C.: National Academic Press, 2006); and Luiza Ch. Savage, "Sleep Crisis: The Science of Slumber," *Maclean's* (June 17, 2013).

9. Kat Duff, *The Secret Life of Sleep* (New York: Atria Books, 2014), 72.

10. In slow wave sleep, spaces between brain cells expand by up to 60 percent, allowing cerebrospinal fluid to flush out toxins.

11. One way to work with insomnia, via the inner yogas, is to engage what the Mahamudra tradition evocatively calls "subterranean *samadhi.*" With this practice you visualize two black pearls at the soles of your feet, one on each sole. By bringing your mind so far down with the visualization, the winds and *bindus* that have gathered at the head chakra (resulting in the insomnia) are also pulled down, and your mind is seduced toward the heart chakra where sleep occurs. (Bindus are like drops of consciousness, and chakras are energy centers where bindus gather to create states of consciousness, as we will see in chapter 5.) It's an application of the "extreme path to the middle" approach, where the middle is your heart center, and the extreme is the bottom of your feet. I've tried this with mixed success.

12. Biographers state that the Buddha slept very little—one hour a night—and took the occasional nap. I have asked several meditation masters, including Khenpo Tsültrim Gyamtso Rinpoche, Sokse Rinpoche, and Choje Rinpoche, about buddhas and sleep, and they assert that buddhas do not sleep. Tulku Urgyen Rinpoche says that the highest stages of spiritual accomplishment "means reaching the point of nondistraction. In other words, one does not sleep at night; one does not fall into the delusory dream state, but is able to recognize dreams as dreams. During deep sleep, there is a continuous long stretch of luminous wakefulness." ("Integrating View and Conduct," in *The Dzogchen Primer: Embracing the Spiritual Path According to the Great Perfection,* compiled and edited by Marcia Binder Smith [Boston: Shambhala, 2002], 65.)

13. It's not just overt grasping that's exhausting, but covert attachment. You may not feel you're grasping after things, but if you believe in things—if you think there's something out there that is solid, lasting, and independent—that very perception is due to your white-knuckled covert grasping, your attachment to the belief that things exist. We'll have much more to say about this throughout the book.

14. In addition to all this grasping, there's a whole lot of splitting going on, which is also draining. Duality is constantly being generated by a relentless fracturing that rips the world into self and other, and an even more subversive splitting that results in "the self divided against itself." The psychotherapist Bruce Tift identifies five successive and persistent levels of unconscious splitting, each serving to disconnect us further from the truth and from who we really are.

   The first split is toward the truth of our experience, refusing to accept our immediate experience as it is. The second split is when we add a disconnect from our immediate embodied experience, which is an ongoing dissociation from the truth that we're embodied beings. The third split is when we add a continuous stream of self-referential commentary to our experience; we have an experience and we instantly make up a story about how it has to do with us. The fourth level of disconnection is when we link moments of experience to one another, creating an illusion of continuity. And the fifth level of disconnect is when we work to "stabilize a state of chronic struggle by maintaining the claim that there's something really important that has to be fixed about 'us' or about life." (*Already Free,* 115–116.)

   Nightmares often reveal unconscious processes, which suggests that (whether you know it or not) in a nightmare, or any other dream where you're being chased or attacked, you are chasing or attacking part of yourself—which is also exhausting. All this chasing and splitting brings about a kind of psychological and spiritual chronic fatigue syndrome that is the signature of a sentient being (an "un-awakened one"), and that forces us to sleep.

   Buddhism has its own set of subliminal processes that describe how the ego creates the exhausting illusion of self and other. Among the most famous of these is the five *skandhas* ("heaps"), discussed in chapter 13.

15. Christine Dell'Amore, "Why Do We Dream? To Ease Painful Memories, Study Hints." *National Geographic.com,* November 30, 2011, news.nationalgeographic. com/news/2011/11/111129-sleep-dreaming-rem-brain-emotions-science-health/.

16. Fariba Bogzaran and Daniel Deslauriers, *Integral Dreaming: A Holistic Approach to Dreams* (New York: State University of New York Press, 2012), 59–60.

17. Ibid, 63.

18. With refined instruments come refined measurements. Two new states have been added to these classic four. At the very low end, *epsilon* 0–05 hertz has been associated with intense meditative states. At the very high end, *gamma* 30–100+ hertz is associated with the coordination of signals across longer distances in the brain, and is connected to complex actions or associations that require the simultaneous use of multiple brain areas. Research is moving away from these fixed stages as more sophisticated measurements of the sleeping brain are developed. With neuroimaging techniques (fMRI, PET scans), high-density EEG, and spectral analysis (which measures the amplitude and phase of electrical activity over wider frequencies and time scales), new models are emerging.

19. The same downshifting occurs in deep meditation, where respiration can decrease to just a few breaths per minute, and brain waves slow down from beta or alpha into theta and even delta (or epsilon) ranges.

20. Also called "sleep starts," which are often marked by sudden muscle contractions and a sense of stepping off into space or a feeling of falling. This sensation of falling is interesting from the point of view of the inner yogas, as we will see, because falling asleep is when the bindus (drops of consciousness) fall from the head chakra into the heart chakra. It's also suggestive that "contraction" is associated with this stage, which could be a defensive response against falling into space. For a thorough look at the hypnagogic state, see Thompson, *Waking, Dreaming, Being*, 107–138.

21. Why so much time at this stage? Recent studies suggest that fact-based memories are temporarily stored in the hippocampus before being sent to the prefrontal cortex, which may have more storage space. The psychologist Matthew Walker at the University of California at Berkeley, who led one study, says, "It's as though the email inbox in your hippocampus is full and, until you sleep and clear out those fact emails, you're not going to receive any more mail. It's just going to bounce until you sleep and move it into another folder. Sleep is sophisticated, it acts locally to give us what we need." See Yasmin Anwar, "An Afternoon Nap Markedly Boosts the Brain's Learning Capacity," *Berkeley News,* February 22, 2010, newscenter.berkeley.edu/2010/02/22/naps_boost_learning_capacity.

22. Duff, *The Secret Life of Sleep,* 50. The sleep scientist Penny Lewis at the University of Manchester talks about "sleep engineering," which is designed to optimize sleep, and sustain slow wave sleep as we age. The aspiration of sleep engineering is to therefore sustain cognitive function, reduce the effects of aging, enhance creativity, and facilitate problem-solving abilities.

23. Narcoleptics enter REM directly, going from stage 1 to REM within seconds. In fatal familial insomnia, one never gets past stage 1. We don't need to bog down in scientific details, but it's helpful to realize that these cycles are not tidy progressive sequences.

CHAPTER 4 Western Lucid Dream Induction Techniques

1. Even though this chapter is devoted to Western methods, the importance of intention is a common ingredient for both Eastern and Western techniques. In the East, intention is referred to as "the power of resolution," and refers to the power of karma. Karma is basically the law of cause and effect. In Tibetan, "karma" is translated by the word *leh,* which means "action," and action is all about cause and effect.

   Fully constituted karma has four aspects: intention, action, successful completion, and rejoicing. These refer to the intention behind an action, the action itself, successful completion of the action, and a sense of satisfaction in having completed the act. Of these four, intention is first and foremost. The point with dream yoga is that through the power of resolution, we're planting karmic seeds that can ripen in the dream and spark lucidity.

2. Robert F. Price and David B. Cohen, "Lucid Dream Induction," in Gackenbach and LaBerge, *Conscious Mind, Sleeping Brain,* 131.

3. Because Western society tends to dismiss dreams, we also dismiss the importance of good dream recall. Other cultures that support dream recall also support what occurs in the night. The Stanford anthropologist Tanya Luhrmann ("To Dream in Different Cultures," *New York Times,* May 13, 2014) spent time in evangelical churches in Accra, Ghana, and Chennai, India, and writes, "One of the more startling differences is that Christians in Accra and Chennai say that God talks to them when they sleep, and in their dreams. He wakes them up by calling their names. American subjects, asked about odd events in the night, were more likely to say things like this: 'I see things, but it's just sleep deprivation.' It seems likely that the way our culture invites us to pay attention to that delicate space in which one trembles on the edge of sleep *changes what we remember of it* [emphasis added]."

4. Patricia Garfield, *Creative Dreaming* (New York: Ballantine, 1974), 200. Chapter 8, "How to Keep Your Dream Diary," offers many tips on increasing dream recall.

5. Ibid.

6. As we will see, dream yoga stresses the opposite: that the waking state is essentially no more real or unreal than the dream state. But this premise does not negate the effectiveness of conducting state checks to trigger dream lucidity. With dream yoga, instead of conducting state checks, you practice viewing *all* waking events as dreamlike.

7. Some innovative devices are available to help you conduct state checks. For example, here's a description from one website: "Worn during the day, Dream Rooster vibrates silently for ten seconds at random intervals. You simply do a dream test whenever you feel the Dream Rooster vibrate in your underwear." It can also help you fulfill certain fantasies in your lucid dreams. Sarah Coughlin, "Why Masturbate When You Can Have Sex Dreams?" Refinery29, Dec 3, 2014, refinery29.com/2014/12/78860/dream-rooster-sex-toy.

8. Daniel J. Boorstin, *The Discoverers: A History of Man's Search to Know His World and Himself* (New York: Random House, 1983), xv.

9. "Karl Popper," spaceandmotion.com/Philosophy-Karl-Popper.htm, accessed April 13, 2015.

10. R. K. Prasad, "'The Illiterate of the 21st Century Will Not Be Those Who Cannot Read and Write, but Those Who Cannot Learn, Unlearn, and Relearn'—Alvin Toffler," ComLab India, September 9, 2009, blog.commlab-india.com/elearning-design/how_can_you_unlearn, accessed May 22, 2014.

11. It's possible he could arise as a vision during the day, but his presence in a dream is more likely. Among other ways to classify dreamsigns, Stephen LaBerge lists these: (1) action-related dreamsigns (flying cars, walking on water); (2) form-related dreamsigns (tiny dog, huge bike); (3) context-related dreamsigns (meeting Christ, becoming president); and (4) inner-related dreamsigns (great fear, intense passion). (Tim Post, "Educational Frontiers of Training Lucid Dreamers," in Hurd and Bulkeley, *Lucid Dreaming: New Perspectives on Consciousness in Sleep*, vol. 1, 132–133.)

12. My friend Patricia Keelin related a lucid dream where she realized she cast no shadow and delighted in the thought of having become "the light." This is a compelling insight from a veteran oneironaut, about the light of the mind that shines in our dreams and illuminates the dream "objects" that are self-illuminating and therefore self-aware (a reflexive awareness we will return to in the conclusion of this book). When you return to the light (the clear-light mind of sleep yoga), or even approximate it (in dreams), shadows (literal and figurative) gradually disappear.

13. Mindfulness meditation, as we will see in chapter 6, is a form of memory exercise. It's about remembering to come back to the present. Memory is key to the nighttime practices, and to spiritual practice in general.

14. Developmental psychologists have discovered that very young children have no sense of object permanence, which is the idea that something exists even when you don't see it. It's one of the first developmental hints of reification (non-lucidity). Children haven't been fully primed to see the world the way we do. It could be argued that this may be one reason why children have more lucid dreams than adults.

15. Stephen LaBerge, *Lucid Dreaming: The Power of Being Awake and Aware in Your Dreams* (New York: Ballantine, 1985), 155–156.

16. For those who relate to apps, some innovative aids can help. Here are a few of the more popular ones: Awoken; Lucid Dreamer; Dream: On; DreamZ; SHADOW; Dreame; Artify; DreamCatcher Project; Lucid Dream Ultimate; CanLucidDream; 10 Steps to Lucid Dreams.

    DreamZ tracks your movements during sleep (using the sensor in your smartphone to determine your sleep cycle), and then plays an audio cue that acts as a dreamsign when you're in REM. *Shadow* is an alarm clock that slowly wakes up the dreamer and transcribes their voice-recorded dreams. This gradual awakening allows dreamers to preserve the hypno-pompic state, allowing them to more easily recall their dreams. These recorded dreams can then be loaded into a vast database that allows researchers to study the dream patterns (of those who obviously give permission to do so). It can address questions like, "What's the world dreaming about? What do women in Paris dream about, or kids in Bogota?" *Dreame* is an app that simplifies dream recording and also links users with psychologists and dream interpreters who can help them analyze their data. *Aritfy* is a project by the founders of *Dreame* that links users with artists who turn descriptions of dreams into illustrations. The sky is the limit with these innovative dream devices. For a review of these apps, go to world-of-lucid-dreaming.com/lucid-dreaming-apps.html.

17. Summarized in Adam Clark Estes, "Scientists Have Induced Lucid Dreaming with Electric Shocks," Gizmodo.com, May 12, 2014, gizmodo.com/scientists-have-induced-lucid-dreaming-with-electric-sh-1575033076; and in Nicola Davis, "Lucid Dreaming Can Be Induced by Electric Scalp Stimulation, Study Finds," *TheGuardian.com*, May 11, 2014, theguardian.com/lifeandstyle/2014/may/11/lucid-dreaming-electric-scalp-stimulation-study. See the original study, Ursula Voss et al., "Induction of Self Awareness in Dreams Through Frontal Low Current Stimulation of Gamma Activity," in *Nature Neuroscience* 17 (2014): 810–812. This study is not without its detractors. Other dream scientists question both the methods and the definitions of lucidity used here.

18. Voss et al., "Induction of Self Awareness in Dreams Through Frontal Low Current Stimulation of Gamma Activity," *Nature Neuroscience* 17 (2014): 810–812.

19. Thomas Yuschak, *Advanced Lucid Dreaming: The Power of Supplements: How to Induce High Level Lucid Dreams and Out of Body Experiences* (2006) is a self-published personal journey of lucid-dream pharmacological induction tips. Some evidence indicates that vitamin B6, which converts tryptophan into serotonin (and plays a role in brain and nerve function), is associated with more vivid dreams. A 100 milligram supplement of B6 seems to help some lucid dreamers. Yuschak's book lists dozens of other tips, many of which I have not tried.

20. Other acetylcholine esterase inhibitors include donepezil, rivastigmin, and huperzine. Some natural substances like sage *(Salvia)*, and especially Spanish sage *(Salvia lavandulaefolia)*, have also shown evidence of being effective in triggering lucidity.

21. In "The Sleep Industry: Why We're Paying Big Bucks for Something That's Free," *Time,* January 28, 2013 (business.time.com/2013/01/28/the-sleep-industry-why-were-paying-big-bucks-for-something-thats-free/), the psychologist Kit Yarrow offers these time-tested tips for good sleep hygiene:

* *Stick to a routine.* Train your body by going to sleep and getting up at the same time every day.

* *Don't multitask in bed.* Associations are powerful. Use your bed for only sleep and sex in order to create a link between your bed and sleep.

* *Get rid of distractions.* Make sure your room is cool (between 60 and 66 degrees Fahrenheit is ideal), dark, and quiet all night long. The "blue light" display of most computers, tablets, and cell phones mocks daylight and suppresses melatonin. If necessary, get a sleep mask and earplugs. Keep your bed tidy too.

* *Clear your mind.* Focus on your breathing and count "one" as you breathe in and "two" as you breathe out. Don't count any higher. Just go back and forth with one and two because people inadvertently stay alert keeping track of higher numbers.

- *Keep a notepad handy.* If you're the kind of person who stays awake ruminating, put the intrusive thoughts down on paper. That way, you can let them go until the morning rather than stressing about them while you're not falling asleep.

- *Avoid stimulants close to bedtime.* Stop drinking caffeine by around noon, and exercise as early in the day as possible. (Alcohol can accelerate the onset of sleep, but takes its toll throughout the rest of the night, usually leading to an increase in the number of times a person temporarily wakes up.)

- *Power down.* People who text and use their computers an hour before bedtime get fewer hours of sleep, are less likely to get quality sleep, and are less likely to wake up refreshed.

CHAPTER 5   Eastern Lucid Dream Induction Techniques

1. Countless books are available on the inner body. From a Kagyu perspective, Rangjung Dorje, *The Profound Inner Principles,* translated by Elizabeth Callahan (Boston: Shambhala, 2013), remains the classic. For East-West perspectives, see Anodea Judith, *Eastern Body Western Mind: Psychology and the Chakra System as a Path to the Self* (New York: Celestial Arts, 2004), and Maureen Lockhart, *The Subtle Energy Body: The Complete Guide* (Rochester, NY: Inner Traditions, 2010).

2. My principal inner yoga practices are inner Vajrayogini, which is where I first started feeling my subtle body directly, and the Six Yogas of Naropa. The "inner heat" yoga of *chandali* (Sanskrit) or *tummo* (Tibetan) is a central inner yoga practice, and shows you how to control the winds and drops. When the inner subtle body opens with the inner yogas, it thaws and softens the outer body; when the outer body "thaws" and softens with the outer yogas, the inner subtle body opens. Outer and inner yogas work on each other, and both in turn open, thaw, and soften the mind.

   Dream and sleep yoga are two yogas in the Six Yogas of Naropa that follow chandali. By learning how to shift the bindus via chandali practice, moving the bindus into my throat chakra (for dream yoga) and heart chakra (for sleep yoga) became feasible. For those who wish to practice dream and sleep yoga in depth, the Six Yogas are very helpful.

3. Even though we're born with our channels configured in certain ways, a configuration that directly affects our conscious experience, these channels are not fixed. We can change. There's an outer correlate for this inner concept. The current rage in neuroscience is "neuroplasticity," which is the discovery that the circuits in our brains are not hardwired. By changing our mind, we can literally change our brain. In a similar fashion, by changing our mind we can change our nadis, what we could call "nadiplasticity." Meditation changes the configuration and texture of our nadis. The inner yogas simply target this process more directly.

   This is helpful to know, in terms of dream yoga, because the configuration of our nadis dictates our talent for lucidity. Some people are just hardwired for lucidity. The good news behind nadiplasticity is that we can change our nadis so that we become more proficient in lucidity.

4. For a thorough look at the many definitions and applications of bindu, see Hatchell, *Naked Seeing*, 134–144.

5. One refinement to this technique is to tuck your thumbs into your palms and close your other four fingers over your thumbs during the inhalation. Placing the tip of the thumb at the base of the ring finger closes a channel associated with discursive thought. When you exhale, splay your fingers out, as a gesture of expelling.

6. Some texts reverse the channels, and their winds, for women, which suggests that women should lie down on their left side and close off the left channel. But studies have shown that both men and women fare better with lucidity by lying down on their right side. See Stephen LaBerge, "Lucid Dreaming and the Yoga of Dream State," in *Buddhism and Science: Breaking New Ground*, edited by B. Alan Wallace (New York: Columbia University Press, 2003), 239.

7. Even though the channels and winds are non-physical, they do have some correlation with the physical, otherwise lying down on your right side wouldn't have an effect on the subtle body.

8. Nyingma variations include visualizing the AH as white, or replacing the AH with the visualization of Guru Rinpoche, or Tara, or any other deity you have a connection to. Another variation is to start whatever visualization you are doing at the throat as a bit larger, then as you progress in your practice you make it smaller.

9. Maria Popova, "Better than Before: A Pyschological Field Guide to Harnessing the Power of Habit," Brain Pickings, brainpickings.org/2015/03/23/better-than-before-gretchen-rubin, accessed February 13, 2015.

10. This tenet is the basis for things like *phowa* or Pure Land Buddhism, and is a core teaching in all the bardo practices.

11. Chökyi Nyima Rinpoche, with David R. Shlim, *Medicine and Compassion: A Tibetan Lama's Guidance for Caregivers* (Boston: Wisdom Publications, 2006), 68.

12. Geshe Tashi Tsering, *Buddhist Psychology: The Foundation of Buddhist Thought*, vol. 3 (Boston: Wisdom Publications, 2006), 160.

13. Guru Rinpoche guarantees it. See Jamgon Kongtrul, *White Lotus: An Explanation of the Seven-line Prayer to Guru Padmasambhava*, translated by the Padmakara Translation Group (Boston: Shambhala, 2007).

14. "Dharma" comes from the Sanskrit root, *dhr*, which means "to hold, bear, support," and has at least three meanings. First, it refers to the teachings of the Buddha; second, it refers to the natural order of the universe; third, it refers to the "atoms of experience," or the elements that make up the empirical world.

These four "dharmas of sleep" are inspired by the famous *Four Dharmas of Gampopa*: "Grant your blessings so that my mind may be one with the dharma. Grant your blessings so that dharma may progress along the path. Grant your blessings so that the path may clarify confusion. Grant your blessings so that confusion may dawn as wisdom." Thanks to Larry Siedel for the idea behind the "Four Dharmas of Dreams."

Here is an aspiration prayer that was given to me by Tulku Thondup Rinpoche: "Tonight, I will practice dream yoga to free myself and all beings from this ocean of samsara. May all beings achieve perfect happiness and complete awakening. Over and over, I repeat my aspiration to recognize dream as dream, illusion as illusion, confusion as confusion, and see Buddha Nature in all. As I fall asleep, I visualize precious Chenrezig at my throat center. I pray again and again, 'Noble Chenrezig, please help me dissolve distractions and obstacles so I recognize dreams as dreams and rest my mind in awareness as I sleep.'"

This "Prayer to Recognize the Dream State" is from His Holiness Dudjom Rinpoche: "The combined essence of all buddhas / Pervading lord of the ocean of mandalas and buddha families, incomparably kind, most precious root lama, please hear me! / Please bless my mind, I pray! / Please grant blessings to recognize dreams as dreams! / Please bless with the power to transform and emanate in dreams! / Please grant blessings so that dreams arise as Clear Light! / Please grant blessings so that bliss and clarity are continuously integrated!"

15. B. Alan Wallace, trans., *Natural Liberation: Padmasambhava's Teachings on the Six Bardos,* with commentary by Gyatrul Rinpoche (Boston: Wisdom Publications, 1998), 151. *Samadhi* means "meditative absorption," or a gathering of the mind fully onto a single object. Samadhi is a state where the subject (consciousness) and object unite in a unitary experience.

16. Andreas Mavromatis, *Hypnagogia: The Unique State of Consciousness Between Wakefulness and Sleep* (New York: Routledge and Kegan Paul, 1987), 79.

17. See Vesna A. Wallace, *The Inner Kalacakratantra: A Buddhist Tantric View of the Individual* (New York: Oxford University Press, 2001), 57.

18. Tenzin Wangyal, *The Tibetan Yogas of Dream and Sleep* (Ithaca, NY: Snow Lion, 1998), 34.

19. Yasmin Anwar, "An Afternoon Nap Markedly Boosts the Brain's Learning Capacity," *Berkeley News,* February 22, 2010. newscenter.berkeley. edu/2010/02/22/naps_boost_learning_capacity.

20. "Nap-Deprived Tots May Be Missing Out on More Than Sleep, Says New CU-Led Study," News Center: University of Colorado Boulder, January 3, 2012, colorado.edu/news/releases/2012/01/03/ nap-deprived-tots-may-be-missing-out-more-sleep-says-new-cu-led-study.

21. Joe Martino, "How Long to Nap for the Biggest Brain Benefits," CollectiveEvolution.com, February 17, 2014, collective-evolution. com/2014/02/17/how-long-to-nap-for-the-biggest-brain-benefits.

22. Studies have shown that morning naps are more favorable than afternoon naps for producing lucid dreams (42 percent versus 12 percent). See Tadas Stumbrys and Daniel Erlacher, "The Science of Lucid Dream Induction," in Hurd and Bulkeley, *Lucid Dreaming: New Perspectives on Consciousness in Sleep,* vol. 1, 87.

23. Roger N. Shepard, *Mind Sights* (New York: W. H. Freeman, 1990), 37–38.

24. Amanda Gardner, "'Power Naps' May Boost Right-Brain Activity," CNN online, September 25, 2013, cnn.com/2012/10/17/health/health-naps-brain.

25. Judith R. Malamud, "Learning to Become Fully Lucid: A Program for Inner Growth," in Gackenbach and LaBerge, *Conscious Mind, Sleeping Brain,* 311.

CHAPTER 6   **A Fundamental Meditation: Mindfulness**

1. Studies have shown that mindfulness meditators have more lucid dreams (see Varela, *Sleeping, Dreaming, and Dying: An Exploration of Consciousness with The Dalai Lama,* 104), and experienced meditators have significantly more lucid dreams (see Jayne Gackenbach, Robert Cranson, and Charles Alexander, "Lucid Dreaming, Witnessing Dreaming, and the Transcendental Meditation Technique: A Developmental Relationship," *Lucidity Letter 5* [1986]: 34–40).

2. Just as the lucidity cultivated in daily life is carried into the dream, the lucidity cultivated in dream is carried into death. This is another way that dream yoga prepares us for death.

3. Translated by Erik Pema Kunsang.

4. For a startling example of inattentional blindness, see theinvisiblegorilla.com/videos.html.

5. A sixteen-hour day has 57,600 seconds. Look at your mind to see if you have one or more distracting thoughts each second. LONI website, "Brain Trivia," loni.usc.edu/about_loni/education/brain_trivia.php.

6. *Lojong,* or "mind training," is a principal Mahayana slogan practice; *bodhichitta,* or "awakened heart-mind," is a Mahayana practice that cultivates compassion; deity yoga, or *yidam* practice, is a meditation we will discuss later, along with the formless meditations of practices like Dzogchen and Mahamudra. In the Dzogchen teachings it is taught that "duality begins with . . . [a] process called 'straying' *('khrul pa),* in the sense that awareness makes an error and strays from itself, into suffering. This strayed portion of awareness comes to constitute our ordinary universe of self-alienation, ignorance, and violence." (See Hatchell, *Naked Seeing,* 58.)

7. Sogyal Rinpoche's comment suggests that to amp distraction is to amp samsara. With all our electronic gadgets, these clever weapons of mass distraction (smartphones, tablets, and so forth), we only need to look at the world to see the truth of this maxim. Many traditions speak of our time as the "Dark Age" (*kali yuga* in Hinduism), or in our terms, "The Age of Sleep." This is the darkness of ignorance in its moment-to-moment expression as distraction. People often associate the darkness of this age with climate change, environmental destruction, religious and political chaos, and the like. But these are just overt manifestations of the covert origin of this darkness. Distraction is the real stealth bomber of our age. Technology is not the issue. Inappropriate relationship to technology is the issue.

8. Detailed instructions and resources can be found in my book *Meditation in the iGeneration: How to Meditate in a World of Speed and Stress* (Lafayette, CO: Maitri, 2014). Pema Chödrön's *How to Meditate: A Practical Guide to Making Friends with Your Mind* (Boulder, CO: Sounds True, 2013) is another valuable resource.

9. Drew Leder, *The Absent Body* (Chicago: University of Chicago Press, 1990), 173.

10. Scientist Candace Pert, PhD, asserted that your body *is* your subconscious mind, which resonates with the fact that the body cannot lie. The science writer Tor Nørretranders says, "An individual who is one with one's body cannot lie—as children know very well . . . It is also said to be very difficult to lie in the sign language used by the deaf." (Tor Nørretranders, *The User*

Illusion: Cutting Consciousness Down to Size [New York: Viking, 1991], 154, 429.) Body language is a truer language.

11. See Bruce Lipton's "Your Unconscious Mind Is Running Your Life," lifetrainings.com, lifetrainings.com/Your-unconscious-mind-is-running-you-life.html.

CHAPTER 7   The Lion's Gaze

1. "Lookin' for Love" was written by Wanda Mallette, Bob Morrison, and Patti Ryan, and recorded by American country music singer Johnny Lee for the soundtrack to the film *Urban Cowboy* (directed by James Bridges, 1980). In terms of the Yogachara, one of the central doctrinal templates of our journey, Trungpa Rinpoche says, "It is the seventh consciousness that reaches out." This is the *klesha* mind (*klishtamanas* in Sanskrit), or "afflicted mentality," that observes the eighth consciousness and mis-takes it to be the self, and simultaneously reaches out to mistake everything else as "other." When one attains buddhahood, the afflicted mentality transforms into the wisdom of equanimity, or equality, which at one level can be defined as realizing the equality or nonduality of self and other, inside and outside.

2. One of the central contemplations in Buddhism are the "four reminders," or the "four thoughts that turn the mind." They're designed to turn the mind from looking out to looking in. Chökyi Nyima Rinpoche says that when you finally take the four reminders to heart, 50 percent of the spiritual path is complete.

   The four thoughts that turn the mind are the preciousness of human life, the reality of impermanence, the repercussions of karma, and the futility of conventional pursuits.

   On deeper level, a central aim of the inner yogas is to bring the winds into the central channel. When one is thus "centered," the winds no longer move in the side channels and therefore no longer propel ordinary thoughts and sense perceptions. We're no longer thrown out of ourselves by the inner winds, and lost in the outer world. The inner yogas are another set of centering practices that turn the mind in.

3. In neuroscientific terms "outsiders" are victims of "sensory capture," which is exactly what it sounds like. Psychologists call it "exogenous attentional capture." Your attention is captured and held hostage by external stimuli. This is part of the identity theft we've been talking about. You come to identify with external things (your house, car, boat, job, and so forth), and the status conferred by those things. The identity theft is this: you feel like you possess those things, but they actually possess you.

   Magicians call sensory capture "passive misdirection," which is how they steal your attention away from what's really happening, thereby generating the illusion of magic. These are all fancy terms for distraction.

4. Peter Kreeft, "How to Win the Culture War," at his blog, peterkreeft.com/topics-more/how-to-win.htm.

5. Martin Lowenthal, *Dawning of Clear Light: A Western Approach to Tibetan Dark Retreat Meditation* (Charlottesville, VA: Hampton Roads, 2003), 6–7. Diabetes, cancer, obesity, depression, and cardiovascular disease have been linked to overexposure to light at night.

6. No one really knows when Christ was born. December 25 was popularized as his birthday because it was already celebrated in pagan religions as the birthday of the sun, the time of the year when light comes back into the world. (It seems December 25 was close enough to the winter solstice.) Christianity is therefore in the family of "solar theology," where the Son of God is associated with the sun of our solar system.

   In Taoism it is said, "When you enter darkness and it becomes total, the darkness soon turns into light." This is represented in the yin-yang image, and is reiterated in our journey into sleep yoga: when you enter the total darkness of deep dreamless sleep, sleep yoga shows you how to turn this darkness into light.

7. *Vipashyana,* literally "insight meditation," is a principal method for looking within. Because we're so infatuated with looking outside, sometimes it helps to turn off the light. The sun does this at the end of each day, we do so when we close our eyes, and many insight meditations do so by inviting us to look within. Approached through this lens, the nighttime yogas invite the deepest meaning of "insight meditation."

8. The distinction between "outsider" and "insider" can help us relate to conventional success and failure in a new way. From a spiritual perspective, conventional success can easily become spiritual failure, because success is so distracting, and because it tends to keep us heading *out* for more. There is no tyranny as great as the tyranny of success. We get lost and addicted to the projections of mind. Conventional failure, on the other hand, can lead to spiritual success, because failure tends to collapse the "outsider" trajectory and turn us within. It all hinges on proper relationship. If we relate to conventional success properly, we won't let it get to our heads. If we relate to conventional failure properly, we can let it lead us to our hearts.

9. Buddhism talks about the omniscience (*sarvajna,* "awareness of all"; or *sarvakarajnata,* "knowledge of all aspects") of a buddha. A buddha is not only the "awakened one," but the Sanskrit root *budh* ("to awake, know, perceive") is also translated as "one who knows." Buddhas are those who have awakened to the true nature of things, who know the difference between appearance and reality. While there are a few scholars who assert this omniscience is literal, that a buddha is someone who knows everything about everything (which is how the term "omniscience" *appears*), the reality is that omniscience refers to knowing the absolute nature of every relative appearance. In other words, it refers to knowing the emptiness of everything. This is the difference between knowledge and wisdom. Knowledge alone will not liberate. Wisdom liberates. Technically, buddhas possess the five wisdoms: *dharmadhatu* wisdom, mirror-like wisdom, discriminating-awareness wisdom, all-accomplishing wisdom, and the wisdom of equanimity.

10. In a Buddhist interpretation, when Dionysius the Areopagite says, "God is invisible from excess of light," he is referring to how the essence of the mind (God, the *dharmakaya*) gets lost (becomes invisible) in the display, or luminosity of the mind (the *rupakayas*). We're blinded by the light, our own light, and mis-take it to be real. The blindness is reification.

11. Carl Jung, *Memories, Dreams, Reflections* (New York: Vintage Books, 1989).

12. Nyoshul Khenpo, *Natural Great Perfection,* translated by Lama Surya Das (Ithaca, NY: Snow Lion, 1995), 136.

13. See Venerable Khenchen Palden Sherab Rinpoche and Venerable Khenpo Tsewang Dongyal Rinpoche, *The Lion's Gaze: A Commentary on Tsig Sum Nedek,* translated by Sarah Harding, edited by Joan Kaye (Boca Raton, FL: Sky Dancer, 1998).

CHAPTER 8   Advanced Meditations and Visualizations

1. Generation stage practice (*kyerim* in Tibetan, *utpattikrama* in Sanskrit; also called deity yoga or *yidam* meditation), which deals with intentionally generating visualized forms, is designed to purify birth. It's the first half of "generation and completion stage" meditation, which arguably constitutes one-third of all Vajrayana meditation (the inner yogas and formless meditation constitute the other two-thirds). At the conclusion of visualization practice, the visualized forms dissolve into emptiness, or "die" back into formlessness. Hence completion stage practice is designed to purify death. Generation stage practice can be used to strengthen dream yoga (because it works with intentionally generating mental forms), and completion stage practice can be used to strengthen sleep yoga (because it works with intentionally dissolving those forms back into emptiness).

2. See Thompson, *Waking, Dreaming, Being: Self and Consciousness in Neuroscience, Meditation, and Philosophy*, 183. Chapter 6 of Thompson's book, "Imagining: Are We Real?" explores the relationship between dreaming and the imagination in great detail, even though Thompson does not address visualization practice directly.

3. See "Video Games Change How You Dream, Increase Lucid Dreaming," January 27, 2014, truthisscary.com/2014/01/video-games-change-how-you-dream-increase-lucid-dreaming/.

4. This is why the art of *thangka* painting, if approached properly, is a powerful spiritual practice. Instead of tracing out a lotus, you are painting an entire deity or mandala. If you then happen to do the *sadhana*, or generation stage meditation, associated with that deity or mandala, you can really bring the sadhana to life, and therefore the energies associated with that deity or mandala. This is also connected to the form of *nirmanakaya* known as "crafted nirmanakaya." The greatest thangka, or *rupa* (statue), artists imbue their art with spirit, bringing it to life. You can feel this in great works of spiritual art. The art is injected and infused with wisdom and can become a source of spiritual refuge, a representation of the awakened mind.

5. Seed syllables (*bijaksara* in Sanskrit; *bija* is cognate with *bindu*) are the condensed essence of a deity, bodhisattva, or Buddha—or ultimately of any phenomenon. They are the irreducible representation of something in sound. Seed syllables are also the ultimate condensation of the Dharma, the quintessence of mantra. In Buddhist and Hindu cosmology, the entire universe is a manifestation of sound and light, and we can therefore capture the essence of that universe in sound, via mantra and seed syllables. Christianity echoes this principle when it says, "In the beginning was the word [sound] and the word was made flesh." The "Big Bang" is an allusion to this principle from a scientific perspective. Singularities are associated with the seed syllable principle, of which there are mathematical singularities, technological singularities, gravitational singularities, and so forth.

6. What neuro-linguistic programming (NLP) calls "anchoring." You anchor (correlate) stages of consciousness with steps around the lotus.

7. The sense of self always seems to have a specific location, which for most people seems to be either in their head, behind their eyes, or in their forehead area (the location of the "third eye"). In our imagination we can see from any position that we like, but most people locate their sense of self/position in the head, which resonates with the idea that waking consciousness is gathered in the head chakra. This location of identity is probably because vision is the dominant sense in humans and our most dualistic sense (we can see farther than we can hear or smell or taste or touch). It's the position by which we literally see the world, and figuratively see ourselves. When we dream, we don't have a head, let alone a body. But because of the force of habit/karma, we think that we do. We still feel like we're viewing the dream from our eyes, eyes that don't exist.

Douglas Harding wrote an innovative book, *On Having No Head: Zen and the Rediscovery of the Obvious* (London: Arkana, 1986), where he talks about the "eight stages of the headless way." It's a clever way to work with the deeper notion of *anatman*, or "no self." No head = no self. Try it. Imagine relating to your world without the reference point of a head. For me, things get open, and then dreamlike, quickly. It's a glimpse into the nonduality of consciousness. This exercise in headlessness/egolessness can ignite a sudden and illuminating change in perspective. Who is seeing what?

8. One variation of this descent approach is to visualize a stack of AHs from your head down to your throat. As you fall asleep, you fall down the visualized AHs, moving your mind closer to your throat, like dominoes falling onto each other.

9. When one becomes a formal Buddhist, one does so through "taking refuge" in the three jewels. One takes refuge in the Buddha, as an example of someone who woke up; in the Dharma, the teachings that show us how to wake up; and the Sangha, the spiritual community that is motivated to wake up. In its own way, ego takes refuge as well. But instead of taking refuge in these three jewels of awakening, ego takes refuge in its own three jewels: sleep, ignorance, and distraction.

10. Quoted in *Shambhala Sun*, March 2014, 32.

11. Psychologically, we hide out in what Carl Jung called "the shadow." Shadows are rejected aspects of ourselves that we project out onto others, or the world. As a summary maxim: whenever something *affects* you more than it *informs* you, you're probably dealing with a projection or shadow element.

In our terminology, shadows lurk in the bandwidth of the substrate mind. When the clear-light mind shines through this unconscious level, which acts as a filter, the natural radiance of the clear-light mind is perverted into projection. Instead of seeing the light, we see filtered shadows. Instead of seeing truth, we witness lies we didn't even know we were telling. In other words, we get lost in the projections of our substrate mind. The clear-light mind continues to radiate below, like a never-setting sun, but we don't see its shine upon our world. We don't see reality as it is. We see a highly colored, filtered, and projected version of that light as it gets distorted by all the residue in the bandwidth of the substrate.

CHAPTER 9   Illuminating the Deeper Mind

1. The following model is an adaptation of the Yogachara ninefold description of mind. Consciousness one through six = psyche; consciousness seven and mostly eight = the substrate; consciousness nine (which is not included in most standard expositions, which stop at eight consciousnesses) = the clear-light mind.

2. The same dropping occurs at death, which is why dream yoga leads to bardo yoga. We drop dead at the end of life the same way we drop dead asleep each night.

3. Elizabeth Lloyd Mayer, *Extraordinary Knowing: Science, Skepticism, and the Inexplicable Powers of the Human Mind* (New York: Bantam, 2008), 216.

4. For serious students, there's a difference between the "substrate consciousness"—what I'm calling the substrate mind here—and the "substrate." It's the difference between *alaya* (wisdom) and *alaya vijnana* (consciousness, or divided/bifurcated wisdom; *vi* = divided; *jnana = wisdom).* See B. Alan Wallace, *Stilling the Mind: Shamatha Teachings from Dudjom Lingpa's Vajra Essence* (Boston: Wisdom Publications, 2011) and Karl Brunnhölzl, trans., *Luminous Heart: The Third Karmapa on Consciousness, Wisdom, and Buddha Nature* (Ithaca, NY: Snow Lion, 2009), for more on the substrate and substrate consciousness.

5. The brain is constantly lying to us, and we buy into its deceit. You don't really "see" anything. You process patterns related to objects "out there," constructing false representations of the world. "You go from detecting points of light in photoreceptors to detecting the presence of contrast, edges, and corners, to building entire objects, including an awareness of their color, size, distance, and relation to other objects. In this process, your visual system makes inferences and guesses from the get-go. You perceive a three-dimensional world despite the fact that a simple two-dimensional image falls on each retina. Your visual circuits amplify, suppress, converge, and diverge visual information. You perceive what you see as something different from reality . . . you make up a lot of what you see . . . you simply cannot trust your eyes." (Stephen L. Macknik, Susana Martinez-Conde, and Sandra Blakeslee, *Sleights of Mind: What the Neuroscience of Magic Reveals about Our Everyday Deceptions* [New York: Picador, 2011], 12–13.)

6. This is an age-old idea famously depicted in the West by Plato in the "allegory of the cave." Imagine a group of prisoners who have lived their entire lives chained to face the wall of a cave. They spend their time watching shadows projected onto the wall of the cave by objects passing in front of a fire that's behind them. The shadows (appearances) are as close as they get to seeing the reality of the objects behind them. For Plato, the philosopher is the one who frees himself from this bondage to shadows, and finally sees the reality that projects them.

7. Sam Harris, *Waking Up: A Guide to Spirituality Without Religion* (New York: Simon & Schuster, 2014), 38.

8. The Karmapa, Ogyen Trinley Dorje, *The Heart Is Noble: Changing the World from the Inside Out* (Boston: Shambhala, 2013), 60.

9. We confuse the satisfaction of want with its temporary transcendence. We think we're happy when we get what we want, but if we look deeply, we'll discover that we're actually happy because we stopped wanting. "In other

words, we ourselves [our desire] are the bigger problem," as the Karmapa says. The Greek philosopher Epicurus said, "Do not spoil what you have by desiring what you have not; but remember that what you now have was once among the things you only hoped for."

10. "Fault," "fail," "fallacy," "fallible," and "false" all share the same Latin root, *fallere,* which means "to deceive, fail."

11. In the bardo teachings of Tibetan Buddhism, there is a point in the afterlife journey where we come across three great chasms, or faults. This is an archetypal experience that represents the three principal fracture lines that emanate from the fundamental fault of duality. In other words, once you fault reality into self and other, you then either want the other (and fall into the passion fault), push it away (and slip into the aggression fault), or couldn't care less (and slide into the ignorance fault). Like the thousands of fracture lines that radiate out from a core crack in reality, our entire "conscious" lives are comprised of constantly slipping into one subsidiary fault (deception) or another.

12. The Dalai Lama, *The Universe in a Single Atom: The Convergence of Science and Spirituality* (New York: Morgan Road, 2005), 125.

13. Just as we arise from our conventional bed in the morning, and return to it each night, the bed of the clear-light mind is what *everything* arises from and eventually returns to. Thoughts arise from this primordial bed and dissolve back into it; our physical form, and therefore life itself, comes from this same bed in the morning of our birth, and dissolves back into it in the evening of our death. The clear-light mind is the womb and the tomb of all manifest reality.

14. The shadow side (near enemy) of "cutting through" is thinking it implies cutting (and throwing) away. "Cutting through" suggests one aspect of the path (the "sudden" path) and the immediacy of accessing the awakened state. Another and more gradual aspect of the path is about befriending and integrating the contents of the psyche and substrate. The end result is the same, but the skillful means are different. Both paths lead to integration and wholeness.

15. Thomas Merton, *The Wisdom of the Desert* (New York: New Directions, 1960), 11.

16. They acknowledge your relative appearance, but also see through it into your buddha nature (clear-light mind). This gives birth to "pure perception," which we'll return to when we discuss the benefits of dream yoga. In public, this acknowledgment is polite. In private it can be wrathful. Devoted students open themselves, willingly, to being "cut through" by compassionate masters. The traditions are replete with stories of masters taking on a wrathful manifestation to cut through the psyche and substrate of their students.

17. Supramundane "eyes" are mentioned throughout Buddhism, including references in the *Nikayas,* the *Abhidharma,* the *Prajnaparamita* ("perfection of wisdom") literature, Dzogchen, and the Kalachakra. In *The Perfection of Wisdom Sutra in Twenty-Five Thousand Lines,* the "divine eyes" allow one to see the effects of karma in others, and the "dharma eyes," which are related to compassionate activity, allow one to see the personal histories of others, their spiritual development, and how to best help them. When we talk

about the X-ray eyes in chapter 18 that allow one to perceive illusory forms, these are connected to the "eyes of insight" that see emptiness.

18. Sogyal Rinpoche, *Glimpse After Glimpse: Daily Reflections on Living and Dying* (New York: HarperOne, 1995), July 16 entry.

19. Until we come to listen to and trust the wise guy inside, the inner guru, we rely on the wise guy outside, the outer guru. But the outer teacher is nothing other than the external embodiment and voice of our inner wisdom. This is why true devotees connect so strongly to a guru. They're fundamentally connecting to the representative of their own wisdom. When we receive teachings from a master in our dreams, the representative now arises as a more direct manifestation of our own clear-light mind. Of the four types of guru (physical guru, text as guru, world as guru, and the guru within) the ultimate guru is the Buddha (guru) within—our own clear-light mind.

20. While the influence from the relative unconscious mind is often negative, the influence from the absolute unconscious mind is always positive. You could argue that anything positive has its origin in this perfectly pure core of our being. Things become more perfect when we learn how to rest in this natural great perfection. It may not be "perfect" from ego's point of view, but it is perfect from reality's point of view.

21. Sogyal Rinpoche, *Glimpse After Glimpse: Daily Reflections on Living and Dying*, November 6 entry.

CHAPTER 10   The Mind's Fuzzy Boundaries

1. In terms of karma, this means that you can create good karma (habits) in your dreams or purify karma altogether. This reiterates a central theme of the spiritual path: we first replace bad karma with good karma, and we then remove or purify karma altogether. This maxim corresponds to the two ways that dream yoga transforms the relative unconscious mind. Our daily meditations also do this, but with dream yoga we do it more directly because we're working with deeper levels of mind, which is where karmic seeds are stored. In other words, because it's more direct, we can empty out the storehouse consciousness more quickly. Dream yoga is part of the Vajrayana, which is often called "the quick path."

2. Traleg Rinpoche says that we can have lucid dreams, which implies the potential for practicing dream yoga, and not recall it upon waking. The work of transformation is being done even if we don't recall it. There is other data that seems to confirm this (see James F. Pagel, "Lucid Dreaming as Sleep Meditation," in Hurd and Bulkeley, *Lucid Dreaming: New Perspectives on Consciousness in Sleep*, vol. 1, 64). The philosopher Evan Thompson writes, "The fact that you have no memory of some period of time doesn't necessarily imply that you lacked all consciousness during that time. You might have been conscious—in the sense of undergoing qualitative states or processes of sentience or awareness—but for one reason or another not been able to form the kind of memories that later you can retrieve and verbally report." (*Waking, Dreaming, Being: Self and Consciousness in Neuroscience, Meditation, and Philosophy*, 252.)

While sleeping, some people walk, talk, text, cook, eat, drive, and even have sex ("sexsomnia" that leads to "snore-gasm") with no recollection upon awakening. In some remarkable cases, they even commit violent crimes, including murder, while asleep. The prefrontal cortex, which watches and controls our impulses, is unplugged in deep sleep, leading to a host of uncensored activity. (For some wild accounts of "sleepwalking," see chapter 8, "Bumps in the Night," in David K. Randall's *Dreamland: Adventures in the Strange Science of Sleep*.) If all this can happen without recollection, surely we can have lucid dreams and not remember them.

3. Western psychologists might argue that when we become lucid in our dreams, it's no longer the unconscious mind that's at work, because you can't be both conscious and unconscious at the same time (awake and asleep). This is why scientists dismissed lucid dreaming as impossible, until it was scientifically proven. One way to resolve this is to say that the unconscious mind continues to create the background or general atmosphere of the dream (you are still dreaming, after all), but the conscious mind (the lucid part) is also at play, working to transform what's being presented by the unconscious mind, the dream content, and again doing so directly.

4. This is resonant with the view that mindfulness is also an innate and therefore natural capacity of the mind. It's very difficult to get meditation masters to talk about their abilities in lucid dreaming, but the few who do address lucid dreaming intimate a high level of frequency and proficiency.

5. Improper relaxation, in this context, is like plopping onto a couch and letting go in a more Western sense. Proper relaxation is the province of meditation.

6. G. Scott Sparrow, *Lucid Dreaming; Dawning of the Clear Light* (Virginia Beach: A.R.E. Press, 1982), 34. See also Andrew Holecek, *The Power and the Pain: Transforming Spiritual Hardship into Joy* (Ithaca, NY: Snow Lion, 2010), for more on the grace of crises.

7. Inayat Khan, *The Sufi Message of Hazrat Inayat Khan: The Art of Being* (Los Angeles: Library of Alexandria, 2001), 189.

8. The Advaita Vedanta school ("Advaita" = nondual; "Veda-anta" = Veda-end, or the end of the Vedas, which refers to the Upanishads, the foundational texts in Hinduism) refers to deep sleep as "seed sleep," or "causal," which means it's the casual source of dreaming and waking consciousness. In Vedanta, as well as Vajrayana Buddhism, awareness identifies with a very subtle, or "causal body" in deep sleep; a subtle, or "mental body" in dreams; and a gross, or "physical body" in the waking state. The point here is that dreaming and waking consciousness both arise out of deep dreamless sleep.

9. Our samsara comes to an end when we finally wake up to things as they are. But samsara altogether never ends, because there will always be others asleep to the true nature of things, lost in the dream of mere appearance.

CHAPTER 11   A Taxonomy of Dreams

1. Modern dream research also has something to say about types of dreams and their relationship to stages of sleep. Hypnagogic dreams occur when you're falling asleep and tend to be very visual and intense, like a hallucination, but lack a narrative. Light sleep dreams tend to ramble and

replay activities from the day. REM stage dreams tend to be long, with story-like narratives that resemble the waking state. And dreams of deep sleep are often bizarre, with extreme body sensations and night terrors. They exhibit intense but undeveloped thought processes. See Lynne Malcolm, "The New Science of Sleep and Dreaming," ABC Radio National, October 29, 2014, abc.net.au/radionational/programs/allinthemind/the-new-science-of-sleep-and-dreaming/5850416.

2. Robert Bly, *Kabir: Ecstatic Poems* (Boston: Beacon Press, 2011).

3. What kinds of other beings? As suggested below, realized beings who seem to have the capacity to "enter" the mind of another at this level. In Tibetan Buddhism, wisdom protectors *(dharmapalas)*, *yidams*, and other *sambhogakaya*-level forms of being would be included. Shamans would have their own list.

4. Treasure them but be careful how you share them. "Telling the dream to one's immediate group can negate dream omens; keeping silent preserves the omen's effectiveness." (Bogzaran and Deslauriers, *Integral Dreaming: A Holistic Approach to Dreams,* 157.)

5. Marcia Binder Schmidt and Michael Tweed, eds., *Perfect Clarity: A Tibetan Buddhist Anthology of Mahamudra and Dzogchen,* translated by Erik Pema Kunsang (Hong Kong: Ranjung Yeshe, 2012), 87, 89.

6. Dzigar Kongtrul Rinpoche says that the experience of déjà vu might arise from an intuitive sense of karmic seeds in the alaya before they ripen into full-blown experience.

7. In the language of Vajrayana Buddhism, this is the union of creation and completion stage practice. From the perspective of the Mahayana, it is the union of form and emptiness. At this lofty level one never leaves the "samadhi of suchness," or what we're referring to as the clear-light mind, and therefore whatever arises in that samadhi is perceived as the perfectly pure expression of the nature of mind. We will return to this important theme when we discuss the fine points of illusory form. Tenzin Wangyal says: "Developing the capacity for clear-light dreams is similar to developing the capacity of abiding in the nondual presence of *rigpa* during the day. In the beginning, rigpa and thought seem different, so that in the experience of rigpa there is no thought, and if thought arises we are distracted and lose rigpa. But when stability in rigpa is developed, thought simply arises and dissolves without in the least obscuring rigpa; the practitioner remains in nondual awareness." (*The Tibetan Yogas of Dream and Sleep*, 63.) When one is fully integrated with the clear-light mind, dreaming ceases altogether. One might argue that dreams may simply not be recalled, but Buddhism asserts that this is not the case. Dreams do indeed stop.

8. See Bogzaran and Deslauriers, *Integral Dreaming,* 89–103.

9. See John Welwood, *Toward a Psychology of Awakening: Buddhism, Psychotherapy, and the Path of Personal and Spiritual Transformation* (Boston: Shambhala, 2000).

10. For a Hindu-based look at dream interpretation, see Swami Sivananda Radha, *Realities of the Dreaming Mind: The Practice of Dream Yoga* (Spokane, WA: Timeless Books, 2013). She uses the term "dream yoga" in a nontraditional way, but her methods of interpretation do eventually guide the dreamer to the Divine within.

11. "Spirituality" is a term I use cautiously, because it denotes experiences removed from daily life and easily leads to an escapist attitude. "Spiritual," by definition, is set in contrast to "material," and therefore often implies something otherworldly. Real spirituality is to unite the spiritual with the material, which is one rendering of the term "nonduality." Real spirituality is fully embodied, lived right here and now. It's about finding heaven on earth, and discovering the inseparability of nirvana and samsara. It's not about running away from our gritty life experiences into some sterile disembodied bliss. It's about waking up to the bliss that is inherent within any experience.

12. For one compelling story, see Oliver Sacks, *The Man Who Mistook His Wife for a Hat* (New York: Harper & Row, 1985), chapter 3, "The Disembodied Lady." Sacks writes elsewhere, "One must assume in such cases [of dream premonition] that the disease was already affecting neural function, and that the unconscious mind, the dreaming mind, was more sensitive to this than the waking mind . . . Patients with multiple sclerosis may dream of remissions a few hours before they occur, and patients recovering from strokes or neurological injuries may have striking dreams of improvement before such improvement is 'objectively' manifest." (*Dreaming and the Self: New Perspectives on Subjectivity, Identity, and Emotion,* Jeannette Marie Mageo, ed. [Albany: State University of New York Press, 2003], 63–64.) Prophetic dreams are also called "prodromic," "prognostic," "proleptic," or "theorematic." (Havelock Ellis, *The World of Dreams* [Boston: Houghton Mifflin, 1911], 157.)

13. Carl Jung, ed., *Man and His Symbols* (London: Aldus Books, 1964), 37.

14. After the mother of a good friend died, and my friend was lamenting the loss, the deceased mother (or her projected image) came to me in a dream and asked me to convey this message: "Dying wasn't so bad, it just took a bit longer than I thought." On another occasion, when my meditation center was involved with intractable administrative problems, I had a dream where crude oil suddenly erupted in the lawn surrounding the center. When I shared this dream at the next council meeting and suggested that the message was about refining our crude inner wealth into refined oil (energy) we could share with others, we were able to finally break through our problems.

15. An elite aspect of this type of dream is when the highest lamas, like His Holiness the Dalai Lama or the Karmapa, are requested to locate *tulkus,* or reincarnated lamas. Disciples from the previous incarnation of the lama they are searching for will supplicate such a master to help them find the new incarnation. The master will "sleep on it," have a dream that identifies where the tulku can be found, and then pass that dream along to the disciples who use the information to locate the tulku.

16. The science of neuroplasticity is resonant with karmic principles. This field of neuroscience asserts that the mind is plastic, and that what we do with our mind can literally change the structure of our brain. With each repetitive thought, word, or deed, we're strengthening neural connections in the brain, metaphorically cutting grooves that make it easier for us to fall into those grooves. See Sharon Begley, *Train Your Mind, Change Your Brain* (New York: Ballantine, 2008).

17. Dreaming also stops in people who have lesions on the right or left parietal cortex and the occipito-temporoparietal junction, which has nothing to do with karma, at least as it's being engaged here. It would be interesting to see if REM-stage sleep also stops when the storehouse consciousness is emptied.

18. Tulku Urgyen Rinpoche, *Blazing Splendor: The Memoirs of Tulku Urgyen Rinpoche, as Told to Erik Pema Kunsang and Marcia Binder Schmidt* (Hong Kong: Ranjung Yeshe Books, 2005), 82.

19. Bardos only exist from the point of confusion. For a buddha, there is no bardo.

CHAPTER 12   Breaking the Frame: An Introduction to Illusory Form

1. Lucid dreamers have a better vestibular system (which is associated with balance and spatial orientation), and from an Eastern perspective they have subtle body channel configurations that predispose them to lucidity. The dream researchers Thomas Snyder and Jayne Gackenbach compiled this data: "Persons with a propensity to dream lucidly can be described as sensitive to tactile/kinesthetic and vestibular cues, as less reliant on an external visual field, as relatively field-independent, as having a well-delineated body boundary, as being androgenous in sex role and open to internal but not external risks, as being more self- rather than socially oriented, and as tending toward introversion and relatively high level of arousal." ("Individual Differences Associated with Lucid Dreaming," in Gackenbach and LaBerge, *Conscious Mind, Sleeping Brain,* 254–255.)

2. Dzogchen Ponlop, *Mind Beyond Death* (Ithaca, NY: Snow Lion, 2006), 67.

3. "False awakenings" is a term that can be applied to many "enlightened" teachers in the West. These are people who have had temporary enlightened *experiences* and think that those experiences constitute *realization.* Spiritual experiences always have a beginning and an end—they never last. They're the "mist" in mystical experiences, which always evaporates. Realization is stable, like a mountain. Many Westerners grasp after their spiritual experiences (and often proclaim them), which doesn't allow the experience to mature into realization. They get stuck, often for an entire life, into thinking they are awake—when they've merely slipped into another level of dream. False awakenings lead to false prophets and highly marketable "masters." See Andrew Holecek, "Just When You Think You're Enlightened," *Buddhadharma: The Practitioner's Quarterly* 12, no. 4 (summer 2014): 31–35.

4. Wendy Doniger O'Flaherty, *Dreams, Illusion, and other Realities,* (Delhi: Motilal Banarsidass, 1987), 197.

5. Which is *exactly* the same quality that defines the awakened way to relate to anything that arises in your mind. In other words, this ability to witness whatever arises in your mind with equanimity is precisely what brings about this awakened relationship to any state of consciousness. For a buddha, an awakened one, waking, dreaming, and dreamless sleep all arise and dissolve in the vast expanse of such an open mind. These states are therefore equivalent for a buddha, for one who has awakened to the unreality, the emptiness, of them all.

6. As cited in Bruce Tift, *Already Free: Buddhism Meets Psychotherapy on the Path of Liberation* (Boulder, CO: Sounds True, 2015).

7. Doniger O'Flaherty, *Dreams, Illusion, and other Realities*, 202.

8. Illusory form is where we can practice the essence of dream yoga even if we never try the nighttime practices, or ever have a lucid dream. If dream yoga doesn't work for you, you can still get to the heart of it through the practice of illusory form. Tsongkhapa, the founder of the Gelugpa tradition of Tibetan Buddhism, and many other masters, says that dream yoga is part of illusory form yoga, which implies that illusory form is the main practice.

9. Flicker fusion is thought to arise because of a process called "persistence of vision." This is associated with the ability of your retina (or in the case of meditation, your mind's eye) to retain an image of an object for up to one-fifth of a second after it is gone from your visual field, a kind of visual echo of the object. Persistence of vision is what creates the illusion of object constancy, and therefore good continuation (see notes 10 and 11 below).

10. Flicker fusion creates "good continuation," a term coined by Gestalt psychologists to refer to the process by which our brains make things seem solid or whole based on limited information. (The etymology of the word "con-fusion" [fuse together] has deep cognitive and spiritual implications.)

11. Good continuation, which is so coveted by the ego, goes bad. In the Abhidharma tradition, each moment, defined as "the time it takes to snap your fingers," is comprised of sixty-four "sub-moments." Advanced meditators are able to perceive these sub-moments and all the other atoms of experience (dharmas) that underlie every appearance.

12. Both inattentional blindness and change blindness are at the root of so many problems, like our inability to see or admit that the climate is changing, that distraction is becoming epidemic, that speed and greed are destroying our world, and so forth.

13. Thompson, *Waking, Dreaming, Being: Self and Consciousness in Neuroscience, Meditation, and Philosophy*, 174.

14. Ken Wilber, *The Spectrum of Consciousness* (Wheaton, IL: Theosophical Publishing House, 1977), 179.

15. Perhaps mental instability is one reason why nature developed sleep paralysis during REM sleep, as a way to protect ourselves and others from unstable minds as they are released unconstrained during dreams. Imagine the physical instability, the chaos, if our dreams—especially those infected with unconscious desire or aggression—could be acted out. It would be interesting to study meditation masters, those with very stable minds, to see if in fact they experience sleep paralysis during their REM sleep, or if that atonia is somehow lessened. Perhaps really stable minds, when they are unleashed, don't need the leash. They don't need to be restrained the same way we do.

16. Lopon Kalsang Dorje, *The Radiance of Possibility Within Bardo* (Kathmandu: Lopon Kalsang Dorje, 2009), 23.

17. This stability becomes everything when the mind is let loose unconstrained in the big dream at the end of this life, which is death. Mind becomes reality after death—because there's nothing else. When the bardo literature talks about the "terrifying experiences of the bardo," the terror is nothing more than our unstable mind unleashed without constraint (without the

body). There's no terror for the stable mind. In the bardo, the stability of your mind virtually becomes your new body, and you take refuge in that. This is why mindfulness is not only a great preparation for dreaming, but for death.

CHAPTER 13   The Practice of Illusory Form

1. Kodo Sawaki Roshi, "Looking Beyond the Lens," *Buddhadharma: The Practitioner's Quarterly* 13, no. 4 (summer 2015): 50.

2. See Macknik, Martinez-Conde, and Blakeslee, *Sleights of Mind: What the Neuroscience of Magic Reveals About Our Everyday Deceptions.*

3. See, for instance, Al Seckel, *The Great Book of Optical Illusions* (Richmond Hill, Ontario: Firefly Books, 2002); E. Richard Churchill, *How to Make Optical Illusion Tricks and Toys* (New York: Sterling, 1989); and Keith Kay, *The Little Giant Book of Optical Illusions* (New York: Sterling, 1997).

4. In a recent study published in *Human Brain Mapping,* researchers including Robin Carhart-Harris from the Department of Medicine, Imperial College, London, discovered that the mind-altering drug psilocybin unlocked brain states usually only experienced when we dream, and invoked changes in activity that could help unlock permanent shifts in perspective—in the way we see the world. Rachel Feltman of the *Washington Post* writes, "Administration of the drug just before or during sleep seemed to promote higher activity levels during Rapid Eye Movement sleep, when dreams occur. An intriguing finding, Carhart-Harris says, given that people tend to describe their experience on psychedelic drugs as being like 'a waking dream.'" Not only do these psycholytic (mind-loosening) drugs invite a dreamlike reality, they tend to suppress an egoic or solid reality: "Our firm sense of self—the habits and experiences that we find integral to our personality—is quieted by these trips. Carhart-Harris believes that the drugs may unlock emotion while 'basically killing the ego,' allowing users to be less narrow-minded and let go of negative outlooks. It's still not clear why such effects can have more profound long-term effects on the brain than our nightly dreams." According to Carhart-Harris (says Feltman), "[These drugs could] be essentially loosening their minds—promoting a permanent change in outlook." (Rachel Feltman, "Psychedelic Mushrooms Put Your Brain in a 'Waking Dream,' Study Finds," *Washington Post,* July 3, 2014.)

   In a July 3, 2014 press release, Carhart-Harris states, "I was fascinated to see similarities between the pattern of brain activity in a psychedelic state and the pattern of brain activity during dream sleep, especially as both involve the primitive areas of the brain linked to emotions and memory. People often describe taking psilocybin as producing a dreamlike state and our findings have, for the first time, provided a physical representation for the experience in the brain." Carhart-Harris continues, "One particular network that was especially affected [in terms of being suppressed] plays a central role in the brain, essentially 'holding it all together,' and is linked to our sense of self." See eurekalert.org/pub_releases/2014-07/icl-nsd070114.php.

5. The Kagyu master Khenpo Tsültrim Gyamtso Rinpoche has his students sing these songs constantly. All of these verses were translated by Ari Goldfield, under the guidance of Khenpo Rinpoche.

6. The five skandhas, or "heaps, aggregates," are the five ingredients that comprise the sense of self: form, feeling, perception, formation, and consciousness.
   In terms of illusory speech, in Buddhism, "imperceptible forms" are part of the skandha (aggregate) of form, which is generally associated with material objects. One of these imperceptible forms is called "form originating from correct commitment," which refers to vows. This means that words, in the shape of vows, are considered to have almost literal form.

7. *Dasa-kusala-karmapatha* in Sanskrit, or the "ten good paths of action." They are the Buddhist version of the Ten Commandments. Three refer to body: not to kill, not to steal, and not to engage in sexual misconduct. And the final three refer to mind: non-greed, non-hatred, and holding right view.

8. Described in Bernard McGrane, *The Un-TV and the 10 mph Car: Experiments in Personal Freedom and Everyday Life* (Fort Bragg, CA: The Small Press, 1994).

9. A 2014 study in the journal *Science* suggested that people hate being alone with their (reified) thoughts so much that they would rather be in pain than be alone with their mind. (Timothy D. Wilson et al., "Just Think: The Challenges of the Disengaged Mind," *Science* 345, no. 6192 [July 2014]: 75–77.) Given the choice between sitting alone with their thoughts for fifteen minutes or being able to distract themselves with electric shocks during that time, a quarter of women and two-thirds of men chose the distraction of the shocks over their own company. One man in this study shocked himself 190 times within a fifteen-minute "thinking session," while most subjects shocked themselves about seven times. From the abstract of this study: "Most people prefer to do something rather than nothing, even if that something is negative."

10. Andrea Miller and the editors of the *Shambhala Sun*. Also, *Buddha's Daughters: Teachings from Women Who Are Shaping Buddhism in the West* (Boston: Shambhala, 2014), 139.

11. Chögyam Trungpa, *The Sadhana of Mahamudra,* translated by the Nalanda Translation Committee (Halifax, NS; Nalanda Translation Committee Publications, 1990), 19.

12. Echolocation is used by blind people (tapping their canes and so forth) in a process called "acoustic wayfinding," to find their way around the world with acoustic rather than visual clues. Bats, dolphins, whales, and other forms of wildlife, as well as human sonar devices, are similarly used to situate self by situating other.

13. You may not feel that you're overtly grasping after thoughts and things, but the covert expression of grasping is attachment and fixation. This is a level of grasping that's been going on for so long that it's now unconscious. Attachment and fixation are usually exposed when something disappears or someone dies. The pain and grief of that loss is in direct proportion to your subliminal fixation. If you really hurt when something is taken away, you were really attached. Imagine having all your muscles in a constant state of contraction, and doing it for so long that you forgot you're doing it. It's exhausting, whether you know it or not.

14. Khenpo Tsültrim Gyamtso, *Stars of Wisdom: Analytical Meditation, Songs of Yogic Joy, and Prayers of Aspiration,* translated, edited, and introduced by Ari Goldfield and Rose Taylor (Boston: Shambhala, 2010), 65–66.

CHAPTER 14   Advancing to Dream Yoga: First Stages and Practices

1. The Eightfold Noble Path, which constitutes the fourth Noble Truth (the path leading to the cessation of suffering), comprises right view, right resolve, right speech, right action, right livelihood, right effort, right mindfulness, and right meditation. These eight "rights" are all about creating the right environment, meaning every aspect of your life becomes the path and is therefore conducive to flashes of enlightenment.

2. Stephen LaBerge writes of the importance of contrast and the perception born from it: "If you don't know a second state of consciousness, the first state of consciousness—your everyday waking state of consciousness— is unconscious to you, you don't know what it is to be in a state of consciousness. Lucid dreaming provides that extra perspective that gives a much broader view of the possibilities of life." (In Lynne Malcolm and Katie Silver, "Tapping into the Power of Lucid Dreaming," ABC Radio National, November 5, 2014, abc.net.au/radionational/programs/allinthemind/tapping-into-the-power-of-lucid-dreaming/5868072). Orgyenpa quote from *A Commentary on The Ocean of True Meaning,* Part Three, by Khenpo Karthar Rinpoche, translated by Lama Yeshe Gyamtso (Woodstock, NY: KTD Monastery, 1994), 41.

3. That flash is called "the path of seeing."

4. Akin to what Jung called "individuation," which is the process of becoming aware of oneself (through dreams or therapy) and discovering one's inner self. It's the process of integrating the conscious with the unconscious on the way to self-actualization. The process of integration is also akin to psychosynthesis, where the emphasis is on making dream images part of your conscious awareness, as distinct from breaking down parts of the dream for the purpose of analysis, as in psychoanalysis.

   Integrate the disparate and therefore divisive elements within yourself and you will spontaneously do so with others. This is what the Dalai Lama refers to as "inner disarmament," the first and most important step to world disarmament. As the anthropologist Kilton Stewart puts it, "work for peace on earth by first establishing peace inside the earth that is [your] body." Or as the Kalachakra Tantra puts it, "As within, so without."

5. One of my favorite teachers is Dzigar Kongtrul Rinpoche, who has a wonderfully wrathful edge. He doesn't buy our Western trips and he often takes his students lovingly to task when they indulge them. In one question-and-answer session, a student went on at length about her psychological problems and how she was working with them. Rinpoche listened patiently, and then like a skilled surgeon, took out his blade. "Western students are always 'processing' their problems. Try some more cutting. Don't indulge so much. Cut." Rinpoche is well aware of the power of Western psychology and its place in human development, but he's also aware of how we can get lost in those methods.

6. This is pure conjecture, with no studies or empirical backing, but I often wonder if the reason so many lucid (and non-lucid) dreamers report flying dreams is because the inner winds that lift the bindus from the heart center up to the throat also lift us into flight, almost as if we continue to "ride" those winds into the dream air.

7. Wangyal, *The Tibetan Yogas of Dream and Sleep*, 121.

8. Malamud, "Learning to Become Fully Lucid: A Program for Inner Growth," in Gackenbach and LaBerge, *Conscious Mind, Sleeping Brain*, 316.

9. Glenn H. Mullin, trans., *Readings on the Six Yogas of Naropa* (Ithaca, NY: Snow Lion, 1997), 127.

10. For generation stage practitioners, these two steps relate to "self-visualization" and "front visualization," respectively. As a more advanced third step, generate in your dream a richly ornamented palace, with yourself in the center surrounded by a divine retinue.

11. Wallace, *Natural Liberation: Padmasambhava's Teachings on the Six Bardos*, 155.

12. "Pride of the deity" is what finally separates sentient beings from buddhas. It is said that at the very highest levels of the path, one of the final obstacles to full awakening is confidence. Confidence that you *really* are the deity, that you truly are a buddha. You just don't believe it. Once you turn the corner of confidence, you're on the final stretch to Buddhahood. But in our degraded culture, this is not easy. Poverty mentality dominates, and when confidence does arise, it often flips into its near enemy of arrogance. We all know people who have been beaten down psychologically, let alone spiritually, by abusive parents, siblings, teachers, and other mentors. Replacing "you can't do it" with "you *can* do it" is a big part of conventional and spiritual success. Erasing doubt (which comes from the root *duo*, originally meaning "wavering between two possibilities") is a fundamental charter of the spiritual path. Stop wavering between who you think you are, the doubting psyche, and who you really are, the doubtless clear-light mind— or the buddha within.

      Many years ago I had a powerful dream about erasing doubt. In this dream I was standing with a crowd of onlookers as Trungpa Rinpoche walked toward an auditorium. It was like a scene from the walkway into the Oscars. Lots of fanfare, with admiring onlookers everywhere. Rinpoche was walking with his limp (he was partially paralyzed), supported by one of his attendants. My head was bowed, out of respect and shyness. As Rinpoche walked past me, he stopped, dismissed the attendant who was helping him, and gestured for me to come forward (which I interpreted later as an invitation for me to come out of my shell). I looked behind me, certain he was gesturing to someone else. I surely wasn't worthy to be summoned. But his gaze assured me he was asking for me, so I walked up hesitantly. He then leaned on me as I took the place of his attendant, and slowly began to walk again, now with my support. After a few steps Rinpoche turned to me, and with a voice of unshakable authority said a few words, virtually a command, that have inspired me for decades. "*You* can do it!" These words were delivered with such force, such unwavering confidence, that I have frequently taken refuge in his mandate when I find myself wracked with doubt. He saw in me what I was unable to see in myself.

13. Hatchell, *Naked Seeing*, p. 29.

14. For those who engage in deity yoga, this becomes another way to work with fear (stage 4). It's amazing what you can find on the Internet: nagual.yuku.com/topic/1735/Stopping-Inorganic-Beings-From-Hijacking-Your-Lucid-Dreams#.UzA-vl4x9ol.

15. Arising as a deity in the bardo of becoming is a key instruction from *The Tibetan Book of the Dead:* "At this time of terror when you are helplessly pursued by the avengers, you should immediately visualize with your whole mind the Blessed Supreme Heruka or Hayagriva or Vajrapani, or your yidam [deity] if you have one, with a huge body and thick limbs, standing in a terrifying attitude of wrath which crushes all evil forces into dust." (Francesca Fremantle and Chögyam Trungpa, trans., *The Tibetan Book of the Dead: The Great Liberation Through Hearing in the Bardo*, [Boston: Shambhala, 1975], 89.) Another instruction from this legendary book is also connected to illusory form; you should see everything that arises in the bardo as unreal: "I believed the nonexistent to exist, the untrue to be true, the illusion to be real; therefore I have wandered in samsara for so long. And if I do not realize that they are illusions, I shall still wander in samsara for a long time and certainly fall into the muddy swamp of suffering. Now they are all like dreams, like illusions, like echoes, like cities of *gandharvas,* like mirages, like images, like optical illusions, like the moon in water; they are not real, even for a moment . . . By concentrating one-pointedly on this conviction, belief in their reality is destroyed, and when one is inwardly convinced in such a way, belief in a self is counteracted. If you understand unreality like this from the bottom of your heart, the womb-entrance will certainly be closed." (page 86.)

    "The womb-entrance will certainly be closed" refers to the very end of the bardo of becoming, when a bardo being is about to take physical birth. This instruction is one way to prevent that samsaric birth. But the inner meaning applies to seeing the illusory nature of things as they appear now, and to close the womb-entrance to birth in a samsaric state of mind right here and now. If you see things as illusory in this very moment, you will prevent rebirth into samsara on the spot.

    If you can't do that, *The Tibetan Book of the Dead* has one final instruction for how to purify your birth. Visualize your future parents, who you will be drawn toward, as your meditation deity, or any sacred form. This purifies your perception of them and helps to purify your birth. Purification, in the bardos or in life, is yet again about seeing the illusory nature, the emptiness, of whatever arises. Remember that dream yoga came about as a way to prepare for death, so with stage 5 you're directly preparing for the bardos.

16. When realized beings serve others on this earth, they do so by spontaneously taking on the forms that are most beneficial to others, depending on the dictates of their environment. For example, when Trungpa Rinpoche came to the West from Tibet, his central purpose was to help others wake up. He tuned in to the Western cultural climate, and then turned into whatever forms were most likely to reach his students. In his case (it's different from tulku to tulku) he dropped the mask of a monk, the role that served him while he was in the East, and put on the mask of a hip Westerner to better relate to his students. He then changed that mask repeatedly throughout the course of his teaching career, sometimes to the consternation of his students, who wanted to keep him securely identified in one limited role. You can't pigeonhole expressions of enlightenment, or freeze it into any solid, lasting, and independent form.

17. This stage also helps prepare for the bardo of becoming, which is also called the bardo of *possibility*. In this bardo it's possible to form your formless awareness into virtually any form. Enlightened beings bring wisdom, the clear-light mind, consciously into form (as a voluntary tulku) as they take birth intentionally to help others; unenlightened beings bring their confusion unconsciously into form (as an involuntary tulku) as they are forced into birth unintentionally by the winds of karma.

Of the four types of tulku (supreme, blessed, variegated, and crafted), the most remarkable is the variegated, or "diversified," tulku. This stupefying level of tulku is when the clear-light mind not only takes on the form of any possible sentient being (including any animal or insect form), but *any* form altogether. This means that the clear-light mind can manifest as seemingly inanimate objects, any object you can think of.

In Buddhism, every time a student matures into a new level of practice, they are given a new name: a refuge name, a bodhisattva name, a "secret" or tantric name, and so forth. This is another skillful means to expand our sense of identity.

CHAPTER 15 Higher Attainment: More Stages of Dream Yoga

1. Paul Tholey, "A Model for Lucidity Training as a Means of Self-Healing and Psychological Growth," in Gackenbach and LaBerge, *Conscious Mind, Sleeping Brain,* 283–284.

2. How do we reconcile this assertion with the central tenet that enlightenment is attained by simply relaxing into it? In Tibetan Buddhism, the Gelugpa tradition often aligns itself with the view that enlightenment must be attained, while the Kagyu and Nyingma traditions are more aligned with the view of relaxation. This is the "immanent versus transcendent" debate. They are both valid. The seeming paradox only exists from a dualistic point of view. One way to approach this issue is to ask: What is the role of effort on the path? From the transcendent side, the role of effort is simple—it takes effort to earn enlightenment. From the immanent side, the role of effort is more subtle—the effort is in creating the environment whereby relaxation can arise. Another way to look at the immanent side is to say that it takes effort to dis-cover the enlightenment within, the irony of "trying to relax."

3. I don't do out-of-body practices, but some readers might see a connection to this practice. On one level, all dreams are "out-of-body" experiences (OBE). You're out of your physical body and into a mental body. People often come to dream yoga events having previously taken courses in OBE at the Monroe Institute. See monroeinstitute.org for more on this unique practice. I can't endorse it because I don't know enough about it. The same can be said for things like astral projection, soul flight, or autoscopy— seeing your own body from a distance.

See Harvey J. Irwin, "Out-of-the-Body Experiences and Dream Lucidity: Empirical Perspectives," and Sue Blackmore, "A Theory of Lucid Dreams and OBE's" in Gackenbach and LaBerge, *Conscious Mind, Sleeping Brain,* for more on this controversial topic. The article by Blackmore is particularly insightful. See also Thompson's *Waking, Dreaming, Being: Self and Consciousness in Neuroscience, Meditation, and Philosophy,* 203–229, for a discerning and healthy skeptical look at out-of-body experiences.

4. Quoted in *Sleeping, Dreaming, and Dying: An Exploration of Consciousness with The Dalai Lama,* 38–39, 125. The Dalai Lama also says, "The practice of developing the special dream body is ultimately aimed at achieving the Sambhogakaya, whereas the ultimate purpose of ascertaining the clear light [of sleep] is achieving the Dharmakaya" (p. 46). Karma Chagme and the previous Dzigar Kongtrul were reputedly highly proficient in the generation of a special dream body.

   The special dream body is also connected to the phenomenon of *delog,* or those who voluntarily go through near-death experiences. See Tulku Thondup, *Peaceful Death, Joyful Rebirth* (Boston: Shambhala, 2005) and Delog Dawa Drolma, *Delog: Journey to Realms Beyond Death* (Junction City, CA: Padma, 1995) for more on delog.

5. One further aspect of this practice connects dream yoga to bardo yoga. Bardo yoga engages an esoteric practice called *phowa,* or "ejection of consciousness." It's beyond our scope to explore phowa, but there are five forms of Vajrayana phowa and many other forms of Sutrayana phowa. One form of Vajrayana phowa is called "celestial phowa," and it's connected to this stage of dream yoga. Instead of sending your dream body to a physical location, with celestial phowa you send it to a Pure Land, usually Sukhavati. So if you can accomplish this stage of dream yoga, you have accomplished celestial phowa, and you're well prepared for death. Speaking within the context of dream yoga, Tsongkhapa says, "Engage in visionary travel by projecting yourself to the various buddhafields, such as Sukhavati, Tushita, Akanishta, and so forth. There you can meet with the buddhas and bodhisattvas, venerate them, listen to their teachings, and engage in many other activities of this nature." (Mullin, *Readings on the Six Yogas of Naropa,* 127.)

6. The CIA has been involved in remote viewing, but I have never come across any mention of research involving the generation of a special dream body. The theme of proper intention, which is key to this stage of practice, would be a central issue in the hands of the CIA. See Mayer, *Extraordinary Knowing: Science, Skepticism, and the Inexplicable Powers of the Human Mind,* 97–131, for a revealing exposé on intelligence-gathering via remote viewing.

7. Namkhai Norbu, *Dream Yoga and the Practice of Natural Light,* edited and introduced by Michael Katz (Ithaca, NY: Snow Lion, 1992), 41.

8. This isn't to say that you can't access the substrate or clear-light mind in daily meditation. You can, but it's equally as subtle. Formless, or non-referential, shamatha is one way to access the substrate during the day, and Dzogchen or Mahamudra are ways to access the clear-light mind during the day. (When you're resting in the nature of mind [clear-light mind] and it eventually "degenerates," it often degenerates, or slips into, the substrate, and therefore into a state of formless shamatha.)

   In the Yogachara system, most of our life as "outsiders" is dictated by the five sensory consciousnesses and the outward-oriented aspect of the sixth consciousness, which is mind as we usually know it (thoughts, emotions, and the like). Meditation cuts our involvement with the five sensory consciousnesses, and turns the lens of our attention onto the sixth consciousness, which is what we experience in heightened form when we meditate (because we're less distracted by the outer five). As our meditation progresses, we shift to the inward-oriented aspect of the sixth, which is when the mind turns directly upon itself. This "insider's" approach continues as our meditation progresses and we gain access to the unconscious seventh and then the eighth (the substrate) consciousness, the ground of samsara. As we've seen, we can then continue inward, cutting through all eight consciousnesses to arrive at the clear-light mind, the groundless ground of both samsara and nirvana.

9. Garfield, *Creative Dreaming*, 94.

10. Thompson, *Waking, Dreaming, Being: Self and Consciousness in Neuroscience, Meditation, and Philosophy,* 163.

11. Traleg Kyabgon Rinpoche, *Dream Yoga* video learning course (New York: E-Vam Buddhist Institute, 2008), disc no. 4.

12. Ziemer, "Lucid Surrender and Jung's Alchemical Coniunctio," in Hurd and Bulkeley, *Lucid Dreaming: New Perspectives on Consciousness in Sleep,* vol. 1, 154.

13. Ryan Hurd, "Unearthing the Paleolithic Mind in Lucid Dreams," in Hurd and Bulkeley, *Lucid Dreaming: New Perspectives on Consciousness in Sleep,* vol. 1, 282.

14. Ted Esser, "Kundalini and Non-Duality in the Lucid Dreaming State," in Hurd and Bulkeley, *Lucid Dreaming: New Perspectives on Consciousness in Sleep,* vol. 2, 237, 255.

15. Namkhai Norbu, *Dream Yoga and the Practice of Natural Light,* 61. Dream yoga is specifically designed to transform the bardo of becoming, which is also called the bardo of opportunity, or possibility. Just as waking up in the bardo of becoming can bring about great opportunity after death, waking up in the bardo of dream can bring about great opportunity during the night.

16. In the spirit of our moniker as dream yoga being "the measure of the path," self-liberation is another way to measure progress on the path. When we first begin the spiritual path, the psyche is in full operation and sticks to everything. We hold on to grudges, can't let go of thoughts, and harbor all sorts of emotional states. The psyche often keeps score and can latch onto a grievance for decades. As we progress on the path and gradually see through the psyche, we may notice that it's easier to let go of things. Instead of being in a foul mood for days, perhaps it's just a few hours, then several minutes, and eventually a few seconds. At the highest levels of spiritual accomplishment, when the sticky psyche has been replaced with the slippery clear-light mind, nothing sticks to you, not even for a second. Thoughts and emotions still arise, but they instantly self-liberate in the light of awareness.

You can observe this firsthand in your meditation. For someone new to meditation, it may take several minutes to realize they've been caught in a fantasy before they "wake up" from the distraction. For a mid-level meditator, they may become lucid to the distraction in a few seconds, and therefore liberate it. For an advanced practitioner who is always lucid, the thought is liberated the moment it arises. It self-liberates on the spot. Things still pop up, but they don't stay up.

Self-liberation, which leaves no trace, means the end of karma. It's the sticky mind, a mind that virtually traces out a thought or emotion over and over as it ruminates, cogitates, worries, or otherwise keeps a thought alive long after it should be dead, that creates karma. Karma is habit, and habits are formed by reiteration. If you let it go the instant it comes, you will simultaneously let go of karma. This is fundamentally what constitutes the path to complete liberation, or enlightenment.

17. Khenpo Tsültrim Gyamtso Rinpoche, "The Eight Kinds of Mastery," trans. Jim Scott, in *Buddhadharma: The Practitioner's Quarterly* 13, no. 2 (winter 2014), 37. This is another example of dream yoga as "the measure of the path."

18. Tsongkhapa says, "[Meditate] upon the suchness of dreams. This stage of the practice can only be undertaken when the training in retaining conscious presence during dreams has become stable. Here meditate upon yourself as the manifest radiant form of the mandala deity. The mantric syllable hum shines with a great light from your heart. This light melts the animate and inanimate dream objects into light, which is absorbed into yourself. Your body then also melts into light, from the head downward and feet upward, and is absorbed into the hum at your heart. The hum then melts into unapprehendable clear light. Rest the mind unwaveringly within this light." (Mullin, *Readings on the Six Yogas of Naropa,* 128.)

CHAPTER 16   Near Enemies and Other Obstacles

1. See Patricia Garfield, "Learn from Senoi Dreams," in *Creative Dreaming,* 80–118.

2. *Random House Dictionary* defines nihilism as (1) total rejection of established laws and institutions; (2) an extreme form of skepticism: the denial of all existence or the possibility of an objective basis for truth; (3) nothingness or nonexistence; (4) annihilation of the self; and, in extreme manifestations, (5) anarchy, terrorism, or other revolutionary activity.

3. John Welwood, "Intimate Relationship as a Spiritual Crucible," *Shambhala Sun* 17, no. 2 (2008), 63.

4. A. H. Almaas, *Facets of Unity: The Enneagram of Holy Ideas* (Shambhala Publications: Boston, 2002), 54.

5. Classically, this is why the Buddha manifested the form (rupa) kayas: the sambhogakaya and nirmanakaya. Someone at the dharmakaya can see and hear those at the sambhogakaya and nirmanakaya levels, but not the other way around. In other words, someone at the nirmanakaya (our level) cannot see or hear those who abide in the higher kayas (you have to attain the first bhumi, or ground of realization, to stably perceive the sambhogakaya, and the tenth bhumi to sustain your perception of the dharmakaya). So out of compassion, the dharmakaya buddhas manifest in sambhogakaya and nirmanakaya forms as a way to communicate with people like us.

6. Transforming the psyche instead of rejecting it is the essence of Vajrayana practice. The Vajrayana is an alchemical tradition, which means it transforms the "lead" of the psyche and substrate into gold. Confusion is transformed into wisdom. Specifically, the substrate is transformed into mirror-like wisdom, and the psyche is transformed into discriminating awareness wisdom.

7. A synonym for the clear-light mind is "basic goodness." Basic goodness is not just our absolute basic nature, it's also a relative practice. In other words, the relative (practice) leads to the absolute (nature) in the following way. We practice basic goodness, and therefore accelerate its actualization, every time we look for the goodness, the enlightened qualities, in ourselves and others (what we'll discuss in terms of the practice of "pure perception," or "sacred world," later). Look *through* the shadow side of a person and you'll find the light within them (like a parent looking through the tantrum of a child and therefore not getting swept away with the emotional upheaval). *Practice* looking for the "near friend" in any adverse (enemy-like) situation. It's always there. This is another instance of taking responsibility for our enlightenment, and actually practicing it. It's also another instance of the maxim: reality is what you attend to.

8. Translated and arranged by Jim Scott, Tegchokling, Boudha, Nepal, 2010.

9. This is the devastating message of the Prasangika Madhyamaka, which will destroy anything you try to say about reality. If you can put it into words, the Prasangikas will annihilate those words—and leave you with nothing. And no-thingness is as close as you can get to the truth. This is called a "non-affirming negation." You negate, but you don't affirm, which leaves you empty-handed and therefore holding the truth. Saying that reality is a dream is a non-affirming negation. The dream negates solidity, but it does not affirm anything to take the place of that solidity.

10. Wallace, *Natural Liberation: Padmasambhava's Teachings on the Six Bardos,* 151, 157.

11. Namkhai Norbu, *Dream Yoga and the Practice of Natural Light,* 56.

12. G. Scott Sparrow, *Lucid Dreaming: Dawning of the Clear Light,* 41.

13. Once again, it's exactly the same way we get distracted—and therefore non-lucid—by our thoughts. Remember that in Buddhism, "thought" is often referred to as the motion of the mind. Consciousness is a motion detector; it thrives on movement.

14. Some dream reports suggest, however, that fixing your gaze on a stationary point in the dream often ends the dream, because it can end the REM characteristic of dreaming. As always, become your own meditation instructor.

15. Harry T. Hunt and Robert D. Ogilvie, "Lucid Dreams in Their Natural Series: Phenomenological and Psychophysiological Findings in Relation to Meditative States," in Gackenbach and LaBerge, *Conscious Mind, Sleeping Brain,* 392.

16. Namkhai Norbu, *Dream Yoga and the Practice of Natural Light,* 56.

CHAPTER 17 An Introduction to Sleep Yoga

1. Varela, *Sleeping, Dreaming, and Dying: An Exploration of Consciousness with The Dalai Lama,* 41.

2. Tulku Urgyen Rinpoche, *Blazing Splendor: The Memoirs of Tulku Urgyen Rinpoche,* as told to Kunsang and Binder Schmidt, 232–233.

3. Ibid, 265.

4. The upper bandwidth of sleep yoga is dropping into the substrate, while the deepest bandwidth is dropping into ultimate reality, or in our terms the clear-light mind. In Yogachara terms, this would be the difference between

alaya vijnana and alaya jnana, respectively. Hindu and Buddhist texts offer different interpretations of dreamless sleep. We're dealing with the most subtle and refined states of mind, and exploring these subtleties in detail is beyond our scope. See B. Alan Wallace, *Stilling the Mind: Shamatha Teachings from Düdjom Lingpa's Vajra Essence* (Somerville, MA: Wisdom Publications, 2011), 160–180, for more on these differences.

5. For a marvelous rendering of light and mind, see *Catching the Light* (New York: Oxford University Press, 1993), by Arthur Zajonc.

6. In many traditions light is closely connected to God. Over one hundred solar deities are connected to the sun, from Ahura Mazda ("Light Wisdom") in Zoroastrianism to Shiwa Okar ("Peaceful White Light") in Shambhala Buddhism. "Solar theology" has been around for millennia. Luminosity yoga is a kind of solar non-theism that points out the god within, the solar deity that resides at the core of your being—*as* the core of your being.

7. Swami Sharvananda, *Kena Upanishad: With Sanskrit Text: Paraphrase with Word-for-Word Literal Translation, English Rendering, and Comments* (Madras: Ramakrishna Math, 1920), 11–14.

8. Dzogchen Ponlop, *Mind Beyond Death*, 86.

9. When we say "thinking" in meditation as thoughts pilfer our awareness, we could also be saying "that's not me."

10. Zajonc, *Catching the Light*, 2.

11. They personally don't want anything for themselves, because there isn't one. They've cut through the illusion of self. This is wisdom. But wisdom automatically expresses itself as compassion, so while they want nothing for themselves, they want happiness for others. This is how passion, or desire, is transformed into compassion.

12. The Tibetan word *nang wa (snang ba)* is provocative when it comes to light, appearance, and death. Nang wa has many meanings. As a verb, it can mean "to appear, to be visible or manifest," and "to exist or occur." As a noun, it can mean "rays of light, an external appearance or circumstance, an internal way of seeing or considering something." It also refers to the specific stage of death in which everything dissolves and one is left with only "a clear sky pervaded by moonlight, empty and radiantly white." Thanks to Jules Levinson for this translation.

13. Swami Sharvananda, *Kena Upanishad*, 7.

14. Lao-tzu, *Tao Te Ching*, translated by Stephen Mitchell (New York: Harper & Row, 1988), 52.

15. Wangyal, *The Tibetan Yogas of Dream and Sleep*, 198.

16. Fariba Bogzaran, "Hyperspace Lucidity and Creative Consciousness," in Hurd and Bulkeley, *Lucid Dreaming: New Perspectives on Consciousness in Sleep*, vol. 2, 213.

17. Waggoner, *Lucid Dreaming: Gateway to the Inner Self*, 81.

18. Ibid, 81–82.

19. Ziemer, "Lucid Surrender and Jung's Alchemical Coniunctio," in Hurd and Bulkeley, *Lucid Dreaming: New Perspectives on Consciousness in Sleep*, vol. 1, 157.

CHAPTER 18   The Practice of Sleep Yoga

1. Chökyi Nyima Rinpoche, "Meditation," in Binder Schmidt, *The Dzogchen Primer: Embracing the Spiritual Path According to the Great Perfection,* 53.
2. B. Alan Wallace, *Dreaming Yourself Awake: Lucid Dreaming and Tibetan Dream Yoga for Insight and Transformation* (Boston: Shambhala, 2012), 60–61.
3. Many books deal with Mahamudra and Dzogchen. The works of Thrangu Rinpoche on Mahamudra (*The Ninth Karmapa's Ocean of Definitive Meaning* [Ithaca, NY: Snow Lion, 2003], *Crystal Clear: Practical Advice for Mahamudra Meditators* [Hong Kong: Rangjung Yeshe, 2003], *An Ocean of the Ultimate Meaning: Teachings on Mahamudra* [Boston: Shambhala, 2004], *Pointing Out the Dharmakaya* [Ithaca, NY: Snow Lion, 2003], *Essentials of Mahamudra: Looking Directly at the Mind* [Boston: Wisdom, 2004]); the works of Tulku Urgyen Rinpoche on Dzogchen (*Rainbow Painting* [Hong Kong: Rangjung Yeshe, 1995], *As It Is,* vols. 1 and 2 [Hong Kong: Rangjung Yeshe, 1999, 2000]); and Tsoknyi Rinpoche on Dzogchen (*Carefree Dignity: Discourses on Training in the Nature of Mind* [Hong Kong: Ranjung Yeshe, 1998], *Fearless Simplicity: The Dzogchen Way of Living Fearlessly in a Complex World* [Hong Kong: Ranjung Yeshe, 2003]) are some of my favorites.
4. Namkhai Norbu, *Dream Yoga and the Practice of Natural Light,* 101.
5. Some lucid dreamers report that closing their dream eyes causes them to return to waking consciousness, not to dreamless awareness. See what it does for you.
6. Varela, *Sleeping, Dreaming, and Dying: An Exploration of Consciousness with The Dalai Lama,* 129.
7. HUM, "the sonorous sound of silence," is one of the most powerful mantras. It's the seed syllable of *Akshobya,* the mind aspect of all buddhas, and regarded as the vajra family seed syllable, capable of shocking us into awakening. Within the HUM the five buddhas are also represented, so HUM invokes the energy of the five buddhas and empowers us so we don't forget (who we are). HUM is in the class of semi-wrathful mantras, designed to penetrate through the psyche and substrate, and therefore one of the great "cutting through" mantras. It's a way of piercing ourselves. Mantra as "mind protector" here means that recitation of HUM not only accesses the clear-light mind, but protects it from distraction/forgetfulness. HUM protects from identity theft. In terms of relative *siddhi,* HUM is used to cut through rocks and the like: in terms of absolute siddhi, it cuts through the even denser strata of the petrified psyche and substrate.

    HUM was used by Padmasambhava in his wrathful aspect to subdue the negative forces in the environment of Tibet. It was by the force of HUM that the fortress of *rudra,* the archetype of the ego, was reduced to dust. HUM is the audible analog to the *phurba,* or *kilaya,* a three-bladed ritual dagger used to penetrate the three poisons of passion, aggression, and ignorance (as embodied in the psyche and substrate). I recite it as the "triple HUM," or "HUM HUM HUM" (which I use to replace my usual samsaric mantra, "me me me"), which represents cutting these three poisons. Trungpa Rinpoche said that the phurba, and therefore HUM, "pierces the heart of confused darkness," and reveals the light. "The abrupt experience of cutting through all thoughts is the action of HUM."

8. The dream researcher Clare Johnson writes, "In nondual lucid dream experiences, we generally have a minimal body-sense, perhaps experiencing ourselves as a 'dot of consciousness.' Sensory perceptions tend to be minimized to an impression of light or darkness, and our thought processes are reduced to a state of nonthought in which we might describe ourselves after the event as having existed as 'pure awareness.' A spatial sense often seems present as an impression of existing in infinite space, and the nondual experience might be described as 'merging with infinite light,' or simply as having no further sense of separate existence. In a sense, we are no longer *in* the gap between dreams; we become it." (Clare R. Johnson, "Magic, Meditation, and the Void: Creative Dimensions of Lucid Dreaming," in Hurd and Bulkeley, *Lucid Dreaming: New Perspectives on Consciousness in Sleep,* vol. 2, 63).

9. This sequence parallels the outer dissolution of the elements that occurs during death, going from gross earth to subtle space. So with this visualization you're also simulating death. When reality starts to take form in the Luminous Bardo of Dharmata after death, this process is reversed. From the pure white light of space arises the green light of wind, the red light of fire, the blue light of water, and the yellow light of earth. If these lights are not recognized for what they are, the clear-light mind refracting into the "colors" of the five buddha families, those lights then gradually freeze or reify into the elements that create the mental body in the Bardo of Becoming, and then further reify into all the elements of the natural world. This world, therefore, is nothing but frozen light, a light that can be revealed with advanced stages in the practice of illusory form.

10. Wallace, *Natural Liberation: Padmasambhava's Teachings on the Six Bardos,* 165–166.

11. Proprioception means "one's own" or "individual" *(proprius)* perception. It's the sense of relative position of neighboring body parts, or the body altogether, brought about by proprioceptors in muscles and joints. Proprioception is distinguished from "interoception," by which we perceive hunger, pain, and other internal senses, and "exteroception," by which we perceive the outside world. Proprioception is what brings us awareness of the position of our body. "Spiritual proprioception" is what brings us (erroneous) awareness of the position of our sense of self altogether. It's principally the function of the seventh consciousness, which looks back upon the eighth and mis-takes it for the ineffable sense of self. It's truly ineffable, because when we bother to take a close look, which is the purpose of insight meditation, we won't find a self. Hence this form of proprioception, as powerful as it is, is an illusion.

12. Holding my dream breath is something that came to me by experimentation, but it makes sense. According to the inner yogas, when the winds are flowing through the two side channels, the resulting experience is one of duality. When the winds enter the central channel, the resulting experience is nonduality. It's literally and figuratively a breath-taking experience. When this happens in life, you can sit in meditation with no discernable respiration. The psyche has died and dissolved into either the deepest substrate (with formless shamatha), or even the clear-light mind (with Mahamudra or Dzogchen meditation), and one outer sign is that you're alive but not breathing. Some

inner yoga practices work with holding the breath as a way to "force" it into the central channel, and therefore into nonduality. (Watch your mind when you come upon something that takes your breath away and you'll often find it takes your thoughts away, offering a snapshot of the clear-light mind during the day. For a quick experiment: straighten your posture, look straight ahead, and gently hold your breath. What happens to your mind?)

Studies have shown that "Voluntary control of the mental image of respiration during lucid dreaming is reflected in corresponding changes in actual respiration," which means that holding your dream breath does indeed result in holding your real breath (LaBerge, *Lucid Dreaming: The Power of Being Awake and Aware in Your Dreams*, 85). Since the dream body is associated with the subtle body, perhaps the subtle breath ("winds") does enter the center channel, resulting in the experience of the clear-light mind. Once again, try it and see it if works for you.

13. Wangyal, *The Tibetan Yogas of Dream and Sleep*, 157.

14. *Manjushri Sadhana*, by Trungpa Rinpoche, says: "In the darkness of frightful existence, all beings are possessed by the [enemy] of ignorance." Taking things to be truly existent (solid, lasting, and independent) is the obscuration to emptiness. It's another instance of appearance (things appear to truly exist) not being in harmony with reality (things are empty of inherent existence).

15. Johnson, "Magic, Meditation, and the Void: Creative Dimensions of Lucid Dreaming," in Hurd and Bulkeley, *Lucid Dreaming: New Perspectives on Consciousness in Sleep,* vol. 2, 60.

16. Technically speaking, it results in "ultra pure" illusory form, which means the perception of illusory form happens spontaneously. You're no longer faking it (as in illusory form), or generating it (as in pure illusory form); you're actually "making it." You've "made it"—you have arrived at the final daytime destination of spontaneously seeing everything as a dream, the "illusion-like samadhi." You now see things with the clear-light eyes of a buddha.

17. Zajonc, *Catching the Light*, xiv.

18. Wangyal, *The Tibetan Yogas of Dream and Sleep*, 208.

CHAPTER 19   The Fruition of Dream and Sleep Yoga

1. Tholey, "A Model for Lucidity Training as a Means of Self-Healing and Psychological Growth," in Gackenbach and LaBerge, *Conscious Mind, Sleeping Brain*, 276–277.

2. Patricia Garfield, "Clinical Applications of Lucid Dreaming, Introductory Comments," in Gackenbach and LaBerge, *Conscious Mind, Sleeping Brain,* 291.

3. This is what training to recognize recurring dreamsigns can do for us in waking life. In life we tend to repeat reactions to recurring events even when those reactions are unwise, ineffective, or hurtful. Until we begin to see the pattern of how this always plays out, we don't see the event as an opportunity to come up with new, creative, and constructive responses.

4. Tarthang Tulku, *Openness Mind* (Berkeley: Dharma Press, 1978), 77.

5. My oneironaut friend Patricia Keelin shared this with me: "During my first workshop with Stephen LaBerge, he offered the idea that frightening images in our dreams hold only the power with which we imbue them.

Realizing the deep truth of his words, I resolved to remember this and to change my response regarding a recurring nightmare. About a week later, I had my chance to do so and experienced a major emotional transformation. My intention triggered lucidity, and I literally tore away at the image to find nothing but emptiness beyond it! I had been needlessly frightening myself for decades. When it came time later to confront the reality of what had contributed to my fear (the actual person behind the dream mask), I was able to do so with considerable clarity and even some compassion."

6. See Mayer, *Extraordinary Knowing: Science, Skepticism, and the Inexplicable Powers of the Human Mind,* for an elegant discussion on relative siddhi (*sadharanasiddhi* in Sanskrit). Ramana Maharshi, and many other masters, warned people repeatedly against attachment to relative siddhi. Vajrayana Buddhism lists eight ordinary siddhis: (1) the sword that renders unconquerable, (2) the elixir for the eyes that make gods visible, (3) fleetness in running, (4) invisibility, (5) the life-essence that preserves youth, (6) the ability to fly, (7) the ability to make certain pills, (8) power over the world of spirits and demons. (Ingrid Fischer-Schreiber et al., eds., *The Encyclopedia of Eastern Philosophy and Religion* [Boston: Shambhala, 1989], 334). Many other powers are listed informally in the literature, things like clairvoyance, clairaudience, and the ability to read minds.

7. Khenpo Tsültrim Gyamtso Rinpoche, *The Practice of Spontaneous Presence: Stages of the Path of the Essence of Wisdom,* seminar at Kagyu Thubten Choling, July 1996, translated by Lama Yeshe Gyamtso, edited by the Vajravairochana Translation Committee (Halifax, Nova Scotia: Vajravairochana Translation Committee, 1999), 54.

8. Sogyal Rinpoche, *Glimpse After Glimpse: Daily Reflections on Living and Dying,* March 31 entry.

9. "You'll Be There" was written by Cory Mayo and recorded by American country music singer George Strait.

10. "The Doors of Liberation," *Shambhala Sun,* May 2014, 58.

11. Quoted in Jack Kornfield, *After the Ecstasy, the Laundry: How the Heart Grows Wise on the Spiritual Path* (New York: Bantam Books, 2000), 122.

12. The Buddhist scholar Christopher Hatchell writes, "In the Great Perfection, the apparently solid external objects that surround us are in fact a kind of solidified knowing: a high-energy gnosis that has become confused and slowed down to the point that it has entered a state of ossified dormancy." The Great Perfection is Dzogchen, which can also be called the Great Purity, and results in seeing the world purified of these three stains. (*Naked Seeing: The Great Perfection, the Wheel of Time, and Visionary Buddhism in Renaissance Tibet,* 56.) Hatchell refers to this form of knowing as "tantric epistemology," "[W]hich tries to establish the plausibility of perceptual models that do not adhere to the dualistic subject/object format . . . [whereby] the objects perceived by a mind are nothing other than the mind's exteriorization of itself . . . just as the manifold rays of the sun are inseparable from the singular sun itself, so the ignorant mind and the apparently solid objects of the world are all the dimmed efflorescence of awareness that has strayed far from its source." (p. 363.)

13. Quoted in Ken McLeod, *Wake Up to Your Life: Discovering the Buddhist Path of Attention* (New York: HarperCollins, 2001), 382.

CHAPTER 20   **Bardo Yoga**

1. For more on bardo yoga, see my book *Preparing to Die: Practical Advice and Spiritual Wisdom from the Tibetan Buddhist Tradition* (Boston: Snow Lion, 2013); see also Dzogchen Ponlop, *Mind Beyond Death*; Sogyal Rinpoche, *The Tibetan Book of Living and Dying* (New York: HarperCollins, 1992); Tulku Thondup, *Peaceful Death, Joyful Rebirth: A Tibetan Buddhist Guidebook* (Boston: Shambhala, 2006); and Francesca Fremantle, *Luminous Emptiness: Understanding the Tibetan Book of the Dead* (Boston: Shambhala, 2001).

2. This assertion extends an insight from LaBerge, one that applies to the post-death experience: "Waking consciousness is dreaming [bardo] consciousness with sensory constraints; dreaming [bardo] consciousness is waking consciousness without sensory constraints." In the Tibetan tradition, six bardos, or states of consciousness, comprise the totality of all possible experience: the bardo of this life, the bardo of meditation, the bardo of dream, the bardo of dying, the bardo of dharmata, and the bardo of becoming. In this context, every state of consciousness is a bardo, or a state between two other states. In its broadest sense, bardo yoga is any practice that bridges all these states of consciousness into a seamless constant consciousness. Being seamless means there are no breaks or gaps, or in our terms *naps*, where we doze off and lose our awareness in the various forms of distraction that otherwise separate (and therefore create) these bardos. This is why, for an awakened one, a buddha, there are no bardos. Bardos only exist for confused sentient beings. For a buddha, constant consciousness bridges all six states. Buddhas are never distracted, which means they never sleep, dream, or die in the conventional sense. They never "lose it." They never lose their clear-light mind as it manifests in these six states. The light of awareness is always on.

3. Anything constituted of form obviously dies, like the body and the psyche. But the clear-light Buddha mind, as formless awareness, is unborn and therefore undying. Identify with that, and "you" have attained immortality. But, of course, to do that you must first die, or let go of, any level of identification to any level of form. To die before you die is the essence of the spiritual path.

4. Sogyal Rinpoche, *Glimpse After Glimpse: Daily Reflections on Living and Dying,* October 14 entry. That "something," of course, is the no-thingness of the clear-light mind.

5. Hunt and Ogilvie, "Lucid Dreams in Their Natural Series: Phenomenological and Psychophysiological Findings in Relation to Meditative States," in Gackenbach and LaBerge, *Conscious Mind, Sleeping Brain,* 398–399.

6. The scholar Thomas McAlpine writes that in the Old Testament "there is a significant lexical relationship between sleep and death. Of the different activity fields identified as sharing a common vocabulary with the human sleep field, the death field has both the largest number of words in common . . . as well as the largest number of occurrences of these words . . . Death could be spoken of in terms of sleep, a sleep from which one did not awake." (*Sleep, Divine and Human, in the Old Testament* [Sheffield, UK: Sheffield Academic Press, 1987], 144, 149.)

7. In more philosophical terms this is sometimes called the "theory of recapitulation." For one example, microgeny (the origin of the moment) recapitulates ontogeny (the origin of a being) recapitulates phylogeny (the origin of a species) recapitulates cosmogeny (the origin of a cosmos). Echoes of this theme can be found in the Hermetic or alchemical adage "As above, so below," or the Kalachakra maxim "As within, so without." The anthropologist Gregory Bateson speaks about "meta-patterns," or the pattern of patterns; chaos and complexity theory talk about "universality," "self-similarity," and of course, "fractals." Douglas Hofstadter's Pulitzer prize–winning book, *Gödel, Escher, Bach: An Eternal Golden Braid,* alludes to this theme (braid) using the work of masters in logic/mathematics, art, and music. It's no surprise that a Universal Process would find universal iterations throughout multiple disciplines.

   There is promise and peril with the idea of universality. The promise is one of unification and reciprocal understanding (using one process to help you understand another). The peril (or near enemy) is facile and erroneous conclusions: "They're all saying the same thing."

8. Varela, *Sleeping, Dreaming, and Dying: An Exploration of Consciousness with The Dalai Lama,* 40.

9. Bokar Rinpoche, Jennifer Pessereau, ed., and Christiane Buchet, trans., *Death and the Art of Dying in Tibetan Buddhism* (San Francisco: ClearPoint Press, 1993), 20.

10. To create a sense of symmetry with the three death bardos, I sometimes refer to the first bardo as the "painful bardo of unbecoming." This connects it to the third bardo, "the karmic bardo of becoming." The third bardo is where we become somebody, based on the force of our karma (habitual patterns). The first bardo is where that body "unbecomes," or dies. It's also a play on how unbecoming and unflattering death is to the ego.

11. This is an allusion to Dylan Thomas and his epic poem, the first stanza of which is: "Do not go gentle into that good night / Old age should burn and rave at close of day / Rage, rage against the dying of the light." With the right view, no need to rage, because the night is good and the light is not dying.

12. The first phase of the bardo of dharmata is the *emptiness* phase, where pure no-thingness, formless awareness, is uncovered. The second and more famous phase is the *luminosity* phase, which itself is described in four phases, the second of these sub-phases being the appearance of the hundred peaceful and wrathful deities. Because sleep is a concordant experience of death, and not actual death, the full expression of these two phases of the bardo of dharmata is not fully evident when we drop into dreamless sleep. In other words, the four phases of the second luminosity phase do not appear when we sleep.

13. Forty-nine days is not a fixed time; it can be much shorter or much longer. The duration is dictated by karma, and by a sorting out of the four forces of transitional karma: heavy, proximate, habitual, and random.

14. These beings are the tulkus, also called "voluntary nirmanakayas." See Tulku Thondup, *Incarnation: The History and Mysticism of the Tulku Tradition of Tibet* (Boston: Shambhala, 2011).

15. Bardo yoga, as typified in *savasana,* or the "corpse pose" that is usually done at the end of a yoga session, is all about helping us relax into death. This isn't

easy, especially when our usual reflex is to contract in ultimate self-defense as our very sense of self is dissolving, or essentially being "forced" to relax.

16. Wallace, *Natural Liberation: Padmasambhava's Teachings on the Six Bardos,* 160–161.

17. Sogyal Rinpoche, *The Tibetan Book of Living and Dying,* 342.

Epilogue

1. Duff, *The Secret Life of Sleep,* 9.

2. Hurd, "Unearthing the Paleolithic Mind in Lucid Dreams," in Hurd and Bulkeley, *Lucid Dreaming: New Perspectives on Consciousness in Sleep,* vol. 1, 278.

3. To show you how quickly we forget things upon waking up: in terms of our dreams, we forget 50 percent of what we dream within the first five minutes of being awake, and 90 percent after ten minutes. How much quicker and more thorough is the amnesia of our true identity, the clear-light mind we so recently left?

4. Coleman Barks, trans., *The Essential Rumi* (New York: HarperOne, 2004), 16.

5. To see others as living buddhas is to see through (cut through) our obscurations, and to see them as they truly are. This is the practice of pure perception, which connects us to their innate purity. By seeing others that way, identifying *them* as buddhas, we help them reconnect and locate their primordial identity. By doing this for yourself first, by reconnecting and relocating your own true identity, you will come to do it spontaneously for others. It's akin to how treating your adolescent son or daughter as a young adult helps them grow into one.

6. Duff, *The Secret Life of Sleep,* 53.

Suggested Reading

Bogzaran, Fariba, and Daniel Deslauriers. *Integral Dreaming: A Holistic Approach to Dreams*. New York: State University of New York Press, 2012.

Gackenbach, Jayne, and Stephen LaBerge, eds. *Conscious Mind, Sleeping Brain: Perspectives on Lucid Dreaming*. New York: Plenum, 1998.

Garfield, Patricia. *Creative Dreaming*. New York: Ballantine, 1974.

Gyatrul Rinpoche, commentary to *Natural Liberation: Padmasambhava's Teachings on the Six Bardos*. Translated by B. Alan Wallace. Boston: Wisdom Publications, 1998.

Hurd, Ryan, and Kelly Bulkeley, eds. *Lucid Dreaming: New Perspectives on Consciousness in Sleep*. 2 vols. Santa Barbara, CA: Praeger, 2014.

LaBerge, Stephen. *Lucid Dreaming: A Concise Guide to Awakening in Your Dreams and in Your Life*. Boulder: Sounds True, 2004.

LaBerge, Stephen. *Lucid Dreaming: The Power of Being Awake and Aware in Your Dreams*. New York: Ballantine, 1985.

LaBerge, Stephen, and Howard Rheingold. *Exploring the World of Lucid Dreaming*. New York: Ballantine, 1990.

Namkhai Norbu. *Dream Yoga and the Practice of Natural Light*. Edited and introduced by Michael Katz. Ithaca, NY: Snow Lion Publications, 1992.

O'Flaherty, Wendy Doniger. *Dreams, Illusion, and Other Realities*. Delhi: Motilal Banarsidass, 1987.

Sparrow, G. Scott. *Lucid Dreaming: Dawning of the Clear Light*. Virginia Beach: A.R.E. Press, 1982.

Thompson, Evan. *Waking, Dreaming, Being: Self and Consciousness in Neuroscience, Meditation, and Philosophy*. New York: Columbia University Press, 2015.

Varela, Francisco J., ed. *Sleeping, Dreaming, and Dying: An Exploration of Consciousness with the Dalai Lama*. Boston: Wisdom Publications, 1997.

Waggoner, Robert. *Lucid Dreaming: Gateway to the Inner Self*. Needham, MA: Moment Point Press, 2009.

Wallace, B. Alan. *Dreaming Yourself Awake: Lucid Dreaming and Tibetan Dream Yoga for Insight and Transformation.* Boston: Shambhala, 2012.

Wangyal, Tenzin. *The Tibetan Yogas of Dream and Sleep.* Ithaca, NY: Snow Lion, 1998.

Young, Serinity. *Dreaming in the Lotus: Buddhist Dream Narrative, Imagery, and Practice.* Boston: Wisdom Publications, 1999.

Index

About the Author

ANDREW HOLECEK is an author, spiritual teacher, and humanitarian. He has been a practitioner of Vajrayana Buddhism for more than thirty years and has completed the traditional three-year retreat. Andrew has a strong scientific background, including a degree in biology, years in the study of physics, and a doctorate in dental surgery. This has instilled in him a healthy skeptical nature, which inspired him to go directly to the source to obtain his education and meditative training in Buddhism. He has studied extensively in Nepal, India, and even Tibet—the geographic wellspring of Buddhism—and has received teachings from many of the greatest living masters.

Andrew is a concert-level pianist with a degree in classical music and a lifelong fervor for the arts. He is also a dedicated athlete who integrates physical health with his spiritual and intellectual endeavors. His passion for full-spectrum living includes his desire to understand consciousness through waking, dreaming, sleeping, and dying, and his love of exercising body, mind, heart, and spirit.

In 1990, Andrew co-founded Global Dental Relief, which provides health care to impoverished children in Nepal, India, Cambodia, Vietnam, Kenya, and Guatemala.

Between his writing regimen, meditation retreats, and international teaching schedule, Andrew finds time to walk his dog and enjoy the pleasures of life along the foothills of Colorado. For more information see andrewholecek.com.

About Sounds True

SOUNDS TRUE is a multimedia publisher whose mission is to inspire and support personal transformation and spiritual awakening. Founded in 1985 and located in Boulder, Colorado, we work with many of the leading spiritual teachers, thinkers, healers, and visionary artists of our time. We strive with every title to preserve the essential "living wisdom" of the author or artist. It is our goal to create products that not only provide information to a reader or listener, but that also embody the quality of a wisdom transmission.

For those seeking genuine transformation, Sounds True is your trusted partner. At SoundsTrue.com you will find a wealth of free resources to support your journey, including exclusive weekly audio interviews, free downloads, interactive learning tools, and other special savings on all our titles.

To learn more, please visit SoundsTrue.com/freegifts or call us toll-free at 800.333.9185.

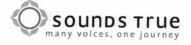